Atlas of
ALLERGIC
DISEASES

Atlas of ALLERGIC DISEASES

Edited by

Phillip L. Lieberman, MD

Clinical Professor of Medicine and Pediatrics
Department of Internal Medicine and Pediatrics
University of Tennessee College of Medicine;
Allergy & Asthma Care
Cordova, Tennessee

Michael S. Blaiss, MD

Clinical Professor of Pediatrics and Medicine
Division of Clinical Immunology and Allergy
University of Tennessee Medical College;
Allergy & Asthma Care
Memphis, Tennessee

With 39 contributors

Developed by Current Medicine, Inc.
Philadelphia

Current Medicine, Inc.
400 Market Street
Suite 700
Philadelphia, PA 19106

Atlas of Allergic Diseases

Although every effort has been made to ensure that drug doses and other information are presented accurately in this publication, the ultimate responsibility rests with the prescribing physician. Neither the publishers nor the authors can be held responsible for errors or for any consequences arising from the use of information contained herein. Products mentioned in this publication should be used in accordance with the prescribing information prepared by the manufacturers. No claims or endorsements are made for any drug or compound at present under clinical investigation.

ISBN 1-57340-182-X

1 2 3 4 5 6 7 8 9 0

DEVELOPMENT EDITOR:
Elise M. Paxson

EDITORIAL ASSISTANT:
Janet Gilmore

COVER DESIGN:
Christine Keller-Quirk

DESIGN AND LAYOUT:
Christine Keller-Quirk

ILLUSTRATORS:
Wieslawa Langenfeld, Maureen Looney

ASSISTANT PRODUCTION MANAGER:
Penny Weisman

INDEXING:
Holly Lukens

For more information, please call 1 (800) 427-1796 or (215) 574-2266 or e-mail us at inquiry@phl.cursci.com
www.current-science-group.com

Printed in Hong Kong by Paramount Printing Group Limited
This book was printed on acid-free paper.
Library of Congress Cataloging-in-Publication Data

Atlas of allergic diseases / edited by Phillip L. Lieberman, Michael S. Blaiss.
   p. ; cm.
 Includes bibliographical references and index.
 ISBN 1-57340-182-X (alk. paper)
 1. Allergy–Atlases.
 [DNLM: 1. Hypersensitivity–Atlases. WD 300 A8805 2001] I. Lieberman, Phil L. II. Blaiss, Michael S.
 RC585 .A87 2001
 616.97–dc21
              2001047167

Dedication

To my children: Ryan, Lee, and Jay.

Phillip L. Lieberman

To my wonderful wife, Terry, and our two magnificent sons, Adam and Joel. Thank you for the support and encouragement you have given me. Words cannot express my love for you.

Michael S. Blaiss

Preface

Allergy–immunology is not, as a rule, a visual specialty. With the possible exceptions of the allergy skin tests, nasal examination, and the reading of nasal eosinophil smears, allergists–immunologists work in a realm of abstract conclusions and concepts rather than palpable, visible problems, such as that which surgeons encounter. Therefore when we began this task, we were somewhat concerned that we could not accumulate enough visual material to flesh out an entire atlas. However, much to our surprise, the ideas began to flow, and we have developed a final product that, at least in our eyes, is a useful and quite striking text that visually depicts the scientific and clinical aspects of our subspecialty.

We are not aware of any text that has approached this specialty in quite the same way. In most textbooks and even other atlases, the immunology and allergy subjects are usually presented as separate entities. For this atlas, our intent was to combine the immunologic basis of our subspecialty with the clinical aspects of the discipline. We believe that the end result is an instructive volume that illustrates the abstract elements of our field quite vividly.

We would like to thank the many authors who spent hours of their time collecting photos and submitting drawings. We knew from the beginning that this would be a difficult task to accomplish, and without the diligent efforts of these contributors it would have been impossible.

Phillip L. Lieberman
Michael S. Blaiss

Contributors

John A. Anderson, MD
Tucson, Arizona

Emil J. Bardana, Jr., MD
Professor of Medicine
Department of Medicine
Oregon Health Sciences University
Portland, Oregon

Fariba Behbod, PharmD
Predoctoral Fellow
Department of Integrative Biology and
    Pharmacology
University of Texas
Houston, Texas

Leonard Bielory, MD
Associate Professor
Departments of Medicine, Pediatrics and
    Ophthalmology
University of Medicine and
    Dentistry–New Jersey Medical School;
Co-Director
Immuno-Ophthalmology Service
University of Medicine and Dentistry–New
    Jersey University Hospital
Newark, New Jersey

Michael S. Blaiss, MD
Clinical Professor of Pediatrics and
    Medicine
Division of Clinical Immunology and
    Allergy
University of Tennessee Medical College;
Staff Physician
Allergy & Asthma Care
Memphis, Tennessee

Wesley Burks, MD
Professor of Pediatrics
Departments of Allergy and Immunology
University of Arkansas School for Medical
    Sciences;
Arkansas Children's Hospital
Little Rock, Arkansas

Rosa Codina, PhD
Assistant Professor
Department of Internal Medicine
University of South Florida Medical School
Tampa, Florida

Nemr S. Eid, MD
Professor
Department of Pediatrics
University of Louisville School of Medicine;
Director
Department of Pediatric Pulmonary
    Medicine;
Director
Cystic Fibrosis Center
Kosair Children's Hospital
Louisville, Kentucky

Stanley Fineman, MD
Clinical Assistant Professor
Department of Pediatrics
Emory University School of Medicine;
Atlanta Allergy and Asthma Clinic
Marietta, Georgia

Jordan Fink, MD
Professor
Department of Pediatrics and Medicine
Medical College of Wisconsin
Milwaukee, Wisconsin

Roger W. Fox, MD
Associate Professor
Department of Medicine and Public Health
Division of Allergy and Immunology
University of South Florida College of
    Medicine and Health Sciences Center
Tampa, Florida

Glenn Furuta, MD
Assistant Professor
Department of Pediatrics
Harvard Medical School;
Attending Physician
Children's Hospital of Boston
Boston, Massachusetts

**Gnanasegaram Gnanakumaran, BM
(Southampton), MRCPCH (UK)**
Clinical Research Fellow
Southampton University Hospital
Southampton, United Kingdom

Deborah A. Gentile, MD
Assistant Professor
Department of Pediatrics
University of Pittsburgh School of
    Medicine;
Children's Hospital of Pittsburgh
Pittsburgh, Pennsylvania

J. Andrew Grant, MD
University of Texas Medical Branch
Galveston, Texas

Jere D. Guin, MD
Professor Emeritus
Department of Dermatology
University of Arkansas for Medical Sciences
Little Rock, Arkansas

Stephen T. Holgate, MD, DSc, FRCP
Professor
Respiratory Cell and Molecular Biology
Southampton Medical School;
MRC Clinical Professor of
    Immunopharmacology
Southampton University Hospital
University of Southampton School of
    Medicine
Southampton, United Kingdom

Stacie M. Jones, MD
Assistant Professor
Department of Pediatrics
University of Arkansas for Medical
    Sciences;
Research Director
Arkansas Children's Asthma Center
Little Rock, Arkansas

Jay M. Kincannon, MD
Associate Professor
Department of Dermatology and Pediatrics
University of Arkansas for Medical
    Sciences;
Chief
Department of Pediatric Dermatology
Arkansas Children's Hospital
Little Rock, Arkansas

Rande H. Lazar, MD
Lebonheur Children's Medical Center
Memphis, Tennessee

Patricia A. Leonard, MD
Fellow Department of Allergy and
    Immunology
University of Texas Medical Branch
Galveston, Texas

D. Betty Lew, MD
Professor
Department of Pediatrics
University of Tennessee Medical College
Memphis, Tennessee

Phillip L. Lieberman, MD
Clinical Professor of Medicine and Pediatrics
Department of Internal Medicine and
    Pediatrics
University of Tennessee College of Medicine;
Allergy & Asthma Care
Cordova, Tennessee

Richard F. Lockey, MD
Department of Internal Medicine
University of South Florida Medical School;
James A. Haley Veter Hospital;
H. Lee Moffitt Cancer Center;
Tampa General Hospital;
Tampa, Florida;
All Children's Hospital
St. Petersburg, Florida

Todd Mahr, MD
Assistant Clinical Professor
Department of Pediatrics
University of Wisconsin Medical School;
Madison, Wisconsin
Director
Department of Pediatric Allergy
Gunderson Clinic
La Crosse, Wisconsin

Gailen D. Marshall, Jr, MD, PhD
Associate Professor
Departments of Medicine and Pathology
University of Texas Medical School;
Chief
Allergy-Immunology Service
Memorial Hermann Hospital
Houston, Texas

Ron B. Mitchell, MD
Assistant Professor
Department of Surgery and Pediatrics
University of New Mexico
Albuquerque, New Mexico

Ronald L. Morton, MD
Assistant Professor
Department of Pediatrics
University of Louisville School of Medicine;
Assistant Professor of Pediatrics
Kosair Children's Hospital
Louisville, Kentucky

James N. Moy, MD
Associate Professor
Department of Immunology and
    Microbiology
Rush Medical College;
Director
Division of Pediatric Allergy and
    Immunology
Cook County Hospital
Chicago, Illinois

Robert P. Nelson, Jr., MD
Indiana Cancer Pavilion
Indianapolis, Indiana

Dennis R. Ownby, MD
Professor
Department of Pediatrics and Medicine
Medical College of Georgia
Augusta, Georgia

Susan Y. Ritter, BA
MD/PhD Student
University of Texas Medical School at
    Houston
Houston, Texas

Joseph L. Roberts, MD, PhD
Assistant Professor
Department of Pediatrics
Duke University Medical Center
Durham, North Carolina

Ketan Sheth, MD, MBA
Assistant Clinical Professor
Department of Pediatrics
Indiana University School of Medicine;
Head
Allergy and Asthma Section
Arnett Clinic
Lafayette, Indiana

Scott H. Sicherer, MD
Assistant Professor
Department of Pediatrics
Mount Sinai School of Medicine
New York, New York

David P. Skoner, MD
Associate Professor
Departments of Pediatrics and
    Otolaryngology
University of Pittsburgh School of
    Medicine;
Chief
Section of Allergy/Immunology
Children's Hospital of Pittsburgh
Pittsburgh, Pennsylvania

Richard W. Weber, MD
Allergist
Austin Allergy Associates
Austin, Texas

Larry W. Williams, MD
Associate Professor
Department of Pediatrics
Duke University Medical Center
Durham, North Carolina

Michael C. Zacharisen, MD
Assistant Professor
Department of Pediatrics and Medicine
Medical College of Wisconsin
Milwaukee, Wisconsin

Contents

Section I:
Immunology and Basic Science

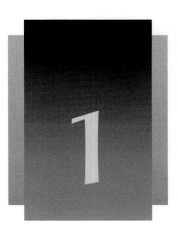

Molecular Biology Techniques for the Investigation of Immune Activation and Immunologic Dysfunction

Fariba Behbod and Gailen D. Marshall, Jr.

Molecular biology involves the study of the structure and function of molecules and various biochemical pathways that work in concert to create a multicellular organism. By employing molecular biology research techniques, scientists have made tremendous progress in understanding how a cell develops, functions, and communicates with other cells and tissues. The purpose of this chapter is to provide examples of molecular biology techniques employed by researchers to investigate and describe pathways involved in immune activation and immunologic dysfunction.

Immune cells such as B and T lymphocytes respond to extracellular antigenic stimuli with varying combinations of activation, differentiation, or proliferation. Upon antigen stimulation, multiple cascades of biochemical reactions are initiated. These pathways lead to different physiologic responses, including cellular proliferation, differentiation, or tolerance. Even though many complex pathways have been identified, relatively little is known about how these pathways communicate with one another or how these pathways lead to specific clinical responses, such as eradication of a pathogen as a normal immune mechanism versus autoimmunity as an abnormal immune response to self.

Researchers in the field of immunology focus greatly on assessing the function of immune cells and identifying intracellular molecules of importance in immune activation. Molecular biology techniques such as SDS-polyacrylamide gel electrophoresis (*see* Fig. 1-4), Western blot (*see* Fig. 1-4), and immunoprecipitation (*see* Fig. 1-5) are commonly used to identify key pathways or molecules mediating various immune responses. T- or B-lymphocyte proliferation (*see* Figs. 1-7 and 1-8) and T-cell cytotoxicity (*see* Fig. 1-6) are techniques used to assess the function of T or B cells in response to antigenic stimuli. These techniques may be used to assess the effect of various pharmacologic or biologic agents in modulating specific cellular functions.

In the near future, two major forces will reshape modern molecular biology: *genomics*, the determination of complete DNA sequence of various organisms, including humans, and *proteomics*, the comprehensive determination of protein structure and function. Furthermore, the development of many molecular biology techniques, such as fluorescence microscopy (*see* Fig. 1-10), fluorescence-tagged antibodies (*see* Fig. 1-11), confocal microscopy, DNA micro-array technology (*see* Fig. 1-12), and many others, have revolutionized our current understanding of immune function. These developments in the field of molecular biology will enable scientists to better understand the mechanisms of immune activation and to discover the role of previously unknown genes in many biologic and pathologic processes. Such discoveries will provide the focus for future development of clinical interventions.

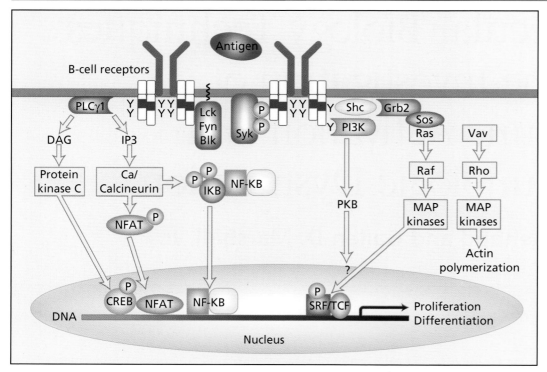

■ Figure 1-1.

B-lymphocyte activation pathway [1–3]. Some surface molecules and regulatory pathways have been omitted for simplicity. Binding of an antigen to a B-cell receptor initiates a cascade of enzymatic reactions catalyzed by two families of tyrosine kinase enzymes: Syk and Src (fyn, lyn, Blk). These enzymes catalyze the transfer of phosphate atoms from ATP to the tyrosine residues (Y) on the intracellular domain of B- cell receptor chains. The receptor chains, when phosphorylated, serve as docking sites for the recruitment of intracellular secondary messengers, *ie*, PLCγ2, PI3K, and Grb2/SOS. These secondary messengers are themselves activated by phosphorylation and initiate cascades of more activation reactions. Each cascade results in the activation of a group of proteins, known as transcription factors, *ie*, SRF/TCF, NFkB, NF-AT, and CREB. Transcription factors, when activated, translocate to the nucleus, bind to specific sites on the chromosome, and initiate transcription of new genes. These new genes encode new proteins and, by mechanisms that are not fully understood, lead to B-lymphocyte responses such as growth and differentiation. An active area of research is the elucidation of how each pathway may lead to a specific antigen-mediated response, *ie*, growth, differentiation to antibody producing cells, survival, or tolerance.

The PLCγ pathway consists of the following: Phospholipase Cγ2 (PLCγ2), an isoform of phospholipase C, is an enzyme that catalyzes the hydrolysis of membrane phospholipids, PIP2 (phosphatidylinositol 4,5-bisphosphate) to IP3 (inositol 1,4,5-triphosphate) and DAG (diacylglycerol). IP3 triggers the release of calcium from the intracellular storage sites, *ie*, endoplasmic reticulum. Calcium release activates calcineurin, a phosphatase, which dephosphorylates a transcription factor, NFAT (nuclear factor of activated T cells). NFAT in its dephosphorylated form is active, enters the nucleus, and initiates gene transcription. DAG activates PKC (protein kinase C). PKC activates a transcription factor, CREB (cyclic adenosine monophosphate, cAMP, response element–binding protein). Calcium elevation may also be involved in activation of another transcription factor, NF-kB (nuclear factor, kB). NF-kB, in an inactive form, is bound to IkB (inhibitor of NF-kB). However, when intracellular calcium levels rise, IkB dissociates from NF-kB. Unbound NF-kB is active, translocates to the nucleus, and initiates gene transcription.

The PI3K pathway consists of the following: PI3K (phosphatidylinositol 3-kinase) is an enzyme that adds a phosphate atom to inositol-containing phospholipids. PI3K activation leads to the conversion of PIP2 (phosphatidylinositol 4,5 bisphosphate) to PIP3 (phos-

phatidyl inositol 3,4,5 triphosphate). PIP3 recruits PKB (protein kinase B) to the membrane and leads to its activation. PKB has been shown to be involved in protection from apoptosis.

A third pathway for B-lymphocyte activation is the Ras pathway. Ras, a secondary messenger protein, is an important mediator of cell growth and differentiation in many cell types. Ras family members (Rac, Rho, Cdc42, Ras) when bound to GDP (guanosine diphosphate) are inactive and when bound to GTP (guanosine triphosphate) are active and function as an activation switch for a number of intracellular pathways. B-cell receptor cross-linking leads to receptor phosphorylation and recruitment of an intracellular adaptor protein, Shc. Shc, when phosphorylated, binds to another adaptor protein, Grb2. Grb2 binds to a nucleotide exchange factor, SOS (Son of Sevenless). SOS facilitates the exchange of GDP for GTP on Ras and therefore leads to the activation of Ras. Active Ras associates with and activates Raf, a serine threonine kinase. Raf activates a group of serine/threonine/tyrosine kinases (*see* next paragraph for definition) known as mitogen-activated protein kinases (MAP kinases). MAP kinases, when activated, activate a group of transcription factors such as SRF/TCF (serum response factors). Vav is another nucleotide exchange factor that is phosphorylated by receptor-associated kinases and becomes activated. Vav in its active form activates Rho (a Ras family member) by facilitating GTP for GDP exchange. Rho in its GTP bound form is active and regulates polymerization of actin cytoskeleton through the activation of MAP kinases. Polymerization of actin in cytoskeleton has an essential role in membrane rearrangements, cellular trafficking, and activation.

Kinases are intracellular enzymes that catalyze transfer of a phosphate on specific amino acid residues by hydrolysis of ATP. Phosphorylation of proteins in most cases leads to their activation. Kinases may catalyze transfer of phosphate groups on tyrosine, threonine, or serine residues and are called tyrosine, threonine, or serine kinases, respectively. Some kinases have a dual role, *ie*, serine/threonine kinases are able to transfer phosphate on serine and threonine residues, whereas some kinases have a specific role and can only transfer phosphate on a serine or a threonine.

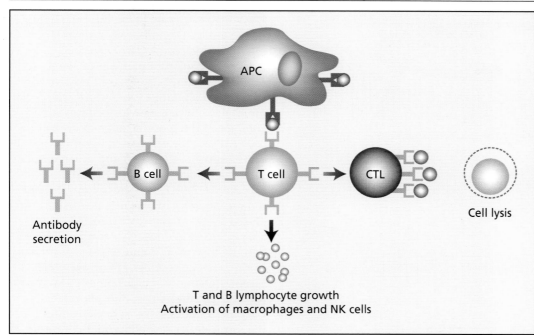

Figure 1-2.

T lymphocyte pathways. Following antigen presentation, T lymphocytes may follow any of the following pathways: 1) T lymphocytes aid in B lymphocyte activation and result in B-lymphocyte differentiation to antibody-producing cells; 2) T lymphocytes differentiate to cytotoxic T lymphocytes and directly kill other cells; and 3) T lymphocytes release cytokines. Cytokines are responsible for the growth and activation of other T lymphocytes, B lymphocytes, and inflammatory cells such as macrophages and natural killer cells [4].

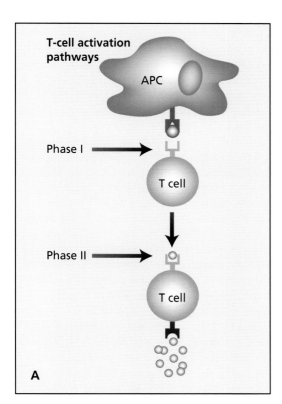

Figure 1-3.

Phases of T-cell activation. **A,** Overview of phases of T-cell activation pathways. An essential step in immune activation is the release of cytokines from T lymphocytes. Cytokines are involved in a number of immune-mediated responses, such as growth and activation of B and T lymphocytes, recruitment of inflammatory cells to the site of inflammation, and activation of macrophages and natural killer cells. Release of cytokines from T cells involves two phases. *Phase I* is initiated when an antigen is presented to T lymphocytes via specialized cells known as antigen-presenting cells, such as macrophages, dendritic cells, or even, in certain cases, B cells. Phase I results in the expression of cytokines and cytokine receptors. Binding of a cytokine to its cognate cytokine receptor initiates phase II of T lymphocyte activation. *Phase II* leads to the expression of new genes that are responsible for specific cytokine-mediated effects, such as T cell growth, differentiation to cytotoxic or helper cells, tolerance, or apoptosis. (*continued on next page*)

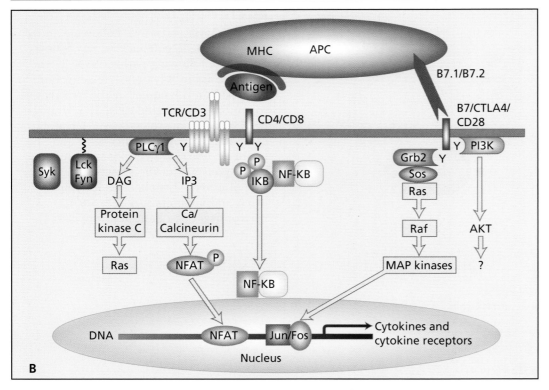

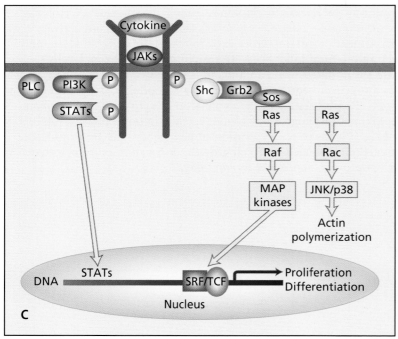

Figure 1-3. *(continued)*

B, Phase I of T-lymphocyte activation [5–10]. Some costimulatory surface molecules and regulatory pathways have been omitted for simplicity. Phase I involves presentation of an antigen to a T cell via special molecules of the major histocompatability complex (MHC) on the antigen-presenting cells (APC). Antigen presentation recruits T-cell receptor (TCR/CD3) and other surface molecules, such as CD4/CD8 and CTLA4/CD28/B7, to form a complex and initiate cascades of enzymatic reactions catalyzed by two families of tyrosine kinase enzymes, Syk and Src. Syk and Src (Lck, Fyn) hydrolyze ATP and transfer phosphate to the tyrosine residues (Y) on the T-cell receptor chains as well as other co-stimulatory surface molecules. Phosphorylated tyrosine residues serve as docking sites for the intracellular secondary messengers, *ie,* PLCγ1, PI3K, and Grb2/SOS/Ras. The secondary messengers, once recruited to their specific docking sites on the receptors, are themselves activated by phosphorylation and initiate cascades of biochemical reactions leading to the activation of transcription factors such as Jun, Fos, NFkB, and NF-AT. These transcription factors, when activated, translocate to the nucleus, bind to specific sites on the chromosome, and initiate transcription of genes for cytokines and cytokine receptors.

The Ras pathway in the T cell is responsible for the activation of two transcription factors, Fos and Jun. Jun/Fos, when activated in a cooperative manner with NFAT (nuclear factor of activated T cells), regulates the transcription of cytokine and cytokine receptor genes.

C, Phase II of T-lymphocyte activation [11]. Phase II involves binding of cytokines to their cognate cytokine receptors and activation of a group of intracellular tyrosine kinase enzymes known as Janus kinases (Jaks). There are four members of Janus kinases: Jak1, Jak2, Jak3, and Tyk2. Janus kinase enzymes are recruited to the cytokine receptors and result in the activation (phosphorylation) of secondary messenger molecules such as STATs (signal transducers and activators of transcription), Shc, and PI3K. The enzymatic reactions activated by Jaks lead to the initiation of cascades of biochemical events, resulting in the activation of transcription factors such as STATs and SRF. These transcription factors, once activated, translocate to the nucleus, bind to specific sites on the chromosome, and initiate transcription of new genes. Cytokines have a wide variety of functions and mediate natural as well as specific immune activation against antigens. P—phosphate moiety; Y—tyrosine residue.

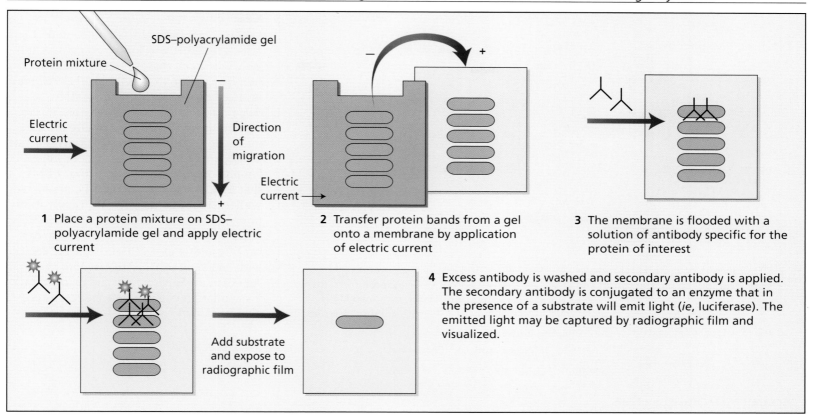

Figure 1-4.

Isolation and identification of intracellular proteins by SDS-poly-acrylamide gel electrophoresis [12]. This technique is commonly used for the identification of intracellular enzymes, secondary messengers or transcription factors involved in T- or B- cell activation. For this purpose, T or B lymphocytes are purified from the whole blood of animal or human and stimulated with an antibody or a chemical agent to mimic T- or B-cell receptor stimulation. After stimulation, the T or B cells are lysed, and the cytoplasmic content is subjected to SDS-polyacrylamide gel electrophoresis (SDS-PAGE).

SDS-polyacrylamide gels are semisolid porous gels. When electrophoresis is applied to an SDS polyacrylamide gel, smaller proteins migrate faster than larger proteins. After applying electric current to the SDS-PAGE gel, proteins are separated based on size (1), separated proteins are then transferred onto a membrane (2), antibody specific to the protein of interest is applied to the membrane (this step is known as Western blot) (3), and the protein bands are visualized on radiographic film (4).

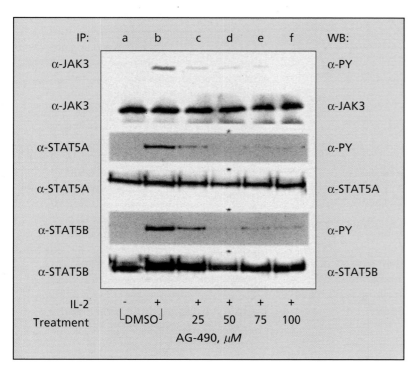

Figure 1-5.

An example of SDS-PAGE for identification of proteins involved in a cytokine-activated pathway. This diagram demonstrates that a pharmaceutical agent, AG490 (A Janus kinase inhibitor), inhibits phosphorylation of an intracellular tyrosine kinase, Jak3 (an enzyme responsible for the phosphorylation of transcription factors, Stat 5a/b). Note that Jak3 is autophosphorylated, a mechanism for self-activation of the enzyme [13].

The methods used include the following steps: 1) Human T lymphocytes are stimulated by a cytokine, IL-2; 2) T cells are lysed and cytoplasmic contents separated by centrifugation; 3) antibodies specific for Jak3, Stat5a, and Stat5b are added to the cytoplasmic content; 4) a complex is formed between the proteins of interest and their specific antibodies; 5) the complex of protein and antibodies are captured using special beads; 6) the captured proteins are denatured in a special buffer (SDS), subjected to SDS-polyacrylamide gel electrophoresis, and transferred to a membrane (as described in Fig. 1-4); 7) The Western blot technique is applied to the membrane, using an antibody specific for the tyrosine phosphorylated proteins; and 8) the tyrosine phosphorylated proteins are visualized on radiographic film.

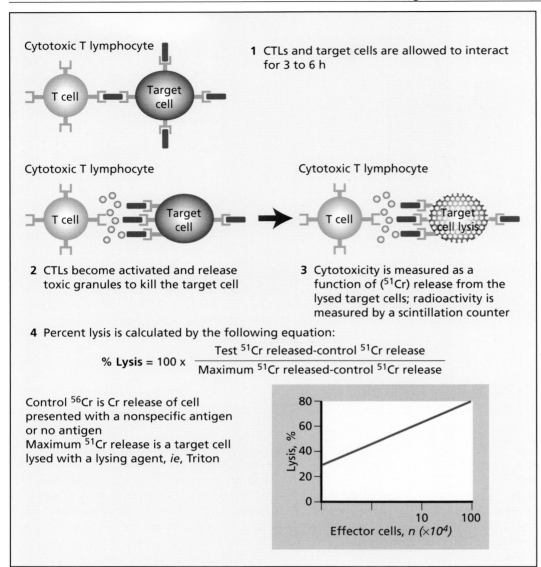

Cytotoxic T lymphocyte

T cell — Target cell

1 CTLs and target cells are allowed to interact for 3 to 6 h

Cytotoxic T lymphocyte

T cell — Target cell

Cytotoxic T lymphocyte

T cell — Target cell lysis

2 CTLs become activated and release toxic granules to kill the target cell

3 Cytotoxicity is measured as a function of (^{51}Cr) release from the lysed target cells; radioactivity is measured by a scintillation counter

4 Percent lysis is calculated by the following equation:

$$\% \text{ Lysis} = 100 \times \frac{\text{Test }^{51}\text{Cr released-control }^{51}\text{Cr release}}{\text{Maximum }^{51}\text{Cr released-control }^{51}\text{Cr release}}$$

Control ^{56}Cr is Cr release of cell presented with a nonspecific antigen or no antigen
Maximum ^{51}Cr release is a target cell lysed with a lysing agent, *ie,* Triton

Effector cells, n (×10⁴) — Lysis, %

Figure 1-6.

Cytotoxicity assay [14]. A function of T cells is to destroy or kill target cells. A target cell is a cell that is targeted for destruction by a cytotoxic T cell. A target cell may be a cell possessing a different MHC molecule or a cell infected with a virus. Target cells are labeled with ^{51}Cr briefly prior to interaction with the cytotoxic T cells. These T cells are known as cytotoxic (or killer) T lymphocytes (CTLs). In this assay, PBMC that are thought to contain CTL are mixed with ^{51}Cr-labeled target cells, usually for 4 hours. If there are target cell–specific CTLs in the PBMC, they will initiate a lytic cascade, resulting in death of the target cell with concomitant ^{51}Cr release into the supernatant. Supernatants are counted in a γ scintillation counter, and the results are expressed as percent lysis.

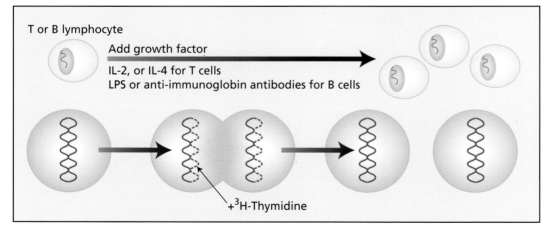

T or B lymphocyte

Add growth factor
IL-2, or IL-4 for T cells
LPS or anti-immunoglobin antibodies for B cells

+^{3}H-Thymidine

Figure 1-7.

Proliferation assay [15]. This test is used to assess proliferation of T or B lymphocytes in response to extracellular stimuli, such as cytokines for T cells or anti-immunoglobulin (anti–B-cell receptor) antibodies for B cells. The process of cell growth or proliferation involves chro-

mosome duplication. In this process, chromosomes are separated into single strands, and each strand synthesizes a new complementary strand by incorporating nucleotides (cytosine, adenine, guanine, and thymidine). The medium containing the growing cells is supplemented with ^{3}H-thymidine, which is incorporated into the newly synthesized chromosomes as cells proliferate.

The method used in this process can be summarized as follows: 1) cells are incubated with a growth factor, *ie,* cytokine IL-2 for 24 hours; 2) in the last 4 hours of incubation, ^{3}H-thymidine is added (0.5 μCi/50,000 cells); 3) growing cells will incorporate ^{3}H-thymidine; and 4) cells are harvested onto a filter paper. The filter papers are placed in scintillation fluid (a solvent) and ^{3}H-thymidine incorporation is measured using a scintillation counter.

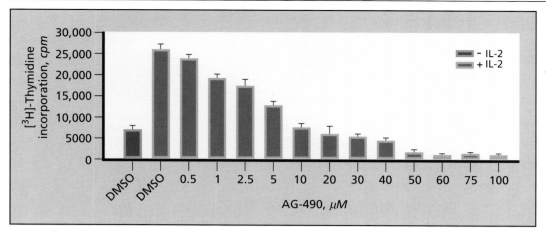

■ Figure 1-8.

An example of proliferation assay. This experiment is performed to assess proliferation of a rat T-cell line in response to IL-2 in the presence or absence of a drug, AG-490. T cells are stimulated with or without IL-2 for 24 hours and incubated with increasing concentrations of AG-490. ^{3}H-thymidine (0.5 μCi/50,000 cells) is added in the last 4 hours of culture. This experiment shows that AG-490 inhibits IL-2–induced proliferation of T cells. The mechanism of action of AG-490 is inhibition of Janus kinase-3 (Jak3) activation, an intracellular enzyme responsible for signal transduction in response to IL-2 [13].

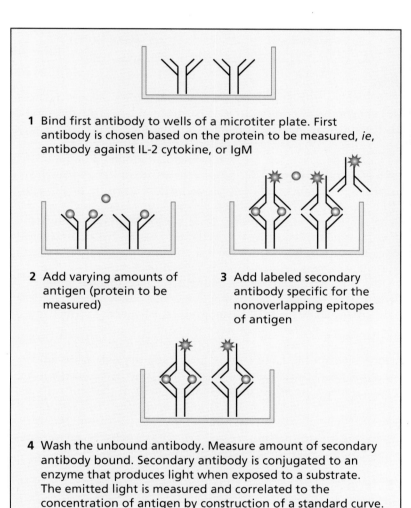

1 Bind first antibody to wells of a microtiter plate. First antibody is chosen based on the protein to be measured, *ie*, antibody against IL-2 cytokine, or IgM

2 Add varying amounts of antigen (protein to be measured)

3 Add labeled secondary antibody specific for the nonoverlapping epitopes of antigen

4 Wash the unbound antibody. Measure amount of secondary antibody bound. Secondary antibody is conjugated to an enzyme that produces light when exposed to a substrate. The emitted light is measured and correlated to the concentration of antigen by construction of a standard curve.

■ Figure 1-9.

Enzyme-linked immunosorbent assay (ELISA). ELISA is a powerful technique for quantitative measurement of proteins produced in biologic systems. The protein of interest is captured by specific antibodies bound to a microtiter plate. A second protein-specific antibody that is conjugated to an enzyme such as horseradish per-oxidase is then added to the mixture. This second antibody also binds to the protein captured by the first. Finally, a substrate for the enzyme is added to all wells. Color develops in proportion to the enzyme present, which is proportional to the concentration of the protein of interest. This test may be used to assess the amount and type of cytokines produced by T lymphocytes in response to certain stimuli, *ie*, an allergen.

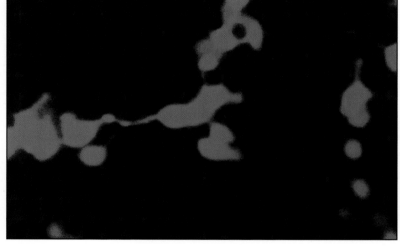

■ Figure 1-10.

Fluorescent microscopy. This technique is used to localize certain proteins in a tissue or cell [17]. A chemical is said to be fluorescent if it absorbs light at one wavelength (excitation wavelength) and emits light at a specific and longer wavelength. Four very useful dyes for fluorescent staining are rhodamine and Texas red (emits red light), Cy3 (emits orange light), and fluorescein (emits green light). A protein conjugated to these dyes may be expressed in cells and visualized using a fluorescent microscope. This figure shows expression of a green fluorescent protein (GFP) in a T cell.

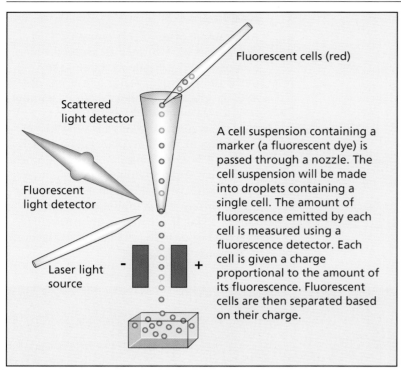

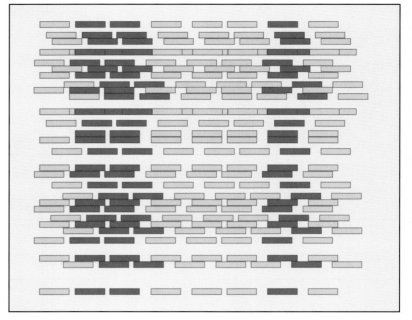

Fluorescent cells (red)

Scattered light detector

Fluorescent light detector

Laser light source

A cell suspension containing a marker (a fluorescent dye) is passed through a nozzle. The cell suspension will be made into droplets containing a single cell. The amount of fluorescence emitted by each cell is measured using a fluorescence detector. Each cell is given a charge proportional to the amount of its fluorescence. Fluorescent cells are then separated based on their charge.

Figure 1-11.

Fluorescence-activated cell sorter (FACS). This technique is used to separate a pure population of cells, *ie*, B lymphocytes or T helper or T cytotoxic lymphocytes. An FACS can separate one cell from a population of thousands of other cells. For example, cells are incubated with a fluorescent conjugated antibody specific to a certain cell surface molecule, *ie*, CD3. Then FACS is used to separate all cells bearing CD3 on their surface. This technique is very effective in separating different types of white blood cells, each expressing a distinct surface molecule, *ie*, CD3 on T lymphocytes or IgM on B cells.

Figure 1-12.

DNA microarray chip. This powerful tool allows the researchers to study expression of thousands of genes simultaneously in response to certain environmental stimuli. Knowing the genomic sequence of an organism, oligonucleotides corresponding to the coding region of each gene of interest are synthesized and mounted on the surface of a glass microscope slide. A tissue or a specific cell type is then exposed to certain conditions (*ie*, allergen stimulation of a T cell). Total cellular mRNA is isolated, reverse-transcribed to cDNA, and labeled with a fluorescent dye. Total mRNA from one condition, (*ie*, unstimulated control) may be labeled with a red fluorescent dye, and total mRNA from the test condition (*ie*, after an antigenic stimulation) may be labeled with a green fluorescent dye. The cDNA mixture of the control and treated cells is incubated to hybridize with the corresponding oligonucleotides on the glass microscope slide. Each DNA spot on the microarray is then analyzed using a scanning laser microscope. The intensity of green or red fluorescence at each DNA spot correlates with the intensity of gene transcription. For example, gene X on the slide with high intensity green fluorescence indicates that gene X transcription is increased in response to antigenic stimulation. If the spot is orange (same intensity red and green), it indicates that the transcription of gene X is unchanged in response to the antigenic stimulation. Therefore, the transcription of all genes in response to an antigenic stimulation may be studied simultaneously.

References

1. Tsubata T: Co-receptors on B lymphocytes. *Curr Opin Immunol* 1999, 11:249–255.

2. Campbell KS: Signal transduction from the B cell antigen receptor. *Curr Opin Immunol* 1999, 11:256–264.

3. DeFranco AL: B lymphocyte activation. In *Fundamental Immunology*. Edited by Paul WE. New York: Lippincott-Raven; 1998:225–261

4. Abbas AK, Lichtman AH, Pober JS: Effector mechanisms of T-cell–mediated immune reactions. In *Cellular and Molecular Immunology*, edn 2. Edited by Abbas AK, Lichtman AH, Pober JS. Philadelphia: WB Saunders; 1994:261–277.

5. Watts TH, DeBenedette MA: T cell co-stimulatory molecules other than CD28. *Curr Opin Immunol* 1999, 11:286–293.

6. Linsley PS, Reth M: Lymphocyte activation and effector functions, multistory progress: increasing organization on all levels. *Curr Opin Immunol* 1999, 11:239–241.

7. Favero J, Lafont V: Effector pathways regulating T-cell activation. *Biochem Pharmacol* 1998, 56:1539–1547.

8. Rincon M, Flavell RA, Davis R: The JNK and P38 Map kinase signaling pathways in T-cell–mediated immune responses. *Free Radic Biol Med* 2000, 28:1328–1337.

9. Serfling E, Berberich-Siebelt F, Chuvpilo S, *et al.*: The role of NF-AT transcription factors in T-cell activation and differentiation. *Biochim Biophys Acta* 2000, 1498:1–18.

10. Weiss A: T-lymphocyte activation. In *Fundamental Immunology*. Edited by Paul WE. New York: Lippincott-Raven; 1998:411–447.

11. Decker S: Introduction: STATs as essential intracellular mediators of cytokine responses. *CMLS Cellular and Molecular Life Sciences* 1999, 55:1505–1508.

12. Lodish H, Berk A, Zipursky SL, *et al.*: Protein structure and function. In *Molecular Cell Biology*. Edited by Lodish H, Zipursky SL, Baltimore D, Darnell J. New York: WH Freeman and Company; 2000:91.

13. Behbod F, Erwin-Cohen RA, Wang Mou-Er, *et al.*: Concomitant inhibition of Jak3 and calcineurin-dependant signaling pathways synergistically prolong the survival of rat heart allografts. *J Immunol* 2001, 166:3724–3732.

14. Abbas AK, Lichtman AH, Pober JS: Antigen processing and presentation to T lymphocytes. In *Cellular and Molecular Immunology*, edn 2. Edited by Abbas AK, Lichtman AH, Pober JS. Philadelphia: WB Saunders; 1994: 116–134.

15. Abbas AK, Lichtman AH, Pober JS: B-cell–activation and antibody production. In *Cellular and Molecular Immunology*, edn 2. Edited by Abbas AK, Lichtman AH, Pober JS. Philadelphia:WB Saunders; 1994:188–203.

16. Abbas AK, Lichtman AH, Pober JS: Antibodies and antigens. In *Cellular and Molecular Immunology*, edn 2. Edited by Abbas AK, Lichtman AH, Pober JS. Philadelphia: WB Saunders; 1994: 34–61.

17. Lodish H, Berk A, Zipursky SL, *et al.*: Biomembranes and the subcellular organization of eukaryotic cells. In *Molecular Cell Biology*. Edited by Lodish H, Zipursky SL, Baltimore D, Darnell J. New York: WH Freeman and Company; 2000:140–168.

18. Lodish H, Berk A, Zipursky SL, *et al.*: Recombinant DNA and genomics. In *Molecular Cell Biology*. Edited by Lodish H, Zipursky SL, Baltimore D, Darnell J. New York: WH Freeman and Company; 2000:248.

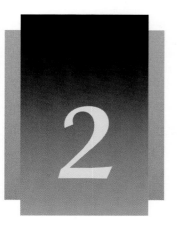

2 Immunoglobulin Structure and Function

Phillip L. Lieberman

Immunoglobulins are products of plasma cells. They are responsible for humoral immunity and are also the effector molecules and antigen receptors for B lymphocytes. All immunoglobulins are glycoproteins. They are found in the serum and also on the surface of certain cells such as natural killer cells, mononuclear phagocytes, and mast cells. In addition, they are present in secretory fluids such as saliva, bronchial and nasal secretions, and colostrum.

Immunoglobulins migrate electrophorectically, for the most part, as γ-globulins during serum electrophoresis. There are five classes of immunoglobulins IgG, IgA, IgM, IgD, and IgE. All immunoglobulin molecules are similar in structure and are composed of polypeptide chains consisting of repeating, homologous units known as domains. Each domain is approximately 110 amino acids in length and is joined by a disulfide bond.

Each immunoglobulin consists of an antibody-combining site (FaB) and a site that determines the effector activity (*eg*, whether the molecule binds to mast cells, crosses the placenta) known as the Fc region. The actual combining site in the FaB region is only a few amino acids in length. It is known as the epitope. There are perhaps as many as 1 billion structurally different immunoglobulin molecules based on epitope variation, each having a unique amino acid sequence at this site.

The antibody-binding site is at the *N*-terminal side of the molecule, and the effector site (the Fc region) is at the carboxy terminal end. Each immunoglobulin molecule is subject to enzymatic digestion. When immunoglobulins are incubated with papain, cleavage occurs at the hinge region on the *N*-terminal side of the disulfide bonds connecting the heavy chains, resulting in the production of three fragments. Two of these fragments are identical to one another and consist of an entire light chain along with the variable region of the heavy chain. These fragments are known as FaB segments. The third segment, which consists of the carboxy end of the molecule, is known as the Fc fragment. When pepsin cleaves the molecule, the enzymatic cut occurs on the carboxy terminal side of the hinge region and the two FaB fragments remain linked. This results in an F(ab)′2 fragment that, in essence, is two FaB fragments linked by disulfide bonds. Papain degrades the Fc fragment, which does not survive after digestion.

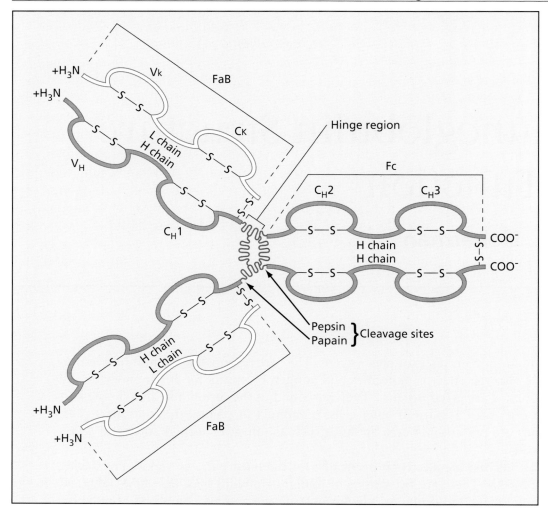

■ Figure 2-1.

Prototype model of the immunoglobulin molecule demonstrating the FaB and Fc fragments and the sites for digestion by papain and pepsin.

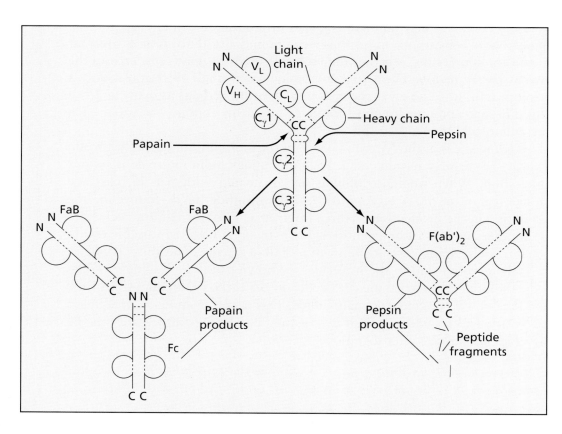

■ Figure 2-2.

The structure of the cleavage products of the immunoglobulin molecule after incubation with papain and pepsin.

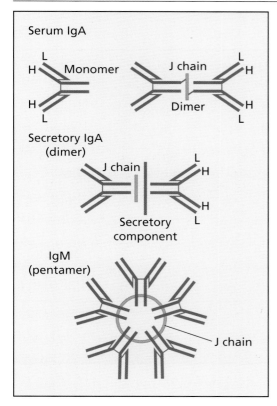

Figure 2-3.

Polymeric human immunoglobulins. Both IgM and IgA exist in polymeric forms. The polymeric form of secretory IgA contains both a J chain and a secretory piece. This secretory piece, unlike the immunoglobulin molecule itself, is produced by epithelial cells and is attached to the molecule after it is synthesized and released from the plasma cell. IgM consists of a pentamer with individual IgM molecules being joined by the J chain (as with IgA).

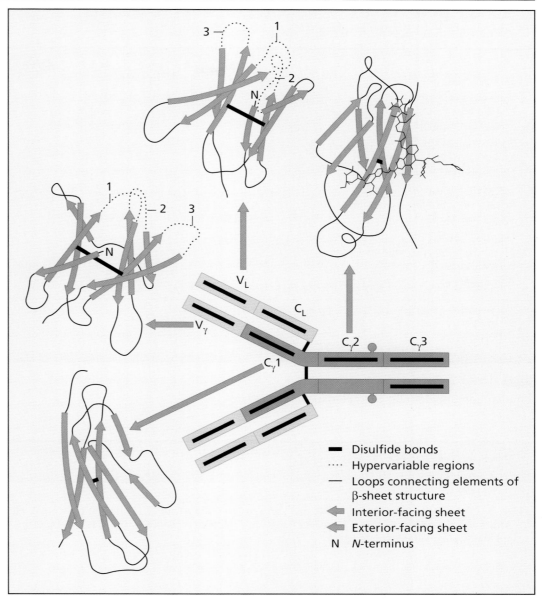

Figure 2-4.

Immunoglobulin domains in IgG. Immunoglobulin peptide chains are folded structures with three-dimensional configurations. The folds of the various domains are depicted. The numbers 1, 2, and 3 indicate the hypervariable regions of the sequence from the *N*-terminus.

Human Immunoglobulin Characteristics

	IgG	IgA	IgM	IgD	IgE
H-chain class	γ	α	μ	δ	ϵ
H-chain subclasses	$\gamma1, \gamma2, \gamma3, \gamma4$	$\alpha1, \alpha2$	–	–	–
L-chain type	κ and λ	κ and λ	κ and λ	κ and λ	κ and λ
Molecular formula	γ_L2	$\alpha_2L_2{}^*$ or $(\alpha_2L_2)SC^\dagger J^\ddagger$	$(\alpha_2L_2)_5J^\ddagger$	δL_2	ϵ_2L_2
Sedimentation coefficient, S	6–7	7	19	7–8	8
Molecular weight (approximate)	150,000	160,000* or 400,000§	900,000	180,000	190,000
Electrophoretic mobility (average)	γ	Fast γ to β	Fast γ to β	Fast γ	Fast γ
Complement fixation (classic)	+	0	++++	0	0
Serum concentration (approximate), *mg/dL*	1000	200	120	3	0.05
Serum half-life, *d*	23	6	5	3	2
Placental transfer	+	0	0	0	0
Mast cell or basophil degranulation	?	0	0	0	++++
Bacterial lysis	+	+	+++	?	?
Antiviral activity	+	+++	+	?	?

*For monomeric serum IgA.
†Secretory component.
§J chain.

Figure 2-5.

Human immunoglobulin characteristics.

Recommended Reading

Abbas A, Lichtman A, Paber J: *Antibodies and Antigens in Cellular and Molecular Immunology*, edn 2. Edited by Abbas A, Lichtman A, Paber J. Philadelphia: WB Saunders; 1994.

Burton D, Woof J: Human antibody effector function. *Adv Immunol* 1992, 51:1–84.

3

The Complement System

Michael S. Blaiss

The complement system is a vital part of the immune system in humans. It is composed of a group of highly coupled proteins that interact with one another to effect inflammation and the humoral immunity [1]. Important aspects of the function of the complement system in triggering action in humans include the following [2]:

1. Opsonization of foreign organisms and particles
2. Cytolysis of invading organisms
3. Rendering immune complexes harmless to the body
4. Generation of complement byproducts that act as chemotactic agents that recruit inflammatory cells
5. Anaphylatoxins, which are complement byproducts that stimulate release of chemical mediators such as histamine from mast cells

Deficiencies and dysfunctions of the complement system can lead to a variety of conditions, some life-threatening, in humans.

Overview of the Complement System

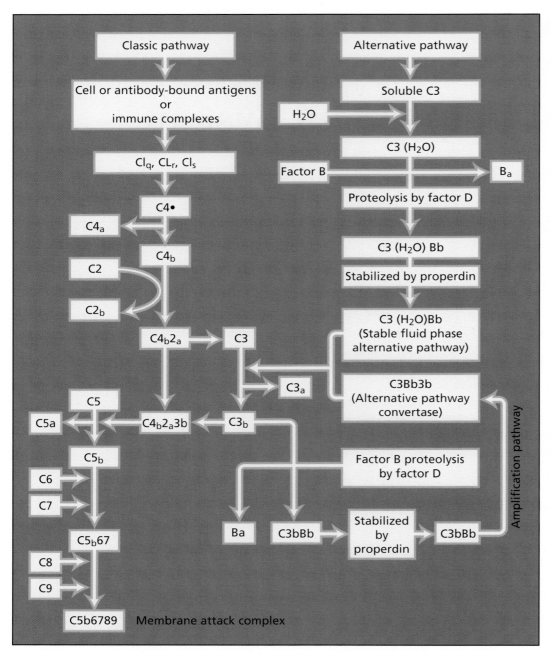

Figure 3-1.

The complement cascade. The complement system is made up of two major pathways: the classic and the alternative pathways [3]. IgG and IgM immune complexes activate the classic pathway. Complement component C1—which is made up of three subunits, C1q, C1r, and C1s—is bound to the Fc portions of antigen–antibody complex and begins the cascade. The complement complex, C1, cleaves and activates C4 and C2. C4 is cleaved into C4a and C4b, and C2 breaks down to C2a and C2b. The components C4b and C2a interact and have enzymatic action in cleaving C3 to create C3a and C3b. The C4b and C2a complex is called the classic pathway C3 convertase. Next the formed C3b and the C4b and C2a have enzymatic activity that triggers the terminal components (C5 to C9) into the membrane attack complex (MAC).

Unlike the classic pathway, the alternative pathway [4] can be activated without antibody and directly triggered by binding to the surface of microorganisms. The first component of the alternative pathway is C3b, which is produced from the classic pathway or nonspecific activation. Factor D then activates C3b, and this complex cleaves factor B. It is the formation of the alternative pathway C3 convertase, involving C3 and factor B, that binds to C5 and results in the formation of the MAC.

The terminal components formed through the classic and alternative pathways are called the MAC. Complement components C5, C6, C7, C8, and C9 are activated and produce pores in the cell surface membrane. These pores allow for the influx of small ions and water into the cell and lead to osmotic lysis of the cell.

Protein Components

Protein Components of the Complementary Cascade

Component	Molecular Size, *kd*	Serum Concentration, *µg/mL*	Molecular Size of Subunit Chains, *kd*	Activation Products	Comments on Function
Classical pathway					
C1 (C1qr$_2$s$_2$)	900				Initiates classical pathway
C1q	410	75	6 of A; 24 6 of B; 23 6 of C; 22		Binds to Fc portion of Ig
C1r	85	50	1	C$\overline{1}$r	C$\overline{1}$r is a serine proteae; cleaves C$\overline{1}$s
C1s	85	50	1	C$\overline{1}$s	C$\overline{1}$s is a serine protease; cleaves C4 and C2
C4	210	200–500	1 of alpha; 90 1 of beta; 78 1 of gamma; 33	C4a C4b	C4a is an anaphylatoxin; C4b covalently binds to activating surfaces, where it is part of C3 convertase
C2	110	20	1	C$\overline{2}$a C2b	C$\overline{2}$a is a serine protease; part of C3 and C5 convertases
C3 (also part of alternative pathway)	195	550–1200	1 of alpha; 110 1 of beta; 85	C3a C3b	C3a is an anaphylatoxin; C3b covalently binds to activating surfaces, where it is part of C3 and C5 convertases and acts as opsonin
Alternative pathway					
Factor B	93	200	1	Ba B$\overline{b}$	B$\overline{b}$ is a serine protease, part of C3 and C5 covertases
Factor D	25	1–2	1	$\overline{D}$	Protease that circulates in active state; cleaves factor B
Properdin	220	25	4; 56		Stabilizes alternative pathway C3 convertase
Terminal lytic components					
C5	190	70	1 of alpha; 115 1 of beta; 75	C5a C5b	C5 is an anaphylatoxin
C6	128	60	1		C5b initiates MAC assembly
C7	121	60	1		Component of MAC
C8	155	60	1 of alpha; 64 1 of beta; 64 1 of gamma; 22		Component of MAC Component of MAC
C9	79	60	1		Component of MAC; polymerizes to form membrane pores

Figure 3-2.

Protein components of the complement system. This table lists the various proteins that make up the complement system along with function and activation products produced. The biologic functions of the complement system occur through two main mechanisms. Effects can be caused by complement activation on immune complexes or cell surfaces. The other major pathway leading to biologic functions is the production of soluble products from complement activation that stimulates receptors on cells throughout the body. MAC—membrane attack complex. (*Adapted from* Abbas *et al.* [2].)

Regulatory Proteins

Soluble and Membrane Proteins that Regulate Complement Activation

Protein	Serum Concentration, µg/mL, or Cellular Distribution	Specifically Interacts With	Function
		Soluble serum proteins	
CI INH	200	C1r, C1s	Serine protease inhibitor covalently binds to C$\overline{1}$r and C$\overline{1}$s and blocks their ability to participate in the classical pathway
			Binds to inactive C1 and prevents spontaneous activation
			Also inhibits kallikrein, plasmin, and factors XIa and XIIa of coagulation system
C4bp	250	C4b	Accelerates decay of classical pathway C3 convertase (C$\overline{4b2a}$)
			Acts as cofactor for factor 1–mediated cleavage of C4b
Factor H	480	C3b	Accelerates decay of alternative pathway C3 convertase (C3bBb)
			Acts as cofactor for factor 1–mediated cleavage of C3b
Factor I	35	C4b, C3b	Proteolytically cleaves and inactivates C4b and C3b, using C4bp, factor H, CRI, or MCP as cofactors
Anaphylatoxin inactivator	35	C3a, C4a, C5a	Proteolytically removes terminal arginine residues and inactivates the anaphylatoxins
S protein	505	C5b-7	Binds to C5b-7 complex and prevents membrane insertion of MAC
SP-40,40	50	C5b-9	Modulates MAC formation
		Integral Membrane Proteins	
CR1 (CD35)	Most blood cells, mast cells	C3b, c4b, iC3b	Accelerates dissociation of classical and alternative pathway C3 convertases
			Acts as cofactor for factor 1–mediated cleavage of C3b and C4b (binds immune complexes and promotes their dissolution and phagocytosis)
MCP (CD46)	Most blood cells (except erythrocytes), epithelial cells, endothelial cells, fibroblasts	C3b, C4b	Acts as cofactor for factor 1–mediated cleavage of C3b and C4b
DAF	Most blood cells	C4b2b C3bBb	Accelerates dissociation of classical and alternative pathway C3 convertases
HRF	Erythrocytes, lymphocytes, monocytes, neutrophils, platelets	C8 C9	Inhibits lysis of bystander cells (reactive lysis)
			Blocks C9 binding to C8, preventing MAC insertion into lipid bilayer of autologous cells and lysis; action restricted to C9, C8 of same species
CD59 (MRLI)	Erythrocytes, lymphocytes, monocytes, neutrophils, platelets	C7 C8	Inhibits lysis of bystander cells (reactive lysis)
			Blocks C7, C8 binding to C5b,6, preventing MAC formation and lysis; action restricted to C7, C8 of same species

■ Figure 3-3.

Regulatory proteins of the complement system. Another important aspect of the complement system is the proteins that are important in regulating the complement cascade [5]. Uncontrolled activation of the complement system may lead to tissue damage by the membrane attack complex and may increase production of inflammatory mediators. These different proteins work at various points in the classic and alternative cascades and the terminal pathway. One group of these proteins consists of the soluble serum proteins; the other group contains the integral membrane proteins. CI INH—C1 inhibitor; CR1—complement receptor type 1; DAF—decay accelerating factor; HRF—homologous restriction factor; MAC—membrane attack complex; MCP—membrane cofactor protein; MIRL—membrane inhibitor reactive lysis.

Complement Deficiencies and Abnormalities

Complement Deficiencies and Abnormalities

Protein	Resulting Complement Activation Abnormalities	Associated Diseases and Pathology	Inheritance
	Classical pathway		
C1q	Defective classical pathway activation	SLE Glomerulonephritis	AR
C1r	Defective classical pathway activation	SLE Glomerulonephritis Pyogenic infections	AR
C1s	Defective classical pathway activation	SLE Glomerulonephritis Pyogenic infections	AR
C4	Defective classical pathway activation	SLE Glomerulonephritis Pyogenic infections	AR
C2	Defective classical pathway activation	SLE Vasculitis Glomerulonephritis Pyogenic infections	AR
C3	Defective classical or alternative pathway activation	Pyogenic infections Glomerulonephritis	AR
	Alternative Pathway		
Properdin	Defective alternative pathway activation	Pyogenic infections	XL
Factor D	Defective alternative pathway activation	Pyogenic infections	?
	Terminal Components		
C5	Defective MAC formation	Disseminated *Neisseria* spp. infections	AR
C6	Defective MAC formation	Disseminated *Neisseria* spp. infections	AR
C7	Defective MAC formation	Disseminated *Neisseria* spp. infections Glomerulonephritis SLE	AR
C8	Defective MAC formation	Disseminated *Neisseria* spp. infections SLE	AR
C9	Defective MAC formation	Disseminated *Neisseria* spp. infections	AR

■ Figure 3-4.

Diseases in humans related to the complement system. Fortunately, such diseases are rare [6]. There are two major ways that the complement system can factor into human disease. First, deficiencies can exist in one of the complement components that are involved in the activation of the classic and alternative pathway, or the membrane attack complex. These conditions are usually inherited as an autosomal recessive trait or by mutated genes that fail to code for the production of adequate quantities of the complement protein or produce a dysfunctional or abnormal protein. The second abnormality that leads to human disease is deficiency or dysfunction of the complement regulatory proteins, which can lead to too much activation of the complement system in the wrong location or time.

Deficiencies of the complement components can be divided on the basis of whether they are part of the classic or alternative pathway. In patients with deficiencies of the classic complement proteins, the most common clinical manifestations are autoimmune or immune complex diseases, such as systemic lupus erythematosus (SLE) and glomerulonephritis [7]. It is estimated that up to 50% of patients with C2 and C4 deficiency have SLE. The exact cause for the increase in autoimmune diseases in patients with deficient classic pathway components is not known. One theory is that it may be caused by the close proximity of the genes coding for complement components C2 and C4 and the DR locus and class I MHC genes. Another possibility is an altered host response to chronic or recurrent viral infection with classical complement component deficiencies. In general, patients with deficiency of a classic complement component are not susceptible to increased infections, but there are reports of increased susceptibility to *Hemophilus influenzae* septicemia in infants with C2 deficiency.

Deficiency of the complement component C3 is associated with increased incidence of pyogenic infections, which highlights the pivot role of C3 in opsonization, phagocytosis, and destruction of microorganisms [8]. The increases in bacterial infections are commonly exhibited by recurrent bouts of pneumonia, otitis, meningitis, and pharyngitis.

Whereas the clinical manifestations seen with deficiencies of alternative complement components result primarily in increased pyogenic infections, the deficiencies of the terminal components (ie, C5, C6, C7, and C8) demonstrate an increased risk with recurrent infections caused by *Neisseria* organisms [9]. Currently there is no evidence of any abnormal clinical effects seen in patients with C9 deficiency. AR—autosomal recessive; MAC—membrane attack complex; SLE—systemic lupus erythematosus; XL—X linked. (*Adapted from* Abbas *et al.* [2].)

Deficiencies and Dysfunction of Complement Regulator Proteins

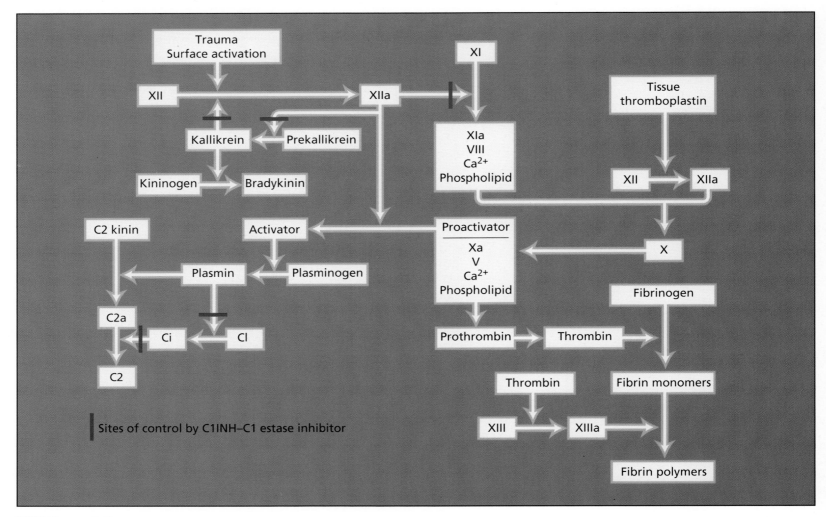

Figure 3-5.

Interaction of clotting, fibrinolysis, kinin system, and complement pathways.

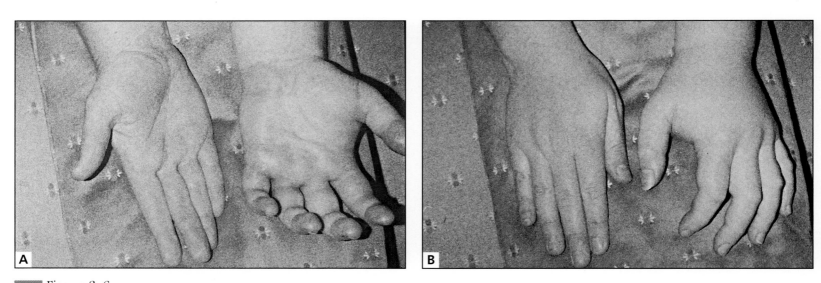

Figure 3-6.

Hereditary angioneurotic edema (HAE). **A** and **B,** Angioedema of the hands. (*continued on next page*)

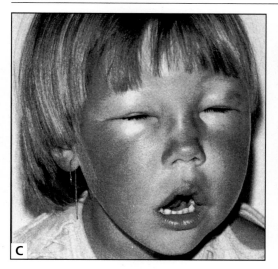

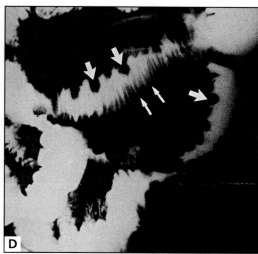

Figure 3-6. *(continued)*

C, Five-year-old girl with a moderate attack of angioedema. D, Small bowel barium radiograph during an acute episode of pain in the proband. Two segments of jejunum have mural edema: "thumbprinting" (*thick arrows*) and spiculation (*thin arrows*).

This condition is one of several that are caused by deficiencies and dysfunction on complement regulator proteins. HAE is an autosomal dominant condition caused by a deficiency or nonfunction of C1 esterase inhibitor [10]. Patients with this abnormality have recurrent episodes of swelling of the soft tissues, primarily of the face, extremities, larynx, and intestinal mucosa. Symptoms usually begin in adolescence, and attacks are commonly triggered by emotional stress and trauma (see *panels A–D*). Without the C1 esterase inhibitor, there is continued activation of the classic complement pathway and dysregulation of the activity of clotting, kinin, and fibrinolysis pathways. The causative factor leading to the angioedema may be C3a, C4a, and C5a; the anaphylotoxins; or C2 kinin from kinin activity. C4 levels are decreased in patients with HAE. Aminocaproic acid is used in the treatment of patients with acute attacks and for prevention before a medical procedure such as surgery. For long-term therapy, androgens such as danazol have been shown to stimulate C1 esterase inhibitor production. (*Panels A* and *B from* Arreaza *et al.* [13], with permission; *panel C* from Weinstock *et al.* [14], with permission; *panel D* from Nielsen *et al.* [15]; with permission.)

Abnormalities and Deficiencies of Regulatory Complement Proteins

Protein	Resulting Complement Activation Abnormalities	Associated Diseases and Pathology
DAF	Deregulated C3 convertase activity	Complement-mediated intravascular hemolysis
HRF	Increased susceptibility of erythrocytes to MAC-mediated lysis	Complement-mediated intravascular hemolysis
CD59 (MIRL)	Increased susceptibility of erythrocytes to MAC-mediated lysis	Complement-mediated intravascular hemolysis

Figure 3-7.

Paroxysmal nocturnal hemoglobinuria. This condition is characterized by repeated episodes of intravascular hemolysis, at least partially caused by complement activation of the surface of the erythrocyte [11]. It is usually caused by a deficiency of decay accelerating factor. This protein is involved in dissociation and inactivation of C3 and C5 convertases for both the classic and alternative complement pathways. Other types of paroxysmal nocturnal hemoglobinuria are from absence of other internal complement regulatory proteins that inhibit the membrane attack complex. In the near future, therapeutic inhibition and manipulation of the complement components may be important tools in clinical medicine [12]. DAF—decay accelerating factor; HRF—homologous restriction factor; MAC—membrane attack complex; MCP—membrane cofactor protein; MIRL—membrane inhibitor reactive lysis.(*Adapted from* Abbas *et al.* [2].)

References

1. Kinoshita T: Biology of complement: the overture. *Immunol Today* 1991, 12:291–295.
2. Abbas AK, Lichtman AH, Pober JS: *Cellular and Molecular Immunology*. Philadelphia: WB Saunders; 1991:262.
3. Winkenstein JA, Fries LF: The complement system. In *Allergy Principles and Practice*. Edited by Middleton E, Reed CE, Ellis EF. St. Louis: Mosby; 1998:58–71.
4. Farries TC, Atkinson JP. Evolution of the complement system. *Immunol Today* 1991, 12:295–300.
5. Parker CJ: Regulation of complement by membrane proteins: an overview. *Curr Opin Microbiol Immunol* 1992, 178:1–6.
6. Holbert JM: Complement deficiency syndromes. *Clin Pract Med* 1999, 2:1821–1827.
7. Sullivan KE: Complement deficiency and autoimmunity. *Curr Opin Pediatr* 1998, 10:600–606.
8. Singer L, Colten HR, Wetsel RA: Complement C3 deficiency: human, animal, and experimental models. *Pathobiology* 1994, 62:14–28.
9. Morris JT, Kelly WJ: Recurrence of neisserial meningococcemia due to deficiency of terminal complement component. *South Med J* 1992, 85:1030–1031.
10. Ebo DG, Stevens WJ: Hereditary angioneurotic edema: review of the literature. *Acta Clin Belg* 2000, 55:22–29.
11. Nishimura J, Murakami Y, Kinoshita T: Paroxysmal nocturnal hemoglobinuria: an acquired genetic disease. *Am J Hematol* 1999, 62:175–182.
12. Makrides SC: Therapeutic inhibition of the complement system. *Pharmacol Rev* 1998, 50:59–87.
13. Arreaza EE, Singh K, Grant JA: Hereditary angioedema: clinical and biochemical heterogeneity. *Ann Allergy* 1988, 61:69–75.
14. Weinstock LB, Kothari T, Sharma RV, Rosenfeld SI: Recurrent abdominal pain as the sole manifestation of hereditary angioedema in multiple family members. *Gastroenterology* 1987, 93:1116–1118.
15. Nielsen EW, Gran JT, Straume B: Hereditary angio-edema: new clinical observations and autoimmune screening, complement and kallikrein-kinin analyses. *J Intern Med* 1996, 239:119–130.

4 Chemokines and Their Receptors

Susan Y. Ritter and Gailen D. Marshall, Jr.

Chemokines are small proteins that promote chemotaxis and activation of cells for inflammatory reactions. Currently more than 50 human chemokines and 18 receptors have been identified. These chemokines are further divided into subfamilies (CXC, CC, CXXXC, and so on) based on their aminoterminal cysteine motifs.

Chemokines could not cause chemotaxis without receptors on target cells. The chemokine receptors are G-protein–coupled receptors present in varying amounts on the cell surface. CXC chemokines bind to one of four CXC receptors (CXCR1-4), whereas CC chemokines are restricted to binding CC receptors. On binding, receptors activate intracellular signaling pathways, such as actin polymerization, to propel the cell toward the stimulus. Receptors may be present constitutively on cells or selectively regulated by cytokines and mitogens. Both Th (T helper)-1 and Th2 lymphocytes have unique chemokine receptor expression; therefore, not only is cytokine production important in determining an immune response, but it has an impact on chemokines and cell trafficking.

Chemokines have been implicated in a variety of diseases such as HIV, in which chemokine receptors are essential for viral infectivity, and cancer, in which, receptor expression has been linked to homing, metastasis, and angiogenesis—all of which promote tumor growth [1]. The functional importance of chemokines in allergy and immunology can be seen in the events associated with inflammatory leukocyte migration. It is the chemotactic gradient that helps direct leukocytes through the vascular endothelium to the antigen-activated cells.

Chemokines of considerable interest to many allergists-immunologists include the CC chemokines such as the eotaxins RANTES and MCPs. These proinflammatory chemokines recruit eosinophils and basophils and promote degranulation and histamine release. For similar reasons, CCR3 has been highly studied because it is the primary receptor for CC chemokines on eosinophils. Whereas eosinophils play a major role in the pathogenesis of asthma and allergy, T lymphocytes and neutrophils also produce and respond to chemokines. Research into the role of chemokines in allergy and asthma consistently finds CC chemokines expressed during periods of clinical exacerbation or experimental allergen challenge. For example, a study of patients with various lung diseases found that eotaxin was upregulated only in the asthma patients [2]. There have been similar findings of increased eotaxin expression in the nasal epithelium of allergic rhinitis patients [3]. Intensive research is currently focused on finding ways to inhibit chemokine production or block binding of chemokines by their receptors to modify their adverse effects on the host.

Role and Functions of Chemokines

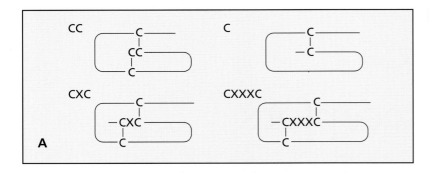

B. Chemokines Involved in Allergy and Asthma

	Receptors	Target Cells
CXC		
GRO-(α, β, γ)	CXCR2	Neutrophil
IL-8	CXCR1, CXCR2	Neutrophil
SDF-1	CXCR4	Resting T cell, dendritic cell, monocyte
IP-10	CXCR3	NK cell
MIG	CXCR3	NK cell
I-TAC	CXCR3	NK cell
CC		
Eotaxin	CCR3	Eosinophil, basophil, lymphocyte
Eotaxin-2	CCR3	Eosinophil, basophil, lymphocyte
MCP-1	CCR2, CCR10	Basophil
MCP-2	CCR2	Basophil
MCP-3	CCR1, CCR3, CCR10	Eosinophil, basophil, lymphocyte
MCP-4	CCR2, CCR3	Eosinophil, basophil, lymphocyte
MDC	CCR4	Dendritic cell, monocytes
MIP-1α	CCR1, CCR5	Eosinophil, lymphocyte, monocyte, dendritic cell
MIP-1β	CCR5, CCR8	NK cell, monocyte, dendritic cell, lymphocyte
MIP-3α	CCR6	Dendritic cell, lymphocyte
MIP-3β	CCR7	Activated T cell
RANTES	CCR1, CCR3, CCR5	Eosinophil, basophil
TARC	CCR4, CCR8	Activated T cells, Th2 cells
C		
Lymphotactin	XCR1	Lymphocyte, NK cells
CXXXC		
Fractalkine	CX3CR1	Monocyte, activated T cell, NK cell

Figure 4-1.

Chemokine families, receptors, and their positions. **A,** Chemokine families are determined by the position of the initial cysteine residues. CXC chemokines have their first two cysteine residues separated by one amino acid, whereas CC chemokines have no break between their first two cysteine residues [4]. **B,** There are four families of chemokines of potential importance in allergy and asthma [5]. Each chemokine can bind to different receptors expressed on particular cell types. For example, CXC chemokines are chemotactic for neutrophils and lymphocytes, whereas CC chemokines attract monocytes, eosinophils, basophils, and lymphocytes. Binding of a chemokine to its receptor can cause chemotaxis, activation, generation of reactive oxygen species, and degranulation of target cells. IL—interleukin; IP—interefon-inducible protein; ITAC—interferon-inducible T-cell α chemoattractant; MCP—monocyte chemoattractant protein; MIG—monokine induced by interferon gamma; MIP—macrophage inflammatory protein; NK—natural killer; RANTES—regulated upon activation normal T cell expressed and secreted; SDF—stromal cell derived factor; TARC—thymus and activation regulated chemokine; T helper—T helper.

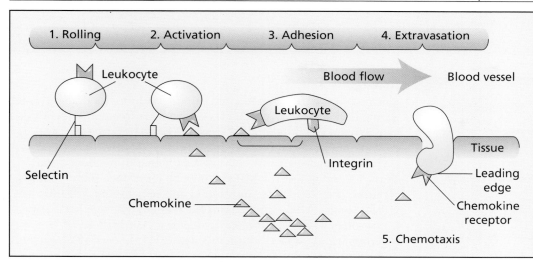

■ Figure 4-2.

The role of chemokines in leukocyte migration. Chemokines are secreted by leukocytes, fibroblasts, and endothelial cells and bound to intracellular matrix and cell-surface proteins, where they will be recognized by chemokine receptors on leukocytes. As leukocytes roll along the vessel wall bound loosely by selectins, they encounter chemokines. Binding of chemokines to their receptors activates cell signaling and cell-surface integrins, which provide tight adherence to the vessel wall. Once the cell has entered the tissue, it again follows the chemotactic gradient to the site of inflammation [4,6].

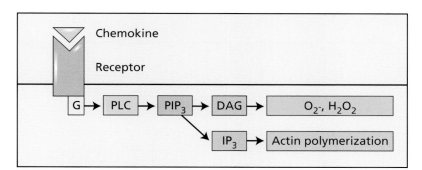

■ Figure 4-3.

Chemokine signaling. Chemokines bind to their cognate, G-protein–linked receptors, resulting in downstream signaling through phospholipase C (PLC). The end result of signaling is actin polymerization, chemotaxis, and release of reactive oxygen species [7]. Actin polymerization helps the cell to move toward the gradient, whereas reactive oxygen species cause tissue damage and inflammation. In addition, some cell types release toxic granules when activated, which contributes to inflammation. DAG—diacylglycerol; IP$_3$—inositol triphosphate; PIP$_3$—phosphatidylinositol triphosphate.

A. Th1/Th2 Cytokine Impact on Chemokine Receptor Expression

	Chemokine Receptors Expressed	Cytokine Regulation of Receptors	Chemokine Ligands
Th1 cells	CCR5	Upregulated by IL-12, IFN-γ, IL-10 Downregulated by IL-4, IL-13	MIP-α, MIP-1β, RANTES, IP-10, MIG, I-TAC
	CSCR3	Upregulated by IFN-γ	
Th2 cells	CCR3	Upregulated by IL-4 Downregulated by TGF-β	Eotaxin, RANTES, MCP-2, -3, -4, TARC, MDC, I-309
	CCR4		
	CCR8		

B. Th1/Th2 Cytokine Impact on Chemokine Synthesis

	IL-12	IFN-γ	IL-4	IL-10	IL-13
IL-8		Downregulated	Upregulated		
IP-10/MIG/I-TAC		Upregulated			
MIP-1α	Upregulated	Upregulated			
RANTES		Upregulated	Downregulated	Downregulated	Downregulated
MDC		Downregulated	Upregulated		Upregulated
Eotaxin			Upregulated		Upregulated

■ Figure 4-4.

The functions of chemokines and cytokines. Not only do cytokines influence the expression of certain chemokines and their receptors (**A**), but chemokines can also function to regulate T helper cell differentiation into Th1 or Th2 by inducing interleukin (IL)-12 or IL-4 production (**B**) [6,8]. Generally speaking, type 1 cytokines upregulate expression of chemokine receptors on Th1 cells and vice versa. IFN-γ—interferon gamma; IL—interleukin; IP—interefon-inducible protein; ITAC—interferon-inducible T-cell a chemoattractant; MCP—monocyte chemoattractant protein; MDC—monocyte-depleted cell; MIG—monokine induced by interferon gamma; RANTES—regulated upon activation normal T cell expressed and secreted; TARC—thymus and activation regulated chemokine; TGF-β—transforming growth factor-β.

Disease Involvement

Chemokines Involved in Allergic Rhinitis, Asthma, Food Allergy, and Atopic Dermatitis	
Disease	**Chemokines**
Allergic rhinitis	MIP-1α, RANTES, IL-8, MCP-1, eotaxin
Asthma	IL-8, eotaxin, MCPs, MDC, MIPs, RANTES, TARC
Atopic dermatitis	RANTES, eotaxin
Food allergy	Eotaxin

Figure 4-5.

Chemokines involved in allergic rhinitis, asthma, food allergy, and atopic dermatitis. CC chemokines have been frequently identified as playing a role in allergic disease [9–12]. The specific chemokines involved in each disease differ slightly; thus whereas a therapeutic agent against eotaxin may help all the above conditions, an antagonist for MIP-1α may be more specific for rhinitis. As more chemokines are discovered and patients studied, this list will likely grow. IL—interleukin; MCP-1—monocyte chemoattractant protein 1; MDC—monocyte-depleted cell; MIP-1α— macrophage inflammatory protein-1α; RANTES— TARC—thymus and activation regulated chemokine; RANTES—regulated upon activation normal T cell expressed and secreted.

Assays

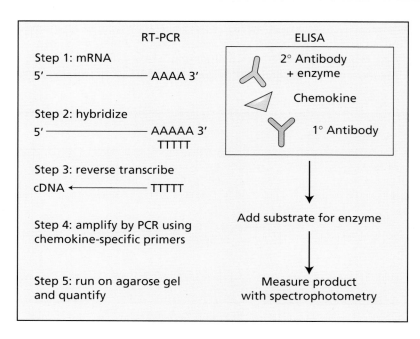

Figure 4-6.

Chemokine assays. Two assays are illustrated: reverse-transcriptase polymerase chain reaction (RT-PCR) and enzyme-linked immunosorbent assay (ELISA). For RT-PCR, one measures the amount of mRNA for a particular cytokine in a cell or tissue. Once the RNA has been isolated, then it is annealed to an oligo-dT primer, which binds the polyA tail. Reverse transcriptase is used to convert the RNA to cDNA, and this is amplified using PCR. By incorporating ^{32}P-labeled dideoxynucleotides during PCR amplification, a semiquantitative measurement of chemokine mRNA can be obtained. The PCR products are run on an agarose gel, then dried and exposed to a phosphorimaging screen. The radiolabeled PCR products are then quantified in phosphorescence units.

Commercial ELISA kits are available for quantification of chemokines. A standard curve is used to determine the amount of chemokine present in a sample. Briefly, antibody specific for the chemokine is bound to the plate by its Fc region. The chemokine-containing solution is added to the well, and binds the antibody. A secondary antibody is added, which recognizes the chemokine and is conjugated to an enzyme. Excess antibody is washed off. On adding the substrate, the enzyme is activated and a colored product, in proportion to the amount of chemokine present, is made that can be read on a spectrophotometer.

Future Therapies

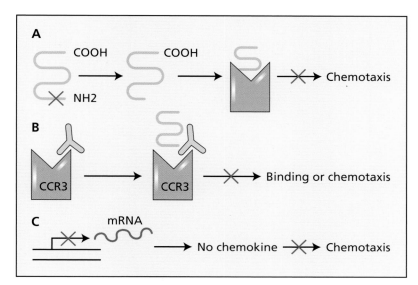

Figure 4-7.

Potential directions for future therapy. By changing the aminoterminus of a chemokine like RANTES, receptor binding can still occur but there will be no signaling activity (A). This will block binding of endogenous chemokine to the receptor [13]. A receptor blockade, either by antibody or a small molecule, will allow specific targeting of a particular receptor, like CCR3, that is relatively specific for allergic inflammation (B) [14]. Blocking the messengers that cause chemokine release, such as antihistamines blocking histamine-induced chemokine production, is a way to minimize the level of chemokines released and prevent massive leukocyte recruitment and subsequent inflammation (C) [15].

References

1. Strieter RM: Chemokines: not just leukocyte chemoattractants in the promotion of cancer. *Nat Immunol* 2001, 2:285–286.

2. Miotto D, Christodoulopoulos P, Olivenstein R, *et al.*: Expression of IFN-gamma-inducible protein; monocyte chemotactic proteins 1,3, and 4; and eotaxin in TH1- and TH2-mediated lung disease. *J Allergy Clin Immunol* 2001, 107:664–670.

3. Minshall EM, Cameron L, Lavinge F, *et al.*: Eotaxin mRNA and protein expression in chronic sinusitis and allergen-induced nasal responses in seasonal allergic rhinitis. *Am J Respir Cell Mol Biol* 1997, 17: 683–690.

4. Luster AD: Chemokines: chemotactic cytokines that mediate inflammation. *N Engl J Med* 1998, 338:436–445.

5. Busse WW, Lemanske RF: Advances in immunology: asthma. *N Engl J Med* 2001, 344: 350–360.

6. Gagner V, Oppenheim JJ: Are chemokines essential or secondary participants in allergic responses? *Ann Allergy Asthma Immunol* 2000, 84:569–578.

7. Elsner J, Petering H, Kimmig D, *et al.*: The CC chemokine receptor antagonist met-RANTES inhibits eosinophil effector functions. *Int Arch Allergy Immunol* 1999, 118:462–465.

8. Luther AS, Cyster JG: Chemokines as regulators of T cell differentiation. *Nat Immunol* 2001, 2:102–107.

9. Ying S, Kay AB, Alam R: *Chemokines in Allergic Disease.* Edited by Rothenberg ME. New York: Marcel Dekker; 2000.

10. Lukas NW, Tekkanat KK: Role of chemokines in asthmatic airway inflammation. *Immunol Rev* 2000, 177:21–30.

11. Morita E, Kameyoshi Y, Hiragun T, *et al.*: The C-C chemokines, RANTES, and eotaxin, in atopic dermatitis. *Allergy* 2001, 56:194–195.

12. Hogan SP, Mishra A, Brandt EB, *et al.*: A pathological function for eotaxin and eosinophils in eosinophilic gastrointestinal inflammation. *Nat Immunol* 2001, 2:353–360.

13. Proudfoot AEI, Power CA, Wells TNC: The strategy of blocking the chemokine system to combat disease. *Immunol Rev* 2000, 177:246–256.

14. Menzies-Gow A, Robinson DS: Eosinophil chemokines and their receptors: an attractive target in asthma? *Lancet* 2000, 355:1741–1743.

15. Fujikura T, Shimsawa T, Yakuo I: Regulatory effect of histamine H1 receptor antagonist on the expression of messenger RNA encoding CC chemokines in the human nasal mucosa. *J Allergy Clin Immunol* 2001, 107:123–128.

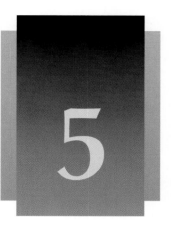

Mast Cell– and Basophil-Derived Mediators

J. Andrew Grant and Patricia A. Leonard

The incidence of allergic disease is increasing. With an estimated 13 million Americans suffering from asthma [1], and another 23 million experiencing symptoms of allergic rhinitis [2], efforts to understand the human allergic response have intensified. Mast cells and basophils are the primary effector cells involved in allergic inflammation; since the 1800s, these cells have been known to participate in allergic reactions. However, recent discoveries of potent cellular mediators have led to exciting new developments in the understanding of the allergic response. This chapter illustrates mast cell and basophil participation in the allergic response through production of cell mediators.

Mast cells and basophils arise from CD34 progenitor cells in the bone marrow and fetal liver [3]. Mast cells circulate in the bloodstream and migrate to anatomic sites, where they are exposed to foreign substances from the external environment. Such sites include the skin, respiratory tract, gastrointestinal (GI) tract, and conjunctiva. They are also found around nerves and blood vessels. In contrast, basophils remain in the circulation, accounting for approximately 0.5% of total leukocytes. They are attracted into peripheral tissue during immune-mediated reactions and other pathologic conditions. When mast cells and basophils become activated, they degranulate and release both preformed and newly synthesized mediators. These cell mediators initiate the allergic response and are responsible for the symptoms of allergic disease. Mast cells and basophils may also be involved in homeostasis, host defense, and inflammatory responses other than allergic.

The allergic response is divided into the early and late phase reaction. Mast cells are the major cells that initiate the early phase allergic reaction. They release preformed (*eg*, histamine) and newly synthesized mediators (*eg*, leukotrienes) into the microenvironment and are responsible for symptoms that occur within the first hour of allergen exposure. This acute phase represents classical immediate-type hypersensitivity. A dramatic example of immediate-type hypersensitivity is anaphylactic shock, a potentially fatal condition. Basophils, acting in concert with eosinophils, Th2 lymphocytes, and other cells, contribute to the late-phase inflammatory response, which appears about 3 to 8 hours after allergen challenge. A group of mediators recently characterized as major participants in the late-phase allergic response are cytokines and chemokines. These proteins are synthesized and released by mast cells, basophils, and other cells, and have effects on the cells of origin as well as other cells involved in allergic inflammation.

Morphology

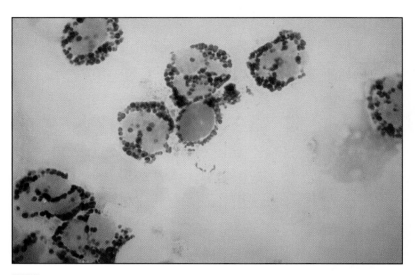

Figure 5-1.

Basophils from peripheral blood with typical multilobulated nuclei and cytoplasmic granules present on staining. The morphologic feature that distinguishes mast cells and basophils from other cells is the presence of cytoplasmic metachromatic granules. These granules store a variety of substances that are released during cell

degranulation. They include biogenic amines (*ie*, histamine), proteoglycans (*ie*, chondroitin sulfate, heparin), and proteins (*ie*, tryptase, chymase).

Mast cells are 9 to 12 μm in diameter with central monolobuled nuclei. The cytoplasm contains membrane-bound secretory granules containing preformed mediators. The most abundant of these mediators include the proteases: tryptase, chymase, and carboxypeptidase. Subclasses of mast cells are described based on differences in their granule protease composition and staining pattern. The subclass containing tryptase (MC_t) is found predominantly in the lung, nose, and small intestines. Chymase and tryptase are both found in the MC_{tc} subclass, and these subtypes can be located in the skin, blood vessels, GI submucosa, heart, and synovium. The cytoplasmic granules of the mast cell also contain histamine, accounting for nearly all the histamine stored in normal tissue of the body.

Basophils are 5- to 7-μm cells with multilobulated nuclei. These cells also contain cytoplasmic granules containing preformed mediators. Chondroitin sulfate A is the predominant proteoglycan found in basophil granules. Charcot-Leyden crystals are also present in these granules. Basophils from nonallergic patients have negligible amounts of tryptase [4], but allergic patients are noted to have detectable levels when challenged with allergens [5]. Basophils provide the main source of histamine in the blood.

Mast Cell and Basophil Mediators

	Mast Cell	Basophils
Mediators preformed		
	Histamine	Histamine
	Tryptase	Charcot-Leyden crystals
	Chymase	Major basic protein
	Chondroitin sulfate	Chondroitin sulfate
	Carboxypeptidase A	Cathepsin G
	Cathepsin G	Tryptase
	Acid hydrolase	
	Heparin	
Newly synthesized lipids		
	$LTC_4, A_4, B_4, D_4, E_4$	LTC_4, D_4, E_4
	PAF	PAF
	PGD_2	
Cytokines		
	IL-3, -4, -5, -6, -8, -10, -13, -16	IL-4, -5, -6, -8, -10, -12, -13
	TNF-α*	TNF-α*
	MIP-1α	MIP-1α*
	GM-CSF	
	β-FGF	RANTES
	SCF	
	TGF-β	
	VEGF, VPF	
	RANTES	
	MCP	

Figure 5-2.

Mast cell and basophil mediators. Mediators may be preformed within the cell or synthesized on cell activation. Although mast cells and basophils share some similarities, they differ in respect to type and quantity of mediators and cytokines they secrete [3,6–8]. Tryptase is found predominantly in mast cells. Whereas circulating α-tryptase reflects the

body's total number of mast cells, levels of β-tryptase reflect acute mast cell activation. This finding has clinical relevance because it serves as a biochemical marker for disease states. Conditions associated with increased mast cells, such as mastocytosis, elevate circulating α-tryptase levels in the blood. β-Tryptase is seen in the serum of patients with anaphylaxis, the nasal secretions of allergic rhinitis patients, and the bronchoalveolar lavage fluid of asthmatics [9]. Prostaglandin D_2 (PGD_2) is recovered from acute allergic reactions and is a product of mast cells, not basophils. Multiple cytokines have been implicated in the pathophysiology of allergic inflammation. Some cytokines play a more critical role than others. GM-CSF—granulocyte macrophage–colony stimulating factor; GM-FGF—fibroblast growth factor; IL—interleukin; LT—leukotriene; MCP—monocyte chemoattractant protein; MIP—macrophage inflammatory protein; PAF—platelet activating factor; PG—prostaglandin; RANTES—regulated on activation, normal T cell expressed and secreted; SCF—stem cell factor; TGF—transforming growth factor; TNF—tumor necrosis factor; VEGF—vascular endothelial cell growth factor; VPF—vascular permeability factor. *Asterisks* indicate mediators that may be both preformed and synthesized within the cell.

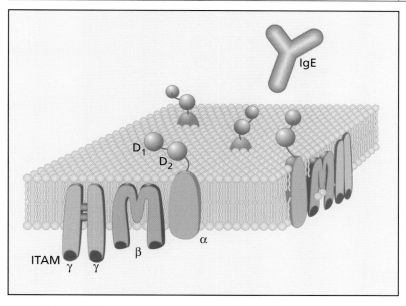

Figure 5-3.

Mast cell and basophil receptors. Mast cells and basophils contain high-affinity receptors for IgE on their cell surfaces. This receptor, FCϵRI, binds IgE at very low concentrations. There are 10^4 to 10^6 FCϵRI receptors per mast cell or basophil [9]. Studies in mice and humans have shown that levels of FCϵRI surface expression in mast cells and basophils can be regulated by levels of IgE [6,10]. High-affinity receptors have also been located on Langerhans cells [11,12], monocytes [13], dermal dendritic cells [14], and eosinophils [15].

Each receptor contains three subunits that act in concert to transduce intracellular signals and activate the cell. Human cells may express two isoforms of ($\alpha\beta\gamma\gamma$ or $\alpha\gamma\gamma$). The α subunit is expressed on the outer surface of the cell, penetrates the membrane, and contains a cytoplasmic tail. The extracellular portion of this subunit has two domains (either D1, D2), the second of which binds to IgE [16]. The β subunit has four transmembrane domains with both amino and carboxy terminals located in the cytoplasm. The two γ subunits are linked by disulfide bonds, transverse the membrane, and have cytoplasmic tails.

The β and γ subunits are responsible for signal transduction. The cytoplasmic domains of the β and γ subunits contain immunoreceptor tyrosine-based activation motifs (ITAM), which recruit and activate tyrosine kinase. This leads to signal transduction and, ultimately, mast cell and basophil degranulation. High affinity receptor for IgG (FCγRI) has recently been shown to be expressed on human mast cells [17].

Activation

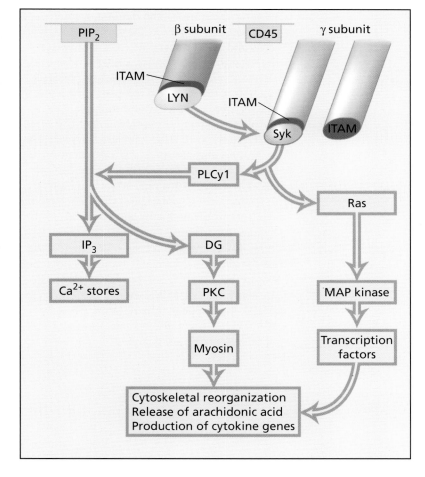

Figure 5-4.

Mast cell activation. The cross-linking of two IgE molecules to FCϵRI receptors initiates cell signaling, which leads to induction of *de nova* synthesis of mediators and subsequent cell degranulation. The src family of kinases is one of many kinases that are activated upon binding of IgE. Lyn kinase is a member of this family and is involved with mast cell and basophil activation. It binds to the immunoreceptor tyrosine-based activation motifs (ITAM) sequence of the β subunit. Lyn then mediates the tyrosine phosphorylation of β and γ ITAMs on the FCϵRI receptor, allowing cytoplasmic tyrosine Syk kinase to aggregate to the γ subunit ITAM. The binding of Syk to the γ subunit activates numerous downstream signaling pathways. CD45 (protein tyrosine phosphatase) regulates the Lyn-Syk union.

Syk activates phospholipase Cy1 (PLCy1), which generates inositol 1,4,5-triphosphate (IP_3) and diacylglycerol (DG) from phosphatidylinositol 4,5-bisphosphate (PIP_2). IP_3 releases stores of intracellular calcium. DG activates and translocates protein kinase C (PKC), which in turn phosphorylates other proteins, including myosin. The activation of myosin results in cell cytoskeletal reorganization, with subsequent granule swelling and fusion of granules with the plasma membranes leading to exocytosis of contents.

Syk also activates Ras, a member of the GTPase family, which then activates the mitogen-activated protein (MAP) kinase pathway. This pathway produces transcription factors (*ie,* cytoplasmic phospholipase A_2) involved in the release of arachidonic acid and production of cytokine genes.

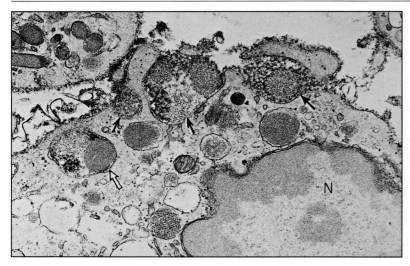

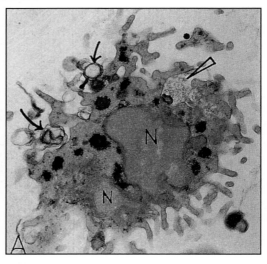

Figure 5-5.

Activated basophil in the degranulation process. *Black arrows* indicate sites around the cell perimeter where granules are fusing with the plasma membranes, releasing both preformed and newly synthesized mediators into the microenvironment. These mediators act on targeted tissues to give rise to the symptoms associated with allergic response.

Figure 5-6.

A completely degranulated human basophil with extruded granules (*open arrow*). When a mast cell or basophil becomes activated, multiple downstream signaling pathways are activated. This process results in activation of proteins that cause derangement in the cell infrastructure leading to marked shape changes. Further cellular activation leads to exocytosis of the secretory granules. *Dark arrows* indicate extruded granules. N—nucleus.

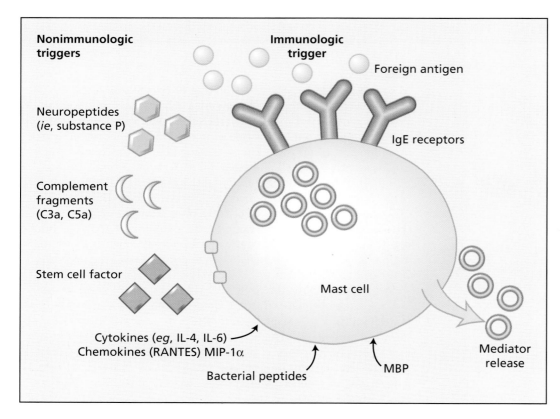

Figure 5-7.

Activation of mast cells and basophils. Mast cells and basophils can be activated by several different stimuli. The binding of multivalent antigens to IgE on the surface of mast cells and basophils initiates the immediate hypersensitivity response. Other modes of cell activation include nonimmunologic triggers such as neuropeptides, complement fragments, stem cell factor, and multiple cytokines. Bacterial peptides and MBP also activate the cell. After they are activated, the mast cells and basophils release potent mediators that act on target tissues. The clinical signs and symptoms that occur in an allergic response vary depending on the differing concentrations of mast cells and basophils in the tissues, the sensitivity of tissue to cell mediators, differing anatomic sites, and the nature of the allergen. Mast cells may also be activated through IgG receptors (FcγRI) [18]. IL—interleukin; MBP—major basic protein; MIP—macrophage inflammatory protein; RANTES— regulated on activation, normal T cell expressed and secreted.

Functions of Mast Cell Preformed Mediators

Mediator	
Biogenic amines	
Histamine	Bronchoconstricts; increases airway mucus secretion; vasodilates; increases smooth muscle contraction; increases vascular permeability; activates nociceptive neurons (*ie*, substance P)
Neutral proteases	
Tryptase	Activates fibroblasts; degrades neuropeptides; cleaves complement 3 and 3a; stimulates collagen synthesis; chemoattracts eosinophils and neutrophils; activates mast cells and induces degranulation [7]; enhances cytokine production [19]
Chymase	Cleaves neuropeptides; converts angiotension I to II; activates matrix metalloproteinases and procollagenase
Carboxypeptidase	Removes carboxyterminal residues from peptides; converts angiotensin I to II; inactivates neuropeptides
Cathepsin G	Chemoattracts proinflammatory cytokines; enhances platelet secretion and aggregation
Acid hydrolases	
Beta-Hexosaminidase	Cleaves β-linked hexosamines from complex carbohydrates and glycoprotein
Beta-Glucuronidase	Cleaves β–linked glucuronic acid from complex carbohydrate chains
Beta-delta-Galactosidase	Cleaves β-linked galactose from complex carbohydrates
Arylsulfatase	Cleaves sulfate esters of aromatic compounds
Oxidative enzymes	
Superoxide desmutase	Converts superoxide anion to hydrogen peroxide
Peroxidase	Catalyzes formation of water from hydrogen peroxide; generates potent lipid mediators
Proteoglycans	
Heparin	Anticoagulates; inhibits complement cascade; binds phospholipase A_2; binds preformed mediators and packages for storage; chemoattracts eosinophils; inhibits cytokine function
Chondroitin sulfate	Activates kinin pathway; stabilizes granule protease; binds phospholipase A_2
Chemotactic factors	
Eosinophil oligopeptides	Chemoattracts eosinophils
Neutrophil chemotactic activity	Chemoattracts neutrophils

Figure 5-8.

Functions of mast cell preformed mediators. Histamine is perhaps the best known stored mediator that plays a prominent role in the early phase allergic response. Elevated levels of histamine are found in the plasma and urine of patients after anaphylactic reactions to allergens, radiocontrast dyes, and other drugs [20]. Histamine found during the late phase allergic response is thought to originate from basophils [21]. Tryptase, a protease, has been used as a marker for severe anaphylactic reactions and remains in the circulation for a few hours. It has been used postmortem to establish anaphylaxis as a cause of death [22]. Acid hydrolases, oxidative enzymes, and chemotactic factors are also found in mast cells. The heavily sulfated proteoglycans heparin and chondroitin sulfate cause the metachromatic staining of human mast cells and basophils. These proteogylcans stabilize the proteases found in the secretory granules.

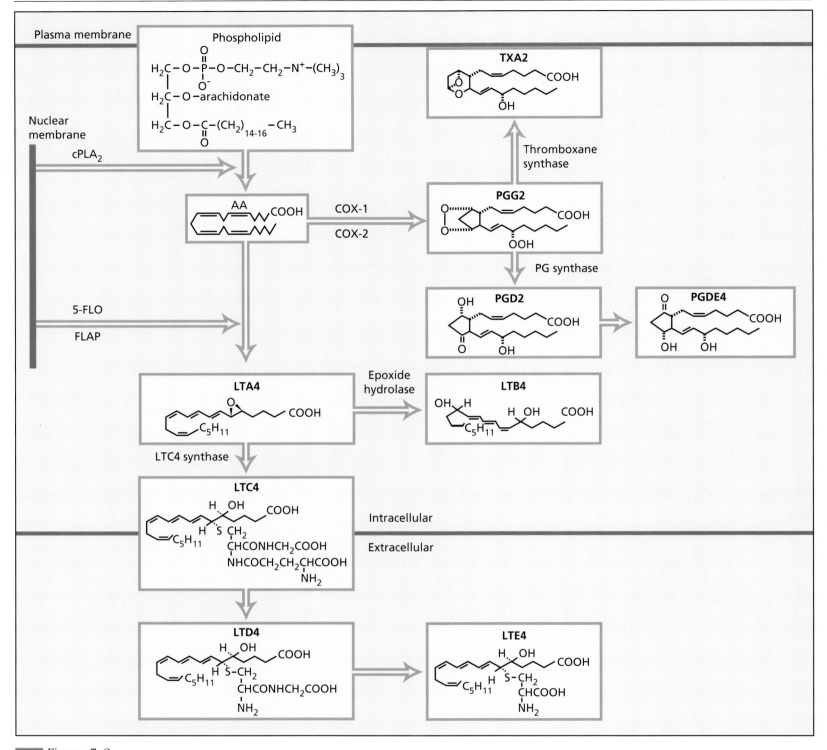

Figure 5-9.

Leukotriene synthesis. Arachidonic acid (AA), an unsaturated fatty acid, is stored as an ester of phospholipid in large quantities in the membranes of mast cells and basophils. After the cell becomes activated by various stimuli, the cytoplasmic enzyme phospholipase A_2 (cPLA$_2$) cleaves arachidonic acid from phosphatidylcholine and other phospholipids. cPLA$_2$, in association with calcium, generates free arachidonate, which is the precursor for the lipid mediators.

The cystineyl leukotrienes are products of a complex biochemical pathway that involves a lipoxygenation enzyme, 5-lipoxygenase (5-LO). 5-LO is located in the cytosol, where, upon cell activation, it translocates to the nuclear envelope energized by calcium and adenosine triphosphate (ATP). There it links with a nuclear membrane-associated protein, 5-LO activating protein (FLAP). Together, FLAP and 5-LO produce an intermediate structure that is quickly converted into leukotriene (LT) A_4. This is the precursor of LTB$_4$

and LTC$_4$. Leukotriene synthase adds a glutathione tripeptide residue to LTA$_4$ to form the cystenyl-LTC$_4$. LTC$_4$ is converted to LTD$_4$ and LTE$_4$ extracellularly by proteases that cleave one amino acid at a time from the glutathione residue.

Cyclooxygenase 1 (COX-1) is the stable isoform of cyclooxygenase. This enzyme is found in all mast cells and basophils and is responsible for maintaining prostaglandin (PG) levels in body tissues, such as the liver, kidney, stomach, and endothelial cells. COX-1 is responsible for eicosanoid production that is induced by IgE dependent mechanisms [23]. Cyclooxygenase-2 (COX-2) is an enzyme not normally detected in resting mast cells or basophils. However, upon immunologic activation by cytokines or cell injury, it rapidly produces prostaglandins (PG). Thromboxane A_2 is formed from prostaglandin G_2.

Functions

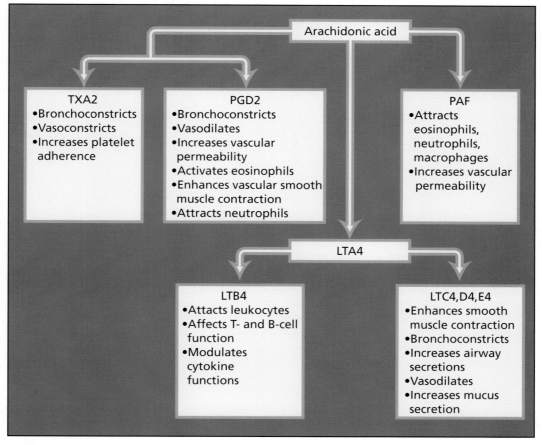

Figure 5-10.

Functions of mast cell lipid mediators. The main products of the lipoxygenase pathway are the leukotrienes LTB_4, LTC_4, LTD_4, and LTE_4. LTB_4 is a potent chemoattractant of leukocytes. LTC_4, LTD_4, and LTE_4 induce smooth muscle contraction, bronchoconstriction, and increase airway secretion. Platelet-activating factor is a product released from activated mast cells and is a powerful eosinophil chemoattractant. Other products contributing to the changes seen in the allergic response are thromboxane A_2 and prostaglandin D_2. Mast cells from the lung, heart, and gastrointestinal tract secrete predominately prostaglandin D_2 (PGD_2) and leukotriene C_4 [21]. Skin mast cells, on the other hand, produce mostly PGD_2. The significance of the different profile of mediators released at varying anatomic sites is currently unknown. LT—leukotriene; PAF—platelet activating factor; PG—prostaglandin; TX—thromboxane.

Mast Cell and Basophil Cytokine Functions

Type of Mast Cell or Basophil Cytokine	Functions
Th2 type cytokines	
IL-4	Critical for IgE synthesis by B lymphocytes
	Eosinophil chemotaxis
	Promotes upregulation of Th2 lymphocytes
	Induces FCεRI expression in mast cells [19]
	Suppresses macrophage activation
	Promotes mast cell proliferation
	Stimulates VCAM-1
	Induces overproduction of mucus
	Promotes fibroblast proliferation
IL-5	Eosinophil protection and maturation
	Airway hyperresponsiveness
IL-9	Enhances B cell response to IL-4
	Promotes mast cell proliferation
IL-13	Induces airway mucus secretion
	Airway hyperresponsiveness
	Promotes upregulation of Th2 lymphocytes
Th1 type cytokines	
IL-2	Stimulates differentiation and proliferation of CD8 T cells
	Promotes activation of neutrophils and endothelial cells
IFN-γ	Downregulates IgE production
	Inhibits Th2 cells, promotes Th1 cells
	Inhibits eosinophilic inflammation
	Stimulates natural killer cells
Both Th1 and Th2	
TNF-α	Upregulates other cytokines
	Recruits neutrophils
	Increases bronchial hyperresponsiveness
	Induces ICAM
IL-3	Induces B cell IgE synthesis
	Prolongs survival of monocytes
IL-10	Potent anti-inflammatory
	Inhibits cytokines and chemokines
GM-CSF	Promotes maturation of neutrophils and macrophages
Other cytokines	
IL-12	Regulates Th1 development
	Promotes secretion of IFN-γ and TNF-α
IL-16	Lymphocyte chemotaxis
TGF-β	Promotes fibroblast activation and proliferation
β-FGF	Promotes fibroblast differentiation
SCF	Promotes mast cell growth, differentiation, and chemotaxin
Chemokines	
RANTES	Mast cell, basophil, and eosinophil chemotaxis
MIP-1α	Mast cell and basophil chemotaxis
MCP-1, 2, 3, 4	Basophil and eosinophil chemotaxis
IL-8	Neutrophil chemotaxis
	Induces production and secretion of LTB$_4$

Figure 5-11.

Mast cell and basophil cytokine functions. Mast cells and basophils generate a wide range of cytokines. Cytokines are small proteins with growth, differentiation, and activation functions. They may have paracrine, autocrine, or endocrine effects. Th1 cytokines are involved in cellular defense against infections and tumor cells, while Th2 cytokines defend against large pathogens (ie, helminths). Most of the features of allergic disease are caused by the effects of type 2 cytokines and are associated with Th2 cells. Studies have shown a similarity between the pattern of cytokines synthesized by mast cells and basophils and those released by Th2 lymphocytes. The cytokine phenotype of allergen-specific Th memory cells is determined very early in life, and it is believed that the imbalance between the Th1 and Th2 systems gives rise to the atopic state. However, the reason for this imbalance is unknown. Chemokines are cytokines that have chemoattractant activity. Chemokines recruit and activate other effector cells involved in the allergic reaction, including eosinophils and lymphocytes. FGF— fibroblast growth factor; GM-CSF—granulocyte macrophage–colony stimulating factor; ICAM—intercellular adhesion molecule; IFN—interferon; IL—interleukin; LT—leukotriene; MCP—monocyte chemoattractant protein; MIP—macrophage inflammatory protein; RANTES—regulated on activation, normal T cell expressed and secreted; SCF—stem cell factor; TGF—transforming growth factor; TNF—tumor necrosis factor; VCAM—vascular cell adhesion molecule.

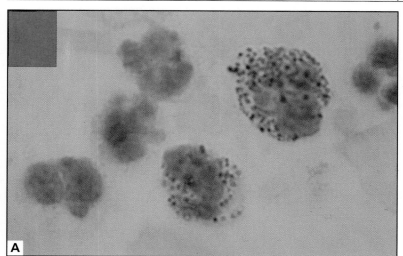

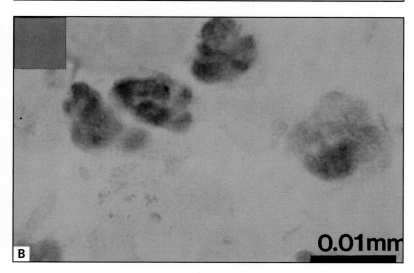

Figure 5-12.

Immunocytochemical staining of intracellular interleukin-4 (IL-4) in basophils. IL-4 is a key cytokine in the allergic response that mediates IgE synthesis and promotes upregulation of Th2 cytokines. Basophils were cultured in the presence and absence of anti-IgE for several hours. **A,** Basophils after stimulation with anti-IgE. **B,** Basophils that were not exposed to anti-IgE. The intracellular yellow-brown staining suggests the presence of IL-4. It also suppresses the induction and function of Th1 cells. IL-4 has become a prime target for treatment of patients with allergic disease. Anti-IL4 monoclonal antibodies, receptor antagonists, and soluble IL-4 receptors are being studied.

Therapeutic Approaches

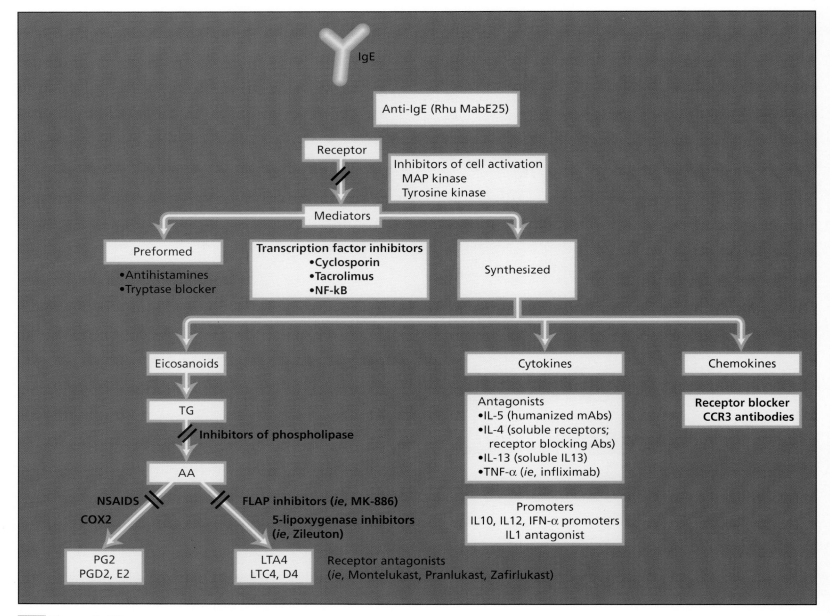

Figure 5-13.

Therapeutic approaches to inhibiting the allergic response through mediators. Advances in the understanding of the cellular and molecular mechanisms involved in the allergic response have identified multiple new targets for therapeutic intervention in atopic disease states [24]. These new therapies are aimed at suppressing components of the allergic inflammatory response. Corticosteroids continue to be the most effective treatment for allergic disease because they suppress inflammation through inhibiting cytokines, enzymes, and other mediators. However, their use is limited because of systemic side effects.

An alternative approach has been to target cell mediators. Antihistamines have been used for many years in the treatment of patients with allergic rhinitis and atopic dermatitis. Tryptase inhibitors are under development [25]. Newer medications that target eicosanoid production have found a role in the treatment of allergic disease. Leukotriene antagonists have become a popular second line treatment option for patients with asthma. FLAP inhibitors and 5-lipoxygenase inhibitors have been used.

A humanized murine monoclonal antibody (rhuMab-E25) against the FCεRI binding domain of IgE has been developed. This antibody has been shown to be effective in lowering IgE

levels in patients with asthma [26] and in decreasing the number of asthma exacerbations and steroid usage [27,28].

Other novel medication approaches are under development. The identification of key cytokines and chemokines in the allergic response has led to the development of drugs that block these mediators. Long-term clinical trials are underway on therapeutic agents that antagonize IL-4, IL-5, IL-13, and TNF-α. Other drugs have been developed to promote the affects of the anti-inflammatory cytokines. Chemokine receptor blockers are also under development. Antibodies to chemokine receptors, such as CCR3, have been developed. Drugs that disrupt key biochemical pathways provide an alternative route of inhibiting the allergic response. Mitogen-activated protein (MAP)–kinase inhibitors, known as cytokine suppressant anti-inflammatory drugs (CSAIDs), inhibit the synthesis of cytokines and chemokines. Tyrosine kinase inhibitors and monoclonal antibodies directed against immunoreceptor tyrosine-based activation motifs (ITAMs) of the high-affinity receptor are also being developed. AA—arachidonic acid; IFN—interferon; IL—interleukin; LT—leukotriene; PG—prostaglandin; TG—triglyceride; TNF—tumor necrosis factor.

References

1. Mannino D, Homa D, Pertowski C, *et al.*: Surveillance for asthma-United States, 1960–1995. *CDC MMWR Surveillance Summaries* April 24, 1998, 47:1-28.

2. Adams PF, Hendershot GE, Marano MA: Current estimates, 1996. National Center for Health Statistics. *Vital Health Statistics* 1999, 10.

3. Grant JA, Huamin L: Biology of basophils. In *Allergy Principles and Practice*. Edited by Middleton E. St Louis: Mosby; 1998:277–283.

4. Castells MC, Irani AM, Swartch LB: Evaluation of human peripheral blood leukocytes for mast cell tryptase. *J Immunol* 1987, 138:2184.

5. Monasterolo G, Rossi R. A simple method to evaluate basophil tryptase after allergen challenge in vitro. *J Allerg Clin Immunol* 1997, 99: 575–577.

6. Williams C, Galli S: The diverse potential effector and immunoregulatory roles of mast cells in allergic disease. *J Allerg Clin Immunol* 2000, 105:847–857.

7. Church M, Holgate S, Shut J, *et al.*: Mast cell derived mediators. In *Allergy Principles and Practice*. Edited by Middleton E. St Louis: Mosby; 1998:146–163.

8. Ott V, Cambier J: Activating and inhibitory signaling in mast cells: new opportunities for therapeutic interventions? *J Allerg Clin Immunol* 2000, 106:429–438.

9. Schwartz L, Huff T: Biology of mast cells. In *Allergy Principles and Practice*. Edited by Middleton E. St Louis: Mosby; 1998: 261–275.

10. Yamaguchi M, Lantz C, Oettgen H, *et al.*: IgE enhances mouse mast cell FC∈RI expression in vitro and in vivo: evidence for a novel amplification mechanism in IgE dependent reactions. *J Exp Med* 1997, 185:663–671.

11. Wang B, Rieger A, Kilgus O, *et al.*: Epidermal Langerhans cells from normal skin bind monomeric IgE via FC epsilon RI. *J Exp Med* 1992, 175:1285–1290.

12. Bieber T, de la Salle H, Wollenberg A, *et al.*: Human epidermal Langerhans cells express the high affinity receptor for immunoglobulin E (FC∈RI). *J Exp Med* 1992, 175:1285.

13. Maurer D, Fiebiger E, Reininger B, *et al.*: Expression of functional high affinity immunoglobulin E receptors (FC∈RI) on monocytes of atopic individuals. *J Exp Med* 1994, 179:745–750.

14. Osterhoff B, Rappersberger C, Wang B, *et al.*: Immunopharmacological characterization of FC epsilon RI- bearing cells within the human dermis. *J Invest Dermatol* 1994, 102:315–320.

15. Gounni AS, Lankhioued B, Ochiai K, *et al.*: High affinity IgE receptor on eosinophils is involved in defence against parasites. *Nature* 1994, 367:183–186.

16. Rigby LJ: Domain one of the high affinity IgE receptor, FC∈RI, regulates binding to IgE through its interface with domain two. *J Biol Chem* 2000, 275: 9664–9672.

17. Okayama Y, Kirshenbaum A, Metcalfe DD: Expression of a functional high-affinity IgG receptor, FCγRI, on human mast cells: up-regulation by IFN-γ. *J Immunol* 2000, 164:4332.

18. Okayama Y, Hagaman D, Metcalfe DD: A comparison of mediators released or generated by IFN-γ-treated human mast cells following aggregation of FCγRI or FCγRI. *J Immunol* 2001, 166:4705.

19. Holgate S: The epidemic of allergy and asthma. *Nature* 1999, 402 (suppl B):2–5.

20. Watkins J: Markers and mechanisms of anaphylactoid reactions. *Monogr Allergy* 1992, 30:108–129.

21. Lie W, Mul F, Roos D, *et al.*: Degranulation of human basophils by picomolar concentrations of IL-3, IL-5, or granulocyte mediated cell stimulatory factor. *J Allerg Clin Immunol* 1998, 101: 683–690.

22. Pumphrey RS, Roberts IS: Postmortem findings after fatal anaphylactic reactions. *J Clin Pathol* 2000, 53: 273–276.

23. Marone G, Casolaro V, Patella V, *et al.*: Molecular and cellular biology of mast cells and basophils. *Internat Arch Allerg Immunol* 1997, 114:207–217.

24. Barnes P: Therapeutic strategies for allergic disease. *Nature* 1999, 402 (suppl B):31–38.

25. Rice KD, Tanaka RD, Katz BA, *et al.*: Inhibitors of tryptase for the treatment of mast cell-mediated disease. *Curr Pharm Des* 1998, 4:381.

26. Milgrom H, Fick R, Su J, *et al.*: Treatment of allergic asthma with monoclonal anti-IgE. *N Engl J Med* 1999, 341:1966–1973.

27. Fick RB, Simm SJ, Su JQ, *et al.*: Anti-IgE (rhumAb) treatment of the symptoms of moderate to severe allergic asthma. *Ann Asthma Allerg Immunol* 1998, 80:80.

28. Metzger WJ, Fick RB: The E25 asthma study group: corticosteroid withdrawal in a study of recombinant humanized monoclonal antibody to IgE (RhumAbE25). *J Allerg Clin Immunol* 1998, 101(suppl):231.

6

The Eosinophil

James N. Moy

Named by Paul Ehrlich more than 120 years ago, the eosinophil is considered to be the central cell in allergic inflammation. Although it is beneficial in the host defense against parasitic infections, the eosinophil is recognized as an effector cell in allergic disorders such as asthma and allergic rhinitis. This chapter uses photomicrographs to show the morphology and ultrastructure of the eosinophil. Tables and drawings are used to detail the immunobiology of the eosinophil.

Tissue or peripheral blood eosinophilia is the hallmark of many allergic conditions. The first section of this chapter lists the clinical conditions that almost always exhibit some degree of eosinophilia. Asthma is a prime example of a disease in which eosinophils have been demonstrated to be a major contributing cell to the pathology of the airways.

The eosinophil is easily recognized because of the vivid staining of the granules with acidic dyes. The section on the morphology of eosinophils and eosinophil products gives examples of the distinctive appearance of the eosinophil and of Charcot-Leyden crystals.

Eosinophil growth and function are regulated by multiple factors such as cytokines, chemokines, and adhesion molecules. In many instances, these factors are specific for eosinophils and not other leukocytes. For example, the chemokine eotaxin is a potent chemoattractant for eosinophils, but eotaxin does not induce chemotaxis of neutrophils. The last section of this chapter contains figures that emphasize the important aspects of the immunobiology of the eosinophil with respect to allergic diseases.

Clinical Conditions with Tissue and Blood Eosinophilia

Eosinophils in Allergic Disorders

Disease Entity	Comments
Asthma	Eosinophils are present in the airways of both atopic and non-atopic asthmatics. Many asthmatics also have peripheral eosinophilia.
Allergic rhinoconjunctivitis	Eosinophils are also found in nasal smears of 15% to 20% of patients with nonallergic rhinitis.
Chronic urticaria	Major basic protein is found in the skin biopsies of 50% of patients, but very few biopsy specimens show intact eosinophils.
Atopic dermatitis	Large quantities of major basic protein, but not intact eosinophils, are found in skin lesions.
Nasal polyposis	Polyps can occur in atopic and non-atopic individuals.
Adverse drug reactions	The major drugs that cause peripheral eosinophilia are phenytoin, ampicillin, sulfonamides, and nitrofurantoin. Methicillin is the most common cause of drug-induced interstitial nephritis.
Eosinophilic gastroenteritis	The esophagus, stomach, and small intestines can be affected.

Figure 6-1.

Eosinophils in allergic disorders. Note that in all of the conditions listed here, intact eosinophils might not be found in affected tissue. The use of antibodies to detect the presence of degranulated eosinophil products, such as major basic protein, is extremely useful for the diagnosis of eosinophil-mediated conditions. Another useful laboratory tool is looking for the presence of Charcot-Leyden crystals by light microscopy in tissues and body fluids.

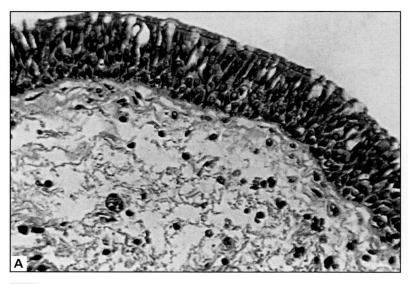
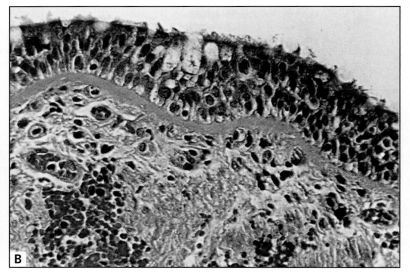

Figure 6-2.

Eosinophils in asthmatic airways. Eosinophils are found in the airways of all asthmatic patients. The eosinophils release granular proteins (especially major basic protein) that damage the respiratory epithelium. Eosinophils also release leukotriene C_4, which causes airway smooth muscle contraction, increases vascular permeability, and increases mucus production.

Compare the light photomicrographs of bronchial biopsies from a person without asthma (**A**) and from a patient with asthma (**B**). The specimen from the patient with asthma shows a pronounced eosinophilic infiltrate in the submucosa and some eosinophils in the epithelium. In addition, epithelial desquamation, goblet cell hyperplasia, and a thickened sub-basement membrane are present. (*From* Busse and Lemanske [1]; with permission).

Morphology of Eosinophils and Eosinophil Products

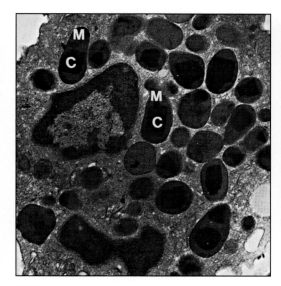

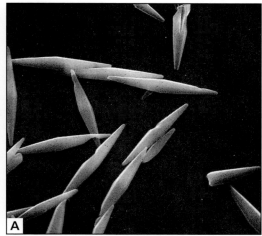

Figure 6-3.

Electron photomicrograph of an eosinophil. Eosinophils contain many granules. Particularly distinctive are the specific or secondary granules. This electron photomicrograph (magnification × 10,000) shows that these granules contain an electron-dense crystalloid core (C) and a less-dense matrix (M). Whereas major basic protein is found in the core, eosinophil cationic protein, eosinophil-derived neurotoxin, and eosinophil peroxidase are found in the matrix. (*From* Gleich [2]; with permission.)

Figure 6-4.

Electron photomicrograph of Charcot-Leyden crystals (CLCs). CLCs are composed of the enzyme lysophospholipase. These electron photomicrographs demonstrate the unique shape of CLCs (**A**, magnification × 400; **B**, magnification × 4000). These unique hexagonal bipyramidal crystals can be found in the sputum of patients with asthma, in the stool of patients with eosinophilic gastroenteritis, and in the urine of patients with drug-induced interstitial nephritis. The presence of CLCs should be pursued when eosinophil-mediated diseases are suspected because, in many instances, the eosinophils have undergone lysis and cannot be detected in biologic specimens.

Immunobiology of Eosinophils

Regulation of Eosinophilopoiesis and Eosinophil Function

Regulatory Factors	Source	Function
IL-5	Th2 cells, mast cells	Stimulates bone marrow production of eosinophils
		Promotes chemotaxis
		Prolongs survival
		Enhances production and secretion of mediators
IL-3	T cells, thymic epithelial cells	Synergistic with IL-5 for bone marrow production
GM-CSF	Macrophages, respiratory epithelial cells, T cells	Synergistic with IL-5 for production and secretion of mediators
Eotaxin	Endothelium, epithelium, monocytes, T cells	Most potent eosinophil chemoattractant
RANTES	Endothelium, epithelium, platelets, T cells	Eosinophil chemoattractant
TGF	Monocytes, T cells	Suppresses eosinophil differentiation
TGF-β	Adrenal glands	Induces apoptosis of eosinophils

Figure 6-5.

Regulation of eosinophilopoiesis and eosinophil function. Eosinophils are constantly under the tight control of many biologic compounds. Shown here are the major substances that regulate eosinophil production and function. Corticosteroids are very effective in the treatment of eosinophil-mediated diseases because they induce apoptosis and inhibit cytokine production. GM-CSF—granulocyte macrophage colony stimulating factor; RANTES—regulated on activation, normal T expressed and secreted; TGF—transforming growth factor.

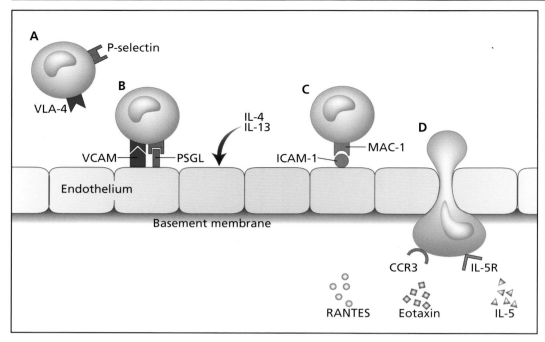

Figure 6-6.

Eosinophil migration to sites of allergic inflammation [3]. The migration of eosinophils into tissue requires the orchestration of cell surface adhesion molecules and chemoattractants. Antigen activation of mast cells leads a cascade of effects that results in the upregulation of adhesion molecules and the production of chemotactic factors. **A,** The eosinophil is flowing unimpeded through the blood vessel. **B,** The eosinphil's velocity is slowed by the interaction of adhesion molecules between the eosinophil and the endothelium. This "rolling" process is initiated by IL-4 and IL-13 upregulation of VCAM-1 (vascular cell adhesion molecule-1) on the vascular endothelium. P-selectin and VCAM-1 and P-selection glycoprotein ligand (PSGL) interact with very late activation antigen-4 (VLA-4) and P-selectin on the eosinophils, respectively. **C,** A different set of adhesion molecules causes the firm binding of the eosinophil to the endothelium. These adhesion molecules are Mac-1 on the eosinophils and ICAM-1 (intercellular adhesion molecule-1) on the endothelial cells. **D,** Attracted by chemoattractants, the eosinophil diapedises through the vessel wall. The chemoattractants include IL-5 and the CC chemokines eotaxin and RANTES (regulated on activation, normal T expressed and secreted). Eosinophils express the CC chemokine receptor (CCR3) and the IL-5 receptor (IL-5R).

Eosinophil-Derived Proinflammatory Products

Eosinophil Product	Comments	Activities Related to Allergic Diseases
Granular proteins		
MBP	From crystalloid core of granules	Toxic to respiratory epithelium
		Stimulates basophils, respiratory goblet cells, neutrophils, and platelets
		Induces bronchial hyperreactivity
Eosinophil cationic protein	From matrix	Degranulation of rat mast cells
EDN	From matrix	Not known
EPO	From matrix	Damages respiratory epithelium
		Induces bronchospasm in primates
		Degranulation of rat mast cells
Lipid mediators		
LTC$_4$	From cell membrane	Smooth muscle contraction, vascular permeability, mucus production
PAF	From cell membrane	Eosinophil chemotaxis, neutrophil and eosinophil activation
Oxidative products		
Superoxide anion	More per cell than neutrophils	Oxidative damage to host tissue
Hydrogen peroxide		
Hydroxyl radicals		
Cytokines and chemokines		
IL-8	CXC chemokine	Synergistic with IL-5 for eosinophilic chemotaxis
MCP-1	CC chemokines	Basophil chemotaxis and degranulation
MIP-1α		

Figure 6-7.

Eosinophil-derived proinflammatory products. Eosinophils synthesize and release many mediators that damage host tissue and propagate allergic inflammation. More than 20 cytokines and chemokines have been reported to be synthesized by eosinophils. Listed here are some of the major ones that are important in the pathophysiology of allergic diseases. More than 20 cytokines and chemokines have been reported to be synthesized by eosinophils. Three of the ones not listed are GM-CSF (granulocyte macrophage–colony stimulating factor), IL-5, and RANTES (regulated on activation, normal T expressed and secreted). The production and release of these three cytokines may have autoregulatory functions. EDN—eosinophil-derived neurotoxin; EPO—eosinophil peroxidase; LTC—leukotriene C; MBP—major basic protein; MCP—monocyte chemoattractant protein; PAF—platelet-activating factor.

References

1. Busse WW, Lemanske RF Advances in immunology: asthma. *N Engl J Med* 2001, 344:350–360.

2. Gleich GJ: Mechanisms of eosinophil-associated inflammation. *J Allergy Clin Immunol* 2000, 105:651–663.

3. Wardlaw AJ: Molecular basis for selective eosinophil trafficking in asthma: a multistep paradigm. *J Allergy Clin Immunol* 1999, 104:917–926.

7

Aerobiology and Aeroallergens

Richard W. Weber

Aerobiology is the broad science of airborne substances of organic origin. In a more restrictive sense, allergists use the term to describe the study of aeroallergens. These may be divided into indoor and outdoor sources, although there is certainly overlap. Additionally, aeroallergens may be characterized as of plant or animal origin: plant sources predominate outdoors while animal sources are most relevant indoors. Allergenic proteins are carried on particles that range greatly in size. Soluble allergens may be found in submicronic droplets. Mold spores range from a few microns to over a hundred in length. Most pollen grains vary between ten to forty microns, although some may be larger. Particles that are five microns and smaller are easily respired into the smaller terminal bronchioles. The sources from which they are derived may be microscopic, as in the case of bacteria, some molds, or dust mites, or as large as horses or cows. The spectrum of aeroallergen sources is delineated in Figure 7-1.

Assessing the intensity of an airborne exposure, with its presumed impact on causing disease, depends on monitoring the numbers of the incriminated particles in a volume of air over a given time. Sampling particles in the air may be as simple as exposing to the air a sticky surface such as a greased microscope slide or a Petri dish and observing what impacts on it. Because such techniques rely on airborne particles settling out of the air by the force of gravity, these are known as "gravimetric" devices. The advantage of these is their simplicity. The disadvantage is being unable to quantify the volume of air sampled. Also, swirling air currents above the device may carry away smaller, light particles, unduly skewing the sample to larger particles. Samplers of choice are "volumetric" devices that either sweep a known volume of air, or pull a fixed volume of air through a collecting device over a defined time. These give a much more accurate estimate of particles, especially those of smaller size. Sampling can also be correlated with meteorological parameters to ascertain the likely conditions for highest exposures [1].

Outdoor allergens play a major role in seasonal allergic rhinitis or rhinoconjunctivitis (hayfever). In certain regions, exposure may be intense, such as with mountain cedar pollen in central and south Texas, ragweed pollen in the Midwest, or rust and smut mold spores during harvesting in the Great Plains. Indoor allergens of primary importance are animal emanations. House dust mites, cat dander, and cockroach allergens have all been linked to allergic asthma. Unless one is dealing with water damage, or excessively damp basements, indoor molds are less important than the above allergens.

This chapter demonstrates typical sampling devices, and results that may be derived, as well as listing some principles of aerobiology. Plant sources are depicted, as well as the appearance of representative pollen grains and mold spores as seen with a light microscope such as would be used at a pollen/mold counting station.

Sampling Devices

Common Biologic Aeroallergen Sources

Source	Particle Type
Plant	
Bacteria, algae	Metabolites in droplets
	Cells, fragments
Fungi	Spores, mycelial fragments
Ferns, club mosses	Spores
Grass, weeds, shrubs, trees	Pollens
Animal	
Protozoa	Metabolites in droplets
Arthropods	Fecal particles, body parts, saliva
Birds	Fecal material
Mammals	Dander, saliva, urine

Figure 7-1.

The spectrum of aeroallergen sources.

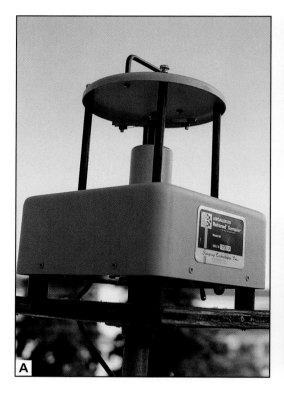
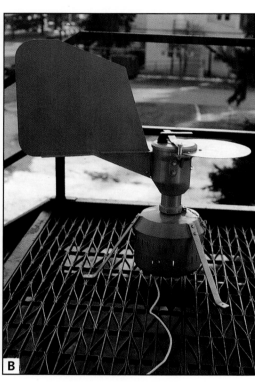

Figure 7-2.

The Rotorod and Burkard sampling devices. **A,** The Rotorod consists of a spinning armature with plastic rods at each end that swing downward into the air by centrifugal force; the rods are retracted by spring traction when the armature stops spinning. The motor is usually programmed to cycle for 1 of every 10 minutes.
B, The Burkard sporetrap draws a volume of air at a defined speed through an aperture to contact a moving drum with an adhesive coating. A rain shield protects the aperture, and the large vane keeps the opening oriented into the wind, which optimizes collection.

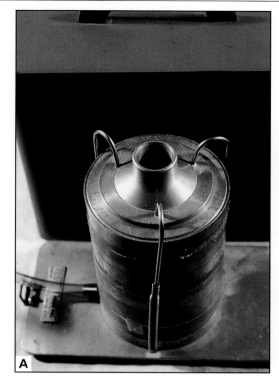
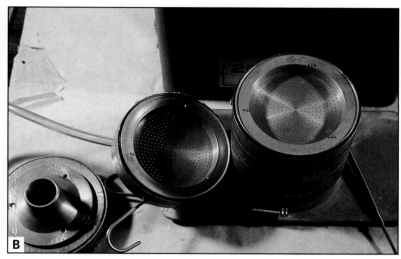

■ Figure 7-3.

The cascade (or sieve) impactor. **A,** The Anderson cascade (or sieve) impactor draws a volume of air through the large aperture on the top at a defined speed. It may be used either indoors or outdoors. **B,** The cascade impactor is multilayered, drawing air through the grids of decreasing diameter holes to impact agar dishes. This allows segregation of the airborne allergens by particle size. Mold spores can then germinate on the agar to allow better identification.

Various Aeroallergen Samplers	
Apparatus Type	**Examples**
Gravimetric	Durham (greased slide)
	Petri dish (culture agar)
Volumetric	
Impaction	
Intermittent rotary	Rotorod
Suction drum	Burkard
	Hirst
	Kramer-Collins
Cascade	Anderson
Filtration	Accu-Vol

■ Figure 7-4.

Types of commonly used samplers. Gravimetric samplers are no longer considered adequate for meaningful study. Intermittent rotary devices may become overloaded due to small surface area. Drum devices allow collection to be segregated into hours of the day, and not just for a total set period such as 24 hours. Filters can be stained with antibodies to detect soluble allergens as well as inspected for discrete particles.

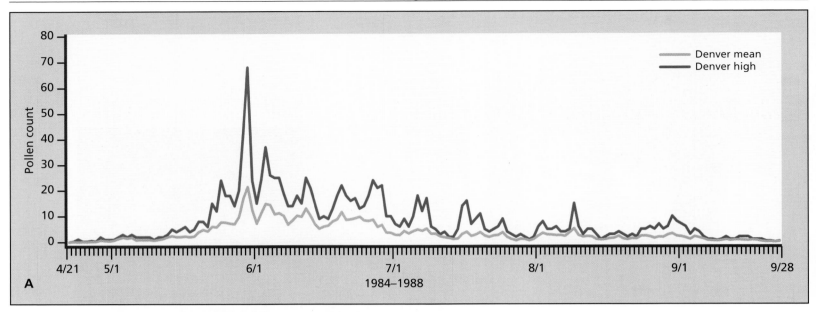

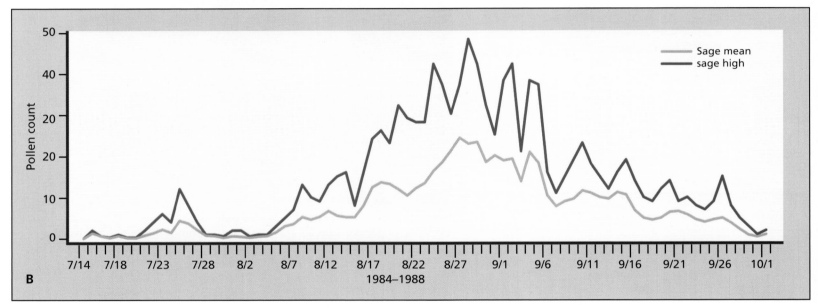

Figure 7-5.

Tracking of outdoor aeroallergen sampling over several years. This technique allows comparisons over several years, and between multiple locales. **A,** Grass pollen (primarily spring-early summer pollination). **B,** Sage pollen, primarily from giant sagebrush (*Artemisia tridentata*). (*Data* from Silvers *et al.* [2]).

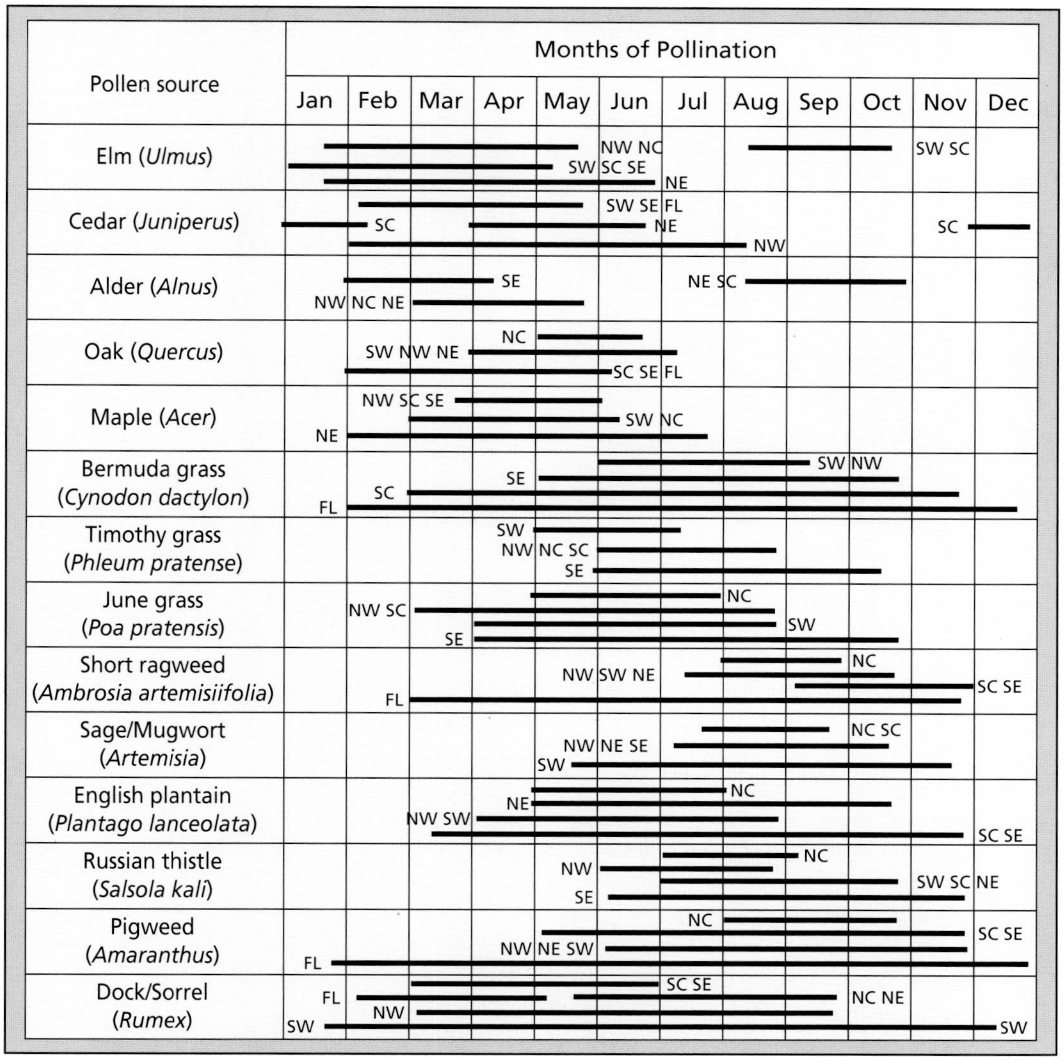

Figure 7-6.

Pollen seasons. Representative tree, grass, and weeds are listed with their respective periods of pollination depicted by the horizontal bars. Periods of pollen anthesis vary depending on the area of the country, as well as particular species endemic to those areas; thus there are several bars for each pollen group or species. FL—South Florida; NC—Northcentral; NE—Northeast; NW—Northwest; SC—Southcentral; SE—Southeast; SW—Southwest. (*Data from* Solomon *et al.* [3] and Lewis *et al.* [4].)

Outdoor Aeroallergens

Thommen's Postulates on Pollen and the Causation of Hayfever

Pollen must contain an excitant of hayfever
Pollen must be anemophilous (wind-pollinated)
Pollen must be produced in sufficiently large quantities
Pollen must be sufficiently buoyant to carry long distances
Plant-producing pollen must be widely and abundantly distributed

Figure 7-7.

Thommen's postulates. First defined in 1931, Thommen's postulates have generally been found to be true, but with some caveats [5]. Some aeroallergen sources, such as Russian olive and linden, are amphiphilous (both insect and wind pollinated). Single plants situated at strategic places, such as outside a bedroom window, may be adequate for sensitization and symptom induction.

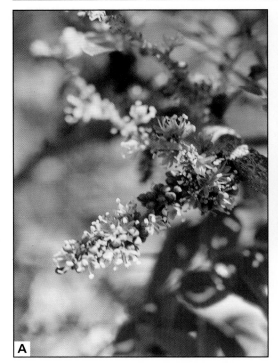

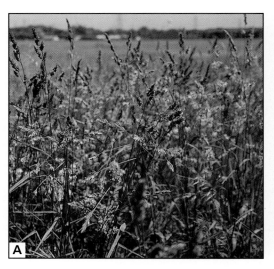

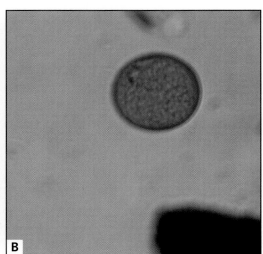

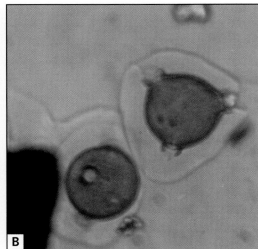 Figure 7-8.

Locust tree anthers and pollen. Locust trees are variably insect or wind pollinated, depending on species. **A,** Pollen-containing anthers. **B,** Locust pollen. Locust pollen is triporate, having three pores, with distinct collared apertures and with a prominent plug, or operculum [6].

Figure 7-9.

Northern pasture grasses and their pollen. **A,** A stand of orchard grass (*Dactylis glomerata*), an introduced species to North America, behind which is a field of Kentucky bluegrass (June grass [*Poa pratensis*]). **B,** Typical monoporate grass pollen grain with single pore. All grasses are monoporate and generally not distinguishable to species by appearance [6].

Characteristics of Wind-pollinated Plants

Flowers are incomplete (spatially separated male and female portions)
Male flowers (pollen producing) exposed to the wind
Petals and sepals are insignificant or absent
Attractants (color, aroma, nectar)
Pollen grains small and dry, with reduced surface ornamentation

Figure 7-10.

Characteristics of wind-pollinated plants. Plants adapted to wind pollination generally have inconspicuous flowers. Conversely, plants with showy flowers are unlikely to have significant amounts of airborne pollen, and airborne sensitization is uncommon but not impossible. Wind-pollinated plants will have pollen-producing anthers dangling in the air on catkins, or on florets that protrude up into airstreams.

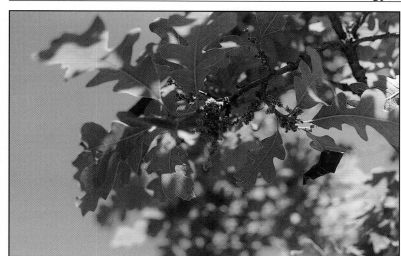

■ Figure 7-11.

Catkins on Gambel oak (*Quercus gambelii*), a common oak of the Rocky Mountains. It is a late pollinator, with anthesis between June and July, overlapping with grasses. Catkins on mature trees will be more prominent in the higher reaches of the tree, for better wind dispersal.

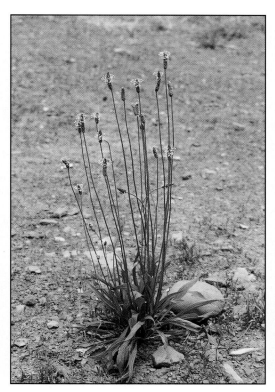

■ Figure 7-12.

English plantain (*Plantago lanceolata*). This common temperate weed produces stalks rising 12 to 18 inches off the ground. Seen here are the typical crown of anthers around the upper portion of the floret.

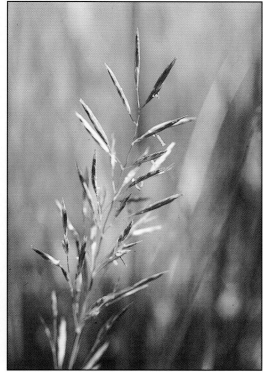

■ Figure 7-13.

Smooth brome (*Bromus inermis*). This introduced temperate climate grass is common throughout the middle to northern states and plains of Canada.

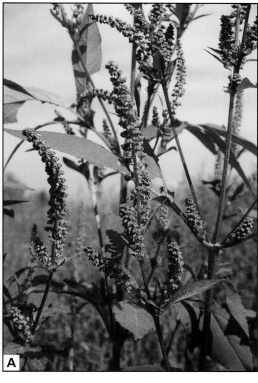

■ Figure 7-14.

Giant ragweed (*Ambrosia trifida*). This plant, along with short ragweed (*Ambrosia artemisiifolia*) are the two major ragweeds of the central and eastern states, accounting for significant late summer hayfever. **A,** Plants with prominent pollen-producing florets on the upper aspects. Leaves near the top are single lobed (as shown); lower leaves are large and trilobed. Giant ragweed can easily reach heights of 8 to 10 feet. (*continued on next page*)

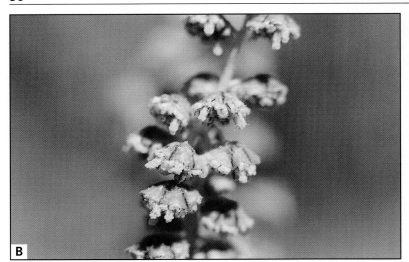

Figure 7-14. (*continued*)
B, Clusters of florets hang like inverted cups. With drying of dew in the early morning, these florets crack open, allowing the anthers to protrude and release copious amounts of pollen.

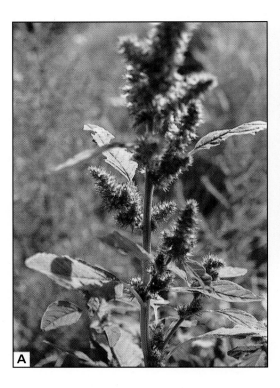

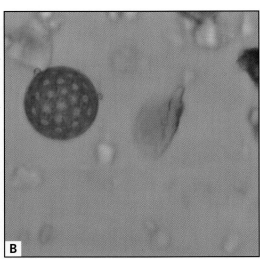

Figure 7-15.
Redroot pigweed (*Amaranthus retroflexus*). This ubiquitous weed is of the Amaranth family. A, Bushy florets are found on the upper portions of the plant. The stems may have some red color, but the main taproot is a distinct magenta red. B, Pollen grains of the related Amaranth and Chenopod weeds are similar in appearance and difficult to tell apart by casual observation. They are periporate, having numerous pores, with the look of a golf ball or whiffle ball [6].

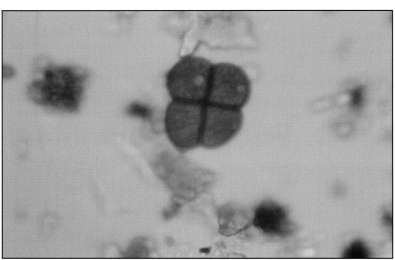

Figure 7-16.
Cattails (*Typhus* species). These plants are related to grasses and have similar single pores (monoporate). However, the pollen grains are usually clumped together in a distinctive tetrad, as seen here [6].

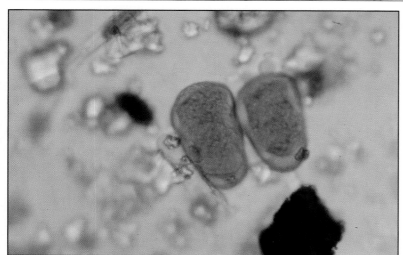

Figure 7-17.

Sedges and bulrushes (*Scirpus* species). These plants are also related to grasses, but have a wedge-shaped grain reminiscent of corn kernels, with a distinctive pore on the flat end [6].

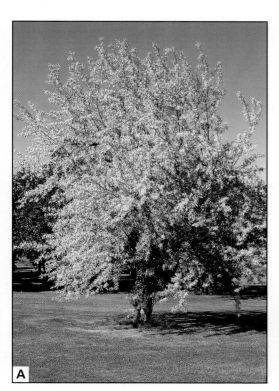

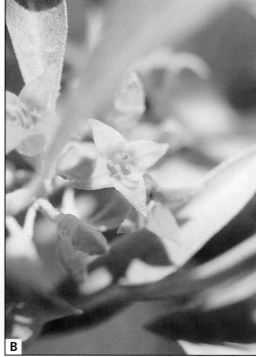

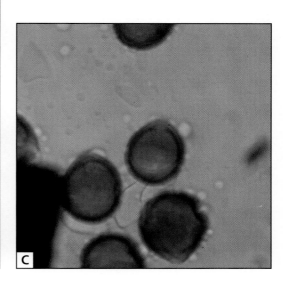

Figure 7-18.

Russian olive (*Elaeagnus angustifolia*). This introduced tree is common in the Great Plains. **A,** The tree has silvery small leaves and dark trunk, and has frequently been used as a wind-break. **B,** The numerous small flowers are primarily insect pollinated but shed sufficient airborne pollen to sensitize people in areas of prevalence. **C,** The grains are tricolporate (having three pores within furrows). The pores have a plug, or operculum.

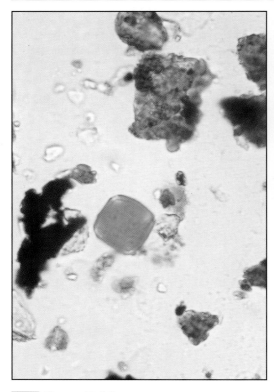

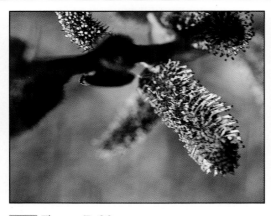

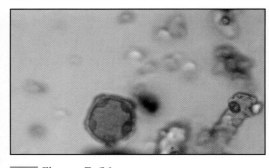

Figure 7-21.
Alder (*Alnus* species). This tree is a member of the birch family, Betulaceae, a native tree especially prevalent in the Rocky Mountains and across the northern forests of Canada. It is also a significant aeroallergen along with birch (*Betula* species) in Scandinavia. Alder pollen has four or five pores, with prominent collars around the pores.

Figure 7-20.
Aspen (*Populus tremuloides*). This dominant deciduous tree of the Rocky Mountains pollinates in April. Pollen is released from short "pussy-willow"–like catkins.

Figure 7-19.
Ash (*Fraxinus* species) trees. These native trees are especially prevalent in the eastern states. The pollen grain is distinctively square with four pores acting as the corners.

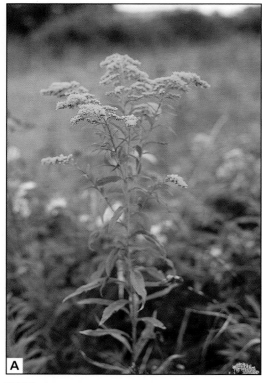

Figure 7-22.
Goldenrod (*Solidago* species). This plant is in the Aster family, related to the ragweeds. **A,** The flashy yellow flowers draw attention not only from insects, but people as well, who falsely attribute their ragweed hayfever to the more obvious goldenrod. Much less goldenrod pollen becomes airborne than ragweed pollen, but sensitization may occur. **B,** The grain has distinct sharp spikes and three less prominent pores with short furrows. Ragweed pollen has much shorter, blunted spikes [6].

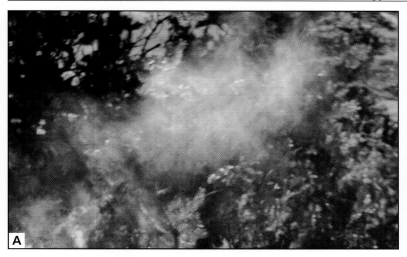

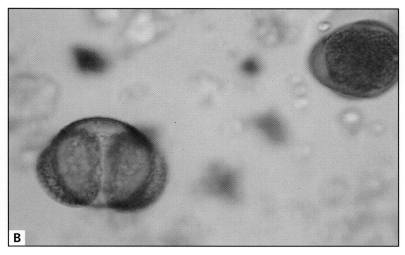

■ Figure 7-23.

Pine and spruce trees (*Pinus* and *Abies* species, respectively). These trees produce copious amounts of pollen. **A,** Pollen cloud rising off of a spruce. Fortunately, pollen from members of the pine family, Pinaceae, is not particularly allergenic, and few persons have appreciable allergic antibodies directed against these pollens.

B, Pine and spruce pollens have two air bladders bracketing a fairly large grain, helping to give the grain greater buoyancy. Depending on the orientation of the grain on the slide, these pollens have a "Mickey Mouse" appearance that is easy to identify. This micrograph also contains a sedge pollen.

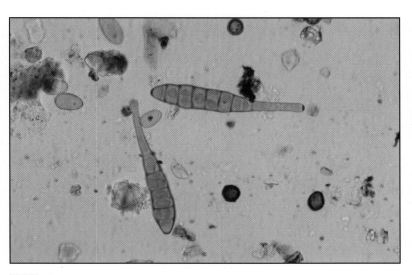

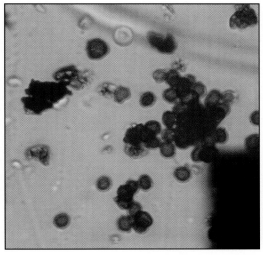

■ Figure 7-24.

Several examples of "dry weather" mold spores. The two larger club-shaped spores with both transverse and longitudinal septations are examples of *Alternaria*. This is a very allergenic saprophytic mold, growing on grasses, grains, wood pulp, and a variety of other substrates. The smaller pale beige elliptical spores are *Cladosporium*, usually present on samplers in at least tenfold higher concentrations than *Alternaria*. They are frequently longer, cigar-shaped, with birefringent endplates. *Cladosporium* species vary greatly in size. The smaller, darker, roughly circular spores are smuts of the Basidiomycete class. All of these spores are more prevalent on dry, windy days [3].

■ Figure 7-25.

Basidiomycete smuts. These organisms frequently grow on grasses and grains, and are especially present in very large numbers in late summer and autumn during harvesting and threshing in farm communities. Fortunately, they appear to be less allergenic than *Alternaria* or *Cladosporium*.

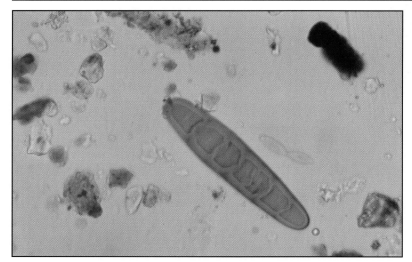

Figure 7-26.
Helminthosporium species. These are elongated spores with pseudoseptations. Although they are perhaps more common with somewhat greater humidity, Helminthosporium and the related Dreschlera may also be prevalent on windy days [3].

Indoor Aeroallergens

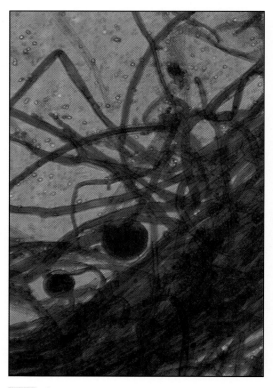

Figure 7-27.
Mucor species. These cosmopolitan molds are found throughout the globe. They are commonly found in house dust samples. High levels of viable organisms may be recovered from air vents, as with this specimen. Mucor has been incriminated in inhalant allergic disease as well as hypersensitivity pneumonitis in occupational settings such as "wood chipper's disease" and "furrier's disease." This micrograph shows many hyphal elements as well as conidia [7].

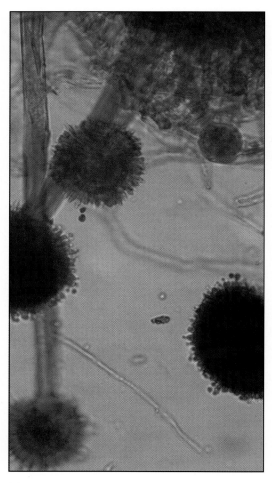

Figure 7-28.
Aspergillus species have likewise been incriminated in inhalant allergy, occupational lung disease in a large variety of settings, and in allergic bronchopulmonary mycoses [7]. Allergic bronchopulmonary aspergillosis (ABPA), caused by *Aspergillus fumigatus*, is the prototype of these latter conditions, presently as severe steroid-requiring asthma with high levels of circulating IgE and pulmonary infiltrates. This specimen was obtained from a contaminated ventilation system, and reveals hyphae and the typical circular beaded conidia.

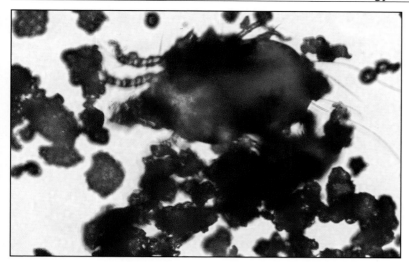

■ Figure 7-29.

House dust mite. Since the late 1960s, house dust mites of the genus *Dermatophagoides* have been identified as the prominent factor in house dust allergy (especially in those homes without pets). The two major species are *Dermatophagoides pteronyssinus* and *Dermatophagoides farinae*, which are found worldwide. There are numerous other types of dust mites and storage mites that are also important in different locales. Although most important in inhalant allergy, there are reports of allergic or anaphylactic reactions following ingestion of mite-contaminated foods. This photograph depicts a mite found in contaminated flour. (*Courtesy of* F. Dan Atkins, MD).

References

1. Glassheim JW, Ledoux RA, Vaughan TR, *et al.*: Analysis of meteorological variables and seasonal aeroallergen pollen counts in Denver, Colorado. *Ann Allergy Asthma Immunol* 1995, 75:149–156.

2. Silvers WS, Ledoux RA, Dolen WK, *et al.*: Aerobiology of the Colorado Rockies: pollen count comparisons between Vail and Denver, Colorado. *Ann Allergy* 1992, 69:421–426.

3. Solomon WR, Weber RW, Dolen WK: Common allergenic pollen and fungi. In *Allergy, Asthma, and Immunology from Infancy to Adulthood*. Edited by Bierman CW, Pearlman DS, Shapiro GG, Busse WW. Philadelphia: WB Saunders Company; 1996:93–114.

4. Lewis WH, Vinay P, Zenger VE: *Airborne and Allergenic Pollen of North America*. Baltimore: Johns Hopkins University Press; 1983.

5. Thommen AA: Which plants cause hayfever? In *Asthma and Hayfever in Theory and Practice*. Edited by Coca AF, Walzer M, Thommen AA. Springfield, IL: Charles C. Thomas; 1931:546–554.

6. Weber RW: Pollen identification. *Ann Allergy Asthma Immunol* 1998, 80:141–145.

7. Gravesen S, Frisvad JC, Samson RA: *Microfungi*. Copenhagen: Munksgaard; 1994.

8 Immunology Laboratory Techniques

D. Betty Lew

This chapter aims to assist readers in understanding the basic principles of commonly applied diagnostic tests in allergic and immunologic diseases. Recent advances in the technology and availability of highly specific immunologic reagents have lessened the burden of the diagnosis and management of patients with allergic and immunologic diseases.

This chapter begins with an illustration of specific IgE measurement in vivo. Allergy skin tests are currently the gold standard in expeditiously diagnosing specific allergy. The radioallergosorbent test (RAST) is an alternative, in vitro, method. The RAST inhibition test for measurement of allergens is illustrated in this chapter.

Commonly used nonradioactive techniques that use immunologic reagents to measure antigen or antibody are presented. These include enzyme immunoassay (EIA), enzyme-linked immunosorbent assay (ELISA), Western blot, direct and indirect immunofluorescence techniques, agglutination, immunodiffusion, and complement fixation.

The gene array technique is useful to detect cytokine and other gene expression. This powerful, although semiquantitative, technique allows us to screen a large number of gene expressions in a relatively short time. Thus, it will prove useful in determining the specific gene defect, monitoring the markers of disease activity, and formulating individual treatment.

Flow cytometry and cell sorter can provide us immunophenotype information rapidly, which can facilitate the diagnosis of immune deficiency. Lymphocyte proliferation response to mitogens in vitro can further provide us information on functional status of lymphocytes. Other techniques that use high-performance light sources, such as nephelometry (used for immunoglobulin and complement measurement), are also included in this chapter.

Finally, basic techniques to determine phagocyte dysfunction, including the quantitative nitroblue tetrazolium (NBT) test and the chemiluminescence test, are illustrated.

Allergy Skin Tests

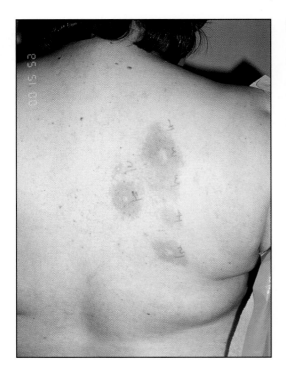

■ Figure 8-1.

Allergy skin test in vivo. Specific IgE reaction to food or inhalant antigens may be detected by epicutaneous skin test (prick, puncture, or scratch test). Skin test results using the DermaPIK (Greer Laboratories, Inc., Lenior, NC) device on the upper back of the subject are shown: **1**, American elm tree pollen. **2**, Perennial rye grass pollen. **3**, Ragweed short pollen. **4**, *Alternaria* spp. mold spore. **5**, *Dermatophagoids farinae* dust mite. **6**, Diluent (negative control). **7**, Histamine (positive control). The average diameter of wheal and flare in millimeters is measured. Positive tests at 1-minute time point to perennial rye, ragweed short, and *Dermatophagoids farinae* are illustrated.

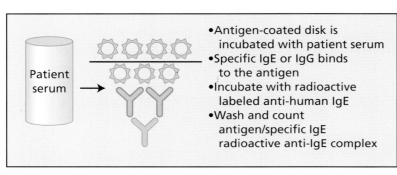

Patient serum →

- Antigen-coated disk is incubated with patient serum
- Specific IgE or IgG binds to the antigen
- Incubate with radioactive labeled anti-human IgE
- Wash and count antigen/specific IgE radioactive anti-IgE complex

■ Figure 8-2.

Radioallergosorbent test (RAST). RAST is a direct radioimmunoassay (RIA). In RIA, radioisotopes are used to measure the concentration of antigen in body fluid samples (*eg*, prostaglandins or leukotrienes) or antibody (*eg*, anti-DNA) in serum. RAST measures antigen-specific IgE antibody. An allergen is covalently bound to a cellulose disk and is allowed to bind to specific IgE antibody in serum, and the antigen–antibody complex is measured by using the anti-IgE antibody radiolabeled ligand.

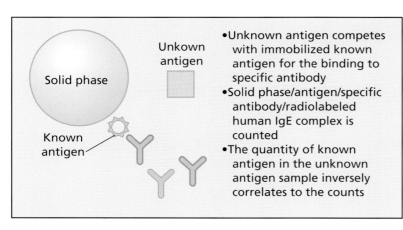

Solid phase

Unkown antigen

Known antigen

- Unknown antigen competes with immobilized known antigen for the binding to specific antibody
- Solid phase/antigen/specific antibody/radiolabeled human IgE complex is counted
- The quantity of known antigen in the unknown antigen sample inversely correlates to the counts

■ Figure 8-3.

Radioallergosorbent test (RAST) inhibition assay. This assay is based on competitive inhibition of binding. In the first phase, known antigen immobilized on a solid phase competes with unknown antigen for the binding to a specific antibody. In the second phase, the antibody bound to the immobilized antigen is measured using radiolabeled ligand. A reduction in radioactivity of the antigen–antibody complex compared with the radioactive counts measured in the control test with no unknown antigen is used to quantitate the amount of unknown antigen.

Nonradioactive Techniques That Use Immunologic Reagents

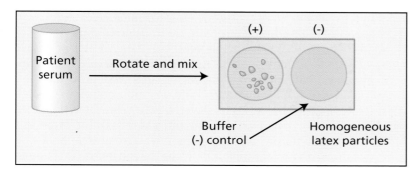

Figure 8-4.

Latex agglutination assay. Latex particles coated with antigen are mixed with dilution buffer or serum on test cards. After adequate rotation and mixing, the results are read macroscopically under a high-intensity incandescent lamp. The presence of specific antibody to the antigen is indicated by agglutinated latex particles. In the absence of a sufficient amount of specific antibody, the latex particles appear smooth and evenly dispersed.

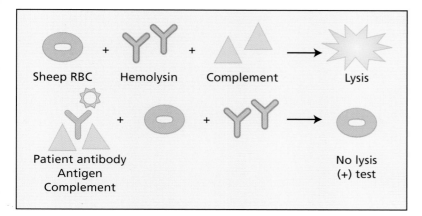

Figure 8-5.

Complement fixation. This method detects specific antibody (*eg*, antistreptolysin O) in serum. Newer methods have replaced this assay in many cases. The first step is to combine sheep red blood cells (RBC), complement-fixing antibody (IgG) directed against sheep RBC, and an exogenous source of complement, guinea pig serum. Hemolysin (*ie*, the antisheep cell antibody) can then bind to the surface of the sheep RBC. Complement can then bind to this antigen–antibody complex and cause cell lysis. The second step is to add a known antigen and patient serum to a suspension of sheep RBC, hemolysin, and a complement. The lack of lysis indicates the binding of complement to antibody and is considered to be a positive test result.

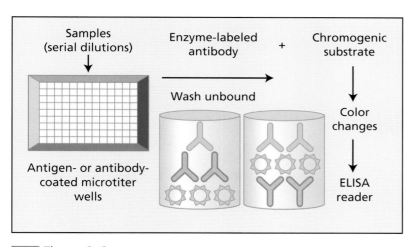

Figure 8-6.

Enzyme immunoassay (EIA). EIA is a sensitive and specific method that uses nonisotopic label. An enzyme-labeled antibody or enzyme-labeled antigen conjugate is used for the quantitative measurement of antigens or antibodies. Horseradish peroxidase, alkaline phosphatase, acetylcholinesterase, or other enzymes are used. For the measurement of antigen, microtiter well plates or beads are coated with specific antibody, to which the antigen in test samples binds. Subsequently, the enzyme-labeled specific antibody binds to the antigen–antibody complex, and the enzyme cleaves its chromogenic substrate, causing a color change. The results are obtained spectrophotometrically and quantitated against a standard curve obtained concurrently.

Various cytokines and lipid mediators (*eg*, prostaglandins and leukotrienes) can be measured by enzyme immunoassay (EIA). Antibody to HIV-1 can be measured with EIA by using microtiter wells coated with antigenic preparation, inactivated and lysed whole virus, and an enzyme-conjugated second antibody specific for human immunoglobulin. Similar to RIA, the EIA procedure is highly sensitive and specific, but the sensitivity and specificity of EIA may vary depending on the quality of the antigen or antibody used in the assay. ELISA—enzyme-linked immunosorbent assay.

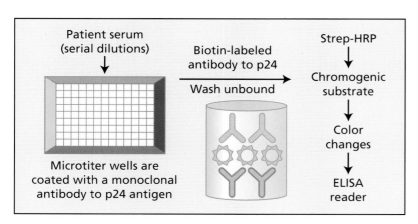

Figure 8-7.

Enzyme-linked immunosorbent assay (ELISA) for p24 antigen. The detection and quantitation of p24 core antigen of HIV-1 uses ELISA. Microtiter wells are coated with monoclonal antibody directed against p24 core antigen. Serum samples are added to the well, incubated, and washed. A probe antibody (biotin conjugate), streptavidin-conjugated horseradish peroxidase, and a substrate (tetramethylbenzidine) are added sequentially with thorough washing procedures between each step. The method is highly sensitive and specific for HIV-1.

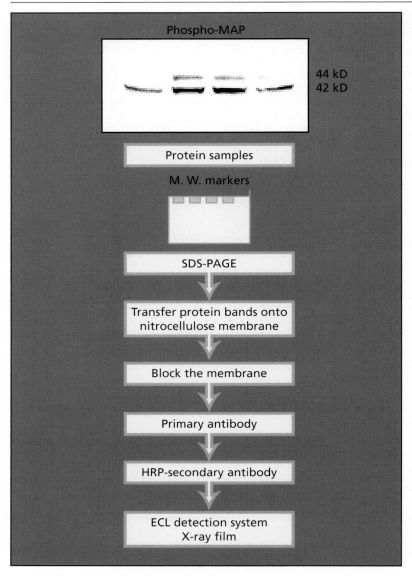

Phospho-MAP

44 kD
42 kD

Protein samples

M. W. markers

SDS-PAGE

Transfer protein bands onto
nitrocellulose membrane

Block the membrane

Primary antibody

HRP-secondary antibody

ECL detection system
X-ray film

■■■ Figure 8-8.

Western blot (also known as immunoblot). This technique may be used to detect antibodies (*eg*, HIV-1 antibody) or to identify unknown antigens by blotting with specific antibody. Antigens are separated by sodium dodecyl sulfate–polyacrylamide gel electrophoresis (SDS-PAGE); the proteins are transferred onto Hybond-ECL nitrocellulose membranes. For Western blot of phospho-p42/44MAPK (mitogen-activated protein kinase) in bovine airway smooth muscle cell lysates, the membranes were probed with antiphospho-p44/42^{MAPK} (Thr202/Tyr204) rabbit polyclonal antibody (New England Biolabs, Inc; Beverly, MA). After washing, the membrane was incubated with a goat antirabbit linked with horseradish peroxidase (HRP), and the immunoreactive protein bands were visualized on radiographic film using an enhanced chemiluminescence light (ECL) detection system (Amersham Pharmacia Biotech Inc.; Piscataway, NJ).

■■■ Figure 8-9.

Immunofluorescence assay. This direct immunofluorescence technique uses a conjugated antibody to detect antigen–antibody reactions in fixed cultured cells, tissue sections, or smears for microorganisms. The indirect immunofluorescence technique is used to detect antigen–antibody complex by conjugated second antibody. A number of conjugates are available: fluorochromes (*eg*, fluorescein isothiocyanate [FITC]); tetramethylrhodamine isothiocyanate (TRITC); and biotin-avidin, which can be complexed to fluorochromes. Indirect immunofluorescence staining of bovine airway smooth muscle α-isoactin detected by TRITC-conjugated second antibody is shown: the primary antibody is mouse monoclonal antibody (1A4 clone: Sigma; St. Louis, MO); the second is rabbit antimouse IgG. Fluorescent signals are detected by epifluorescence microscope (magnification, × 400). Immunofluorescent assay is frequently applied to detect viral antigens (*eg*, herpes simplex) and autoantibodies (*eg*, antinuclear antibody [ANA]).

The Gene Array Technique

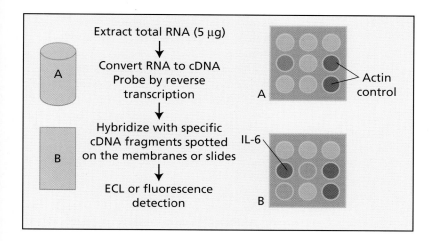

Figure 8-10.

The gene array technique illustrated. This technique may be used to detect gene expression of various cytokines and cytokine receptors. Total RNA isolated from cells or tissue is converted to cDNA probes by reverse transcription. cDNA is then hybridized with gene-specific cDNA fragments spotted on the membranes or slides. The specific gene expression may be detected by one of the three systems: fluorescent detection system, radioactive detection system, or nonradioactive detection system. Interleukin-6 gene expression in bovine airway smooth muscle cells is shown (GEArray system; SuperArray, Inc., Bethesda, MD). An enhanced chemiluminescence light (ECL) detection system (Amersham Pharmacia Biotech Inc.; Piscataway, NJ) was used as described in Figure 8-8.

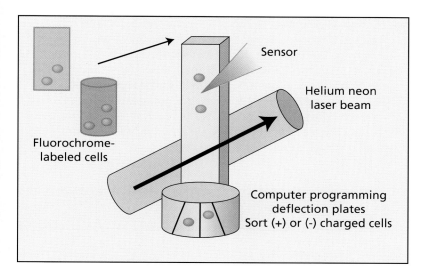

Figure 8-11.

Flow cytometry. The flow cytometry technique allows analyzing properties of single cells as they pass through an orifice at high velocity. Highly specific fluorochrome-coupled antibodies for cell-surface markers may be used for cell sorting with the aid of pre-programmed computer information. Electrostatically positive or negative charge is emitted to the stream containing the target cell. Two or more colors may be used to separate different cell population. Flow cytometric measurement may be applied for cell size, volume, refractory index, viscosity, chemical features (*eg*, content of DNA, RNA, proteins, and enzymes), and cross-matching.

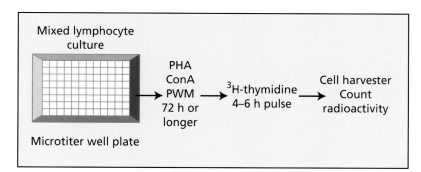

Figure 8-12.

Lymphocyte proliferation assay by ^{3}H-thymidine incorporation. Lymphocytes are purified from anticoagulated peripheral blood by Ficoll-Hypaque density gradient centrifugation. Cells are counted and suspended at 1×10^6 per mL density. Lymphocyte function is assessed by its ability to synthesize DNA in response to mitogens: phytohemagglutinin (PHA), concanavalin A (Con A), pokeweed mitogen (PWM), and so on. Patient lymphocytes or control (immunocompetent) lymphocytes in microtiter well plates are stimulated with one of the above mitogens and incubated at 37°C (95% air; 5% CO_2) for 72 hours in growth medium supplemented with serum (10% to 20%, vol/vol). The cultures are pulse-labeled with ^{3}H-thymidine. The rate of DNA synthesis is measured by counts per minute (CPM) or corrected for quenching to disintegrations per minute (dpm) of ^{3}H-thymidine incorporated into newly synthesized DNA in liquid scintillation spectrophotometer.

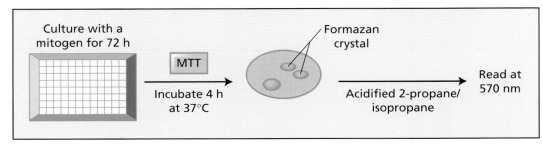

Figure 8-13.
Lymphocyte proliferation assay by MTT (3-[4,5-dimethylthiozol-2-yl]-2,5 diphenyl tetrazolium bromide). To assess cell counts and cytotoxicity, tetrazolium salt reduction colorimetric assay may be used; tetrazolium ring is cleaved in active mitochondria and, therefore, the reaction occurs only in living cells. The lymphocytes are stimulated in microtiter wells as described previously for 72 hours. MTT dissolved in phosphate buffer saline is added to the cells in microtiter wells. After a 4-h incubation at 37°C, acidified (0.04 M HCl) 2-propane/isopropanol is added to wells to dissolve formazan crystals. The plates are left at room temperature for 30 minutes and are read on an enzyme-linked immunosorbent assay (ELISA) reader at a 570-nm wavelength. The values for the cell blank are obtained similarly except for MTT, which is substituted with buffer. Cell numbers are derived from a standard curve generated from known cell numbers. If the serum content is high ($\geq 5\%$), however, optical density is altered and the results are not reliable.

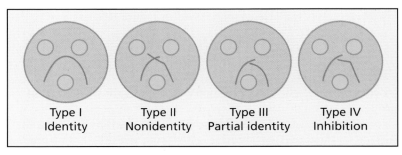

| Type I Identity | Type II Nonidentity | Type III Partial identity | Type IV Inhibition |

Figure 8-14.
Immunodiffusion assay, Ouchterlony type. The precipitation pattern of Ouchterlony type of immunodiffusion is shown.

Commercial immunodiffusion plates (1% agarose with precut wells) are used to perform the test. Specific antisera is added to the brim of the well and patient serum or known antigen is added to the peripheral wells. Plates are incubated with lid on for 18 to 48 hours at 37°C or longer at room temperature. Four types of identity are shown: type I, the reaction of identity, in which the precipitin band forms a single smooth arc; type II, the reaction of nonidentity, in which the precipitation lines cross each other; type III, the reaction of partial identity, in which the precipitation lines merge with spur formation; antigens are nonidentical but possess common determinants; and type IV, the reaction of inhibition, in which the antigens carry unrelated determinants and the antibody contains separate components.

Techniques That Use High-performance Light Sources

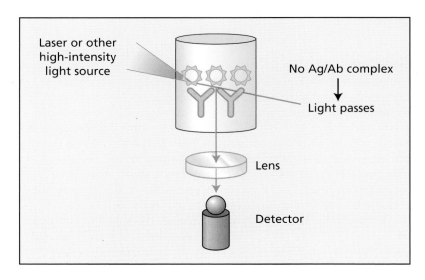

Figure 8-15.
Nephelometry. Nephelometry is based on the principle of light-scattering particles. A laser or another high-performance light source is used. Scattered light rays are collected in a focusing lens and ultimately can be related to the antigen–antibody complex concentration in a sample. For the measurement of antigen, highly purified and optically clear specific antiserum is added to form antigen–antibody complex. Examples of immunologic assays performed by nephelometry are α_1-antitrypsin, α_2-macroglobulin, C1 esterase inhibitor, complement components (C1r, C1s, C2-C8), C-reactive protein, cryoglobulins, and immunoglobulins.

Techniques to Determine Phagocyte Dysfunction

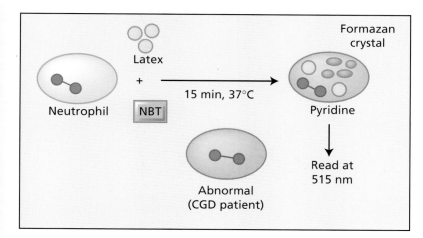

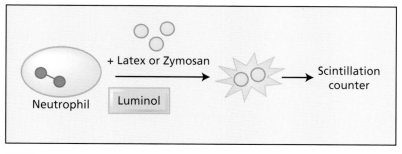

Figure 8-16.

Nitroblue tetrazolium (NBT) dye reduction test. NBT (yellow) compound is reduced in neutrophils undergoing a metabolic burst generated through the hexos monophosphate shunt. Latex particles are added to neutrophils for 15 minutes at 37 C to stimulate phagocytosis and metabolic burst. The dye forms formazan crystals (deep blue) on reduction. The dye is extracted with the organic solvent pyridine and is measured photometrically at a 515-nm wavelength. The test results are strikingly abnormal when chronic granulomatous disease is present.

Figure 8-17.

Chemiluminescence. The chemiluminescent technique is based on the fact that neutrophils emit a small amount of electromagnetic radiation after ingesting microorganisms. During the respiratory burst, reactive oxygen species along with bacteria or other intralysosomal elements form an electronically unstable carboxy group. As these groups relax to ground state, light energy is emitted. There seems to be a precise correlation between light emission and microbicidal activity. Neutrophils are incubated with latex or zymosan particles. Luminol, an intermediate fluorescent compound, can be added to intensify the light emission. The emission of photons of light is measured as counts per minute (CPM) in a scintillation counter over the next 10 minutes at 2-minute intervals. The test is markedly abnormal in chronic granulomatous disease (patients and carriers) and in myeloperoxidase-deficient patients. The test is more sensitive than the quantitative nitroblue tetrazolium test and requires very small numbers of cells.

Recommended Reading

Fleisher TA, Tomar RH: Introduction to diagnostic laboratory immunology. *JAMA* 1997, 278:1823–1834.

Section II:
Allergy and Clinical Immunology

Urticaria and Angioedema

Roger W. Fox

Urticaria and angioedema occur in approximately 20% of the population. Chronic urticaria and/or angioedema are idiopathic or autoimmune in most cases. The differential diagnosis of urticaria and angioedema is extensive, and includes allergic, immunologic, and nonimmunologic causes. The laboratory evaluation must be directed by the history and physical examination, and only appropriate, cost-effective studies should be ordered. Antihistamines are the mainstay of treatment for acute and chronic urticaria and angioedema. Both classic and newer antihistamines are effective in controlling some or all symptoms. Corticosteroids are often used in the management of urticaria and angioedema, but the risk-benefit ratio must be strongly considered in the cases of chronic urticaria and angioedema.

Urticaria

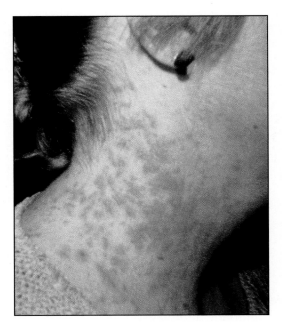

■ Figure 9-1.

Cholinergic (heat-induced) urticaria. Note the 1- to 3-mm punctate hives with large erythematous flare. Urticarial reactions are characterized by pale, localized swellings of the skin with a surrounding border of erythema. These pruritic lesions range from 1 or 3 mm (shown here) to several centimeters (*see* Fig. 9-2) in diameter, and each may be round to serpiginous in configuration (*see* Fig. 9-3). A single hive or a generalized outbreak (*see* Fig. 9-4) may occur in an individual patient. Urticaria is typified by the wheal-and-flare reaction induced by injection of histamine into the superficial dermis, or by cutaneous mast cell degranulation. The individual lesions of urticaria arise suddenly, and persist for a brief period, usually less than 24 hours. The hives can recur in episodes, or continuous outbreaks of groupings of urticaria can develop until treatment intervenes or spontaneous remission occurs. With a few exceptions, such as physical urticaria and urticaria pigmentosa, the cause of urticaria cannot be identified by its physical appearance.

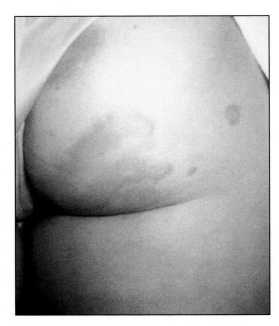

■ Figure 9-2.

Typical, large urticaria with smaller satellite hives occurring in acute or chronic urticaria.

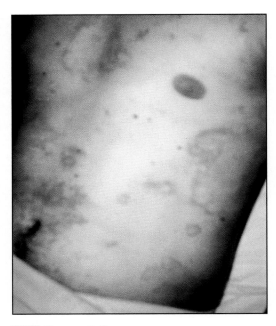

■ Figure 9-3.

Large, serpiginous urticaria. These urticaria are associated with a serum sickness reaction to an antibiotic.

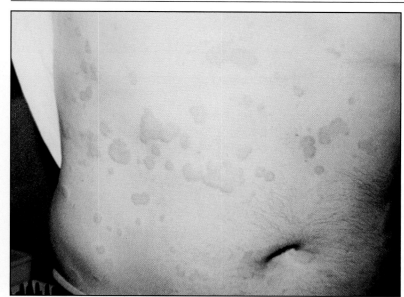

Figure 9-4.

Characteristic, generalized urticaria in an exacerbation of chronic idiopathic urticaria.

Angioedema

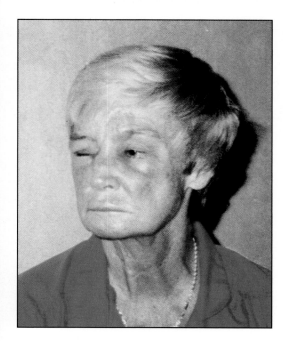

Figure 9-5.

Angioedema of the face. Angioedema, in most cases, is a manifestation of the same pathogenic process as urticaria, although angioedema is characterized by well-demarcated swelling of deeper cutaneous tissues. The sites of predilection are the palms, soles, face, and oral area. The overlying skin appears to be erythematous, and the lesion is nonpruritic. The associated discomfort is described as a burning or pins-and-needles sensation. Angioedema persists longer than urticaria due to the greater quantity of accumulated tissue fluid. Urticaria and angioedema may coexist, or each may appear alone.

Classification

Classification of Urticaria and Angioedema

Immunologic mechanisms		Nonimmunologic mechanisms	Hereditary forms
IgE-mediated	Thyroiditis	**Direct mast cell-releasing agents**	Familial cold urticaria
Allergic reactions	Transfusion-related reactions	Opiates and muscle relaxants	Vibratory angioedema
Foods	ABO mismatched reactions	Radiocontrast media	C3b inactivator deficiency
Drugs	IgA deficiency (IgG–IgA	Others	Amyloidosis, deafness, and urticaria
Hymenoptera venom	immune complexes)	**Alteration of arachidonic acid**	Hereditary angioedema (HAE)
Physical urticaria	Hereditary angioedema and	**metabolism (aspirin and**	
Cholinergic urticaria	C1INH deficiencies	**other nonsteroidal**	
Cold-dependent urticaria	Absent C1INH (I)	**anti-inflammatory drugs)**	
Delayed pressure urticaria and	Nonfunctional C1INH (II)	Acute urticaria	**Chronic idiopathic urticaria**
angioedema	Acquired C1INH deficiency (I)	Chronic idiopathic urticaria	
Solar urticaria	Autoantibodies to C1INH (II)	exacerbations	
Dermatographism	Infections	**Systemic diseases manifesting with**	
Aquagenic urticaria	Hepatitis B, C	**urticaria/angioedema**	
Vibratory angioedema	Mononucleosis	Urticaria pigmentosa/systemic	
Local heat urticaria	Other viral infections (mostly	mastocytosis	
Complement-mediated/autoimmune	in children)	Angioedema associated with	
Collagen vascular diseases	Parasites	eosinophilia	
Systemic lupus erythematosus	Malignancies		
Chronic cutaneous vasculitis	Serum sickness		
Hypocomplementemic urticarial	Paraproteinemias		
vasculitis syndrome			
Chronic autoimmune urticaria			

Figure 9-6.

Classification of urticaria and angioedema. The cumulative prevalence rate of urticaria and/or angioedema in the general population is approximately 15% to 20%, and all ages are affected [1]. Urticaria and angioedema are classified as acute or chronic, based on whether the episodes persist for more or less than 6 to 8 weeks. Acute urticaria and angioedema are short-lived, and are generally associated with allergic reactions to foods, Hymenoptera venom, or medications such as penicillin. Acute urticaria and angioedema occur more frequently in children and young adults, and represent the most common types of hives. In addition to the immediate, IgE-mediated hypersensitivity reaction, urticaria and angioedema are clinical manifestations of other immunologic and nonimmunologic etiologies, as shown here [2]. Immunologic urticaria and angioedema include the classic allergic reaction resulting in acute hives, physical urticaria, and complement-mediated urticaria and angioedema, and urticarial vasculitis. An IgE mechanism has been implicated in several of the physical urticaria (*see* Fig. 9-7), including dermatographism (*see* Fig. 9-8), cold-induced (*see* Fig. 9-9), and solar urticaria (*see* Fig. 9-10) [3]. These types of urticaria can be passively transferred to a normal skin site of a volunteer by injecting a serum sample from an affected patient. However, not all physical urticaria are IgE-mediated and passively transferred with serum; examples include delayed-pressure urticaria, cholinergic urticaria, and four of six types of solar urticaria (*see* Fig. 9-7). Urticaria pigmentosa, a mast cell disorder of the skin, must be considered in the patient with dermatographia.

The skin disorders listed here that result from autoimmunity and the activation of the complement cascade with subsequent generation of anaphylotoxins—C3a, C4a, and C5a—and other mediators, such as bradykinin, are a diverse group [4,5]. Autoantibodies associated with systemic lupus erythematosus (SLE) and thyroiditis, and immune complex formation associated with serum sickness,

hepatitis B or C, and mismatched transfusion reactions result in urticaria and cutaneous vasculitis [6]. In some patients, cutaneous leukocytoclastic vasculitis is a rare cause of chronic urticaria. Unlike the typical hive, the individual lesions of urticarial vasculitis may persist for 1 to 3 days [7]. Some of the cutaneous vasculitis lesions are described as palpable purpura, which are more often localized on the lower extremities. Constitutional symptoms associated with cutaneous vasculitis include myalgias, arthralgias, fever along with the laboratory findings of a leukocytosis, elevated erythrocyte sedimentation rate, and low total complement level (CH_{50}). A skin biopsy can be used to confirm the diagnosis. Hypocomplementemic urticarial vasculitis syndrome (HUVS) is associated with low complement levels and a low molecular weight precipitin (monomeric IgG), which binds to C1q. Other systemic symptoms and organ involvement (*eg*, lung, joints, and kidneys) are associated with HUVS, and this disorder must be differentiated from SLE. Cutaneous vasculitis responds to corticosteroids, dapsone, and hydroxychloroquine.

Hereditary and acquired C1 esterase inhibitor (C1INH) deficiencies are characterized clinically by recurrent attacks of angioedema involving the extremities, upper airway, or gastrointestinal tract [8]. Attacks abate spontaneously, lasting up to 24 to 72 hours. Upper airway obstruction may become life-threatening. Often the swelling is induced by tissue trauma, but episodes may occur spontaneously.

Hereditary angioedema (HAE) is treated with oral, attenuated androgens, stanozolol 1 to 4 mg/d or danazol 50 to 300 mg/d, which stimulates the hepatic synthesis of C1INH [9]. Intravenous C1INH is available in clinical trials.

Idiopathic and delayed-pressure angioedema can be differentiated as hereditary or acquired angioedema by the clinical criteria and by normal levels of C1INH and C4 complement studies.

(*continued on next page*)

■ Figure 9-6. (*continued*)

Two types of hereditary angioedema exist: HAE I has decreased synthesis of a normal C1INH, and HAE II has a dysfunctional C1INH. There are two types of acquired angioedema (AAE) and both I and II have low levels of C1INH and depressed C4 levels. The C1q level is also low secondary to activation and consumption of the initial components of the complement cascade. AAEI is associated with lymphoproliferative disorders and AAEII has an autoantibody against C1INH. AAE are less responsive to the attenuated androgens, and treating the underlying disorder results in resolution of the angioedema attacks.

Among the nonimmunologic causes are drugs that directly perturbate the mast cell to degranulate. Opiates, some general anesthetics, dextran, and conventional radiocontrast materials are the best examples of medication and diagnostic agents that cause hives by a nonallergic mechanism. The nonsteroidal anti-inflammatory drugs (NSAIDs) alter arachidonic acid metabolism, which generates vasoactive substances such as leukotrienes, causing the formation of urticaria and angioedema in susceptible subjects. NSAIDs may exacerbate chronic urticaria/angioedema (CU/A) in some patients.

Chronic CU/A (longer than 6 to 8 weeks duration) are idiopathic in most cases (70% to 95%) [10–12], but recent reports indicate an autoimmune mechanism in fewer than 50% of the cases. CU/A occurs in 0.1% of the population; when extrapolated to the US population, 270,000 Americans have CU/A. Women are affected twice as often as men (*see* Fig. 9-10), and CU/A is uncommon in childhood. The average duration of such hives is 6 months in one large population of patients, but based on other observations, the average duration of CU/A is 3 to 5 years and 20% of the patients have hives spanning a 20-year period. The hives may be daily or sporadic with remissions to exacerbations. Some women have menstrual cycle worsening of their CU/A. Exacerbations of CU/A at night and early morning follow the diurnal circadian rhythm. Individual urticaria persist for hours, and typically less than 24 hours. Angioedema may persist for days as the tissue fluid is absorbed. The clinician can usually identify allergic types of urticaria, physical urticaria and urticaria associated with connective tissue diseases by a thorough history and physical exam. The physical urticaria can be reproduced with the appropriate cutaneous stimulus. CU/A is rarely a manifestation of a chronic allergy such as a "hidden" food allergen or from a collagen vascular disease with an incidence of less than 1%. CU/A patients are generally healthy and represent a heterogeneous group of patients, some whom experience mild symptoms while others have severe hives that are refractory except when on moderate doses of corticosteroids.

Forty percent of the patients with chronic urticaria experience only urticaria; 49% have both urticaria and angioedema, and the remaining 11% have only angioedema. The histopathology of CIU is different from acute urticaria in that there is a mixed cellular perivascular infiltration of the dermal postcapillary venules. Unlike cutaneous vasculitis, necrotizing changes of the venule or leukocytoclasis are not identified (Fig. 9-11). The infiltration of CU/A consists predominantly of CD4+ T cells, monocytes, and mast cells and mixed cellular infiltration of eosinophils and neutrophils (Fig. 9-11) [13]. Chronic idiopathic urticaria (CIU) represents a dynamic process involving a complex interplay of a number of mediators, cytokines, chemokines, adhesion molecules, and cellular interactions. The mast cell has a central role in the initiation of the process by releasing is mediators and cytokines and by activating and interacting with resident cutaneous cells and infiltrating cells which amplify the process. An initiating event that results in a chronic cutaneous inflammation in CU/A has been elusive, but histamine-releasing autoantibody has been identified in 20% to 50% of studied cases of chronic urticaria [14].

In 1986, Grattan *et al.* [15] demonstrated that autologous serum from CU/A patients injected into an intradermal site of these subjects caused a significant wheal-and-flare reaction. Autologous sera from

patients who were in remission were found to be inactive. Biopsy analysis of the positive autologous serum skin reaction was similar to the histology of the late phase allergic reaction, which closely resembles the histology of chronic idiopathic urticaria [16]. These investigators carried out a series of in vitro experiments that further delineated the IgG autoantibody to be specific for the alpha subunit of the IgE receptor. The monoclonal antibody 6F7, which reacts specifically with the alpha subunit, was used in competitive inhibition assays of basophils with sera from CIU patients. In 35 CIU patients, most patients' sera contained both types of autoantibodies [14]. These investigators indicated that the IgG against IgE receptor represents a likely mechanism in the pathogenesis of some CU/A patients [17,18]. IgG anti-IgE receptor autoantibodies are functionally important in CU/A based on the clinical observations that plasmapheresis and intravenous gammaglobulin have induced temporary remissions or improvement in CU/A patients who are autoantibody positive. These immunomodulating procedures would lower the level of the IgG autoantibody. The IgG subtypes in CU/A are predominantly, IgG1 and IgG3, which bind complement. Complement activation and production of C5a is necessary along with the anti-IgE receptor antibody for mast cell histamine release to occur. Only cutaneous mast cells have the receptor for C5a, explaining why mast cells in the lung or GI tract are not activated in CU/A. Less than 50% of CU/A patients react to an autologous serum skin test. Of these patients, 80% have a positive immunoblot test demonstrating the presence of IgG to the alpha subunit of the IgE receptor. Therefore, another histamine releasing factor (HRF) is proposed to stimulate the mast cell in CU/A. The two subsets of CIU patients, those with and those without functional autoantibodies, were investigated histologically and immunochemically at 4 hours and at 12 hours. There was little difference in the cellular infiltration between the two subsets. These findings suggest that a similar pattern of mediator release from mast cells occurs in both subsets of CIU patients [19]. About 17% to 27% of euthyroid CU/A patients have thyroid autoantibodies (TA); antithyroglobulin and/or anti-peroxidase. TA are found in less than 6% of the general population. The precise role for these IgG autoantibodies in CU/A is unclear. Some experts believe that the TA are only a marker of autoimmunity in CU/A and not pathologic, but clinical observations that some TA (+) CU/A patients improve on thyroid hormone implicates some causative role of these autoantibodies in CU/A.

Mast cells are generally viewed as the key cell of the typical wheal-inducing pathology. Human mast cells have been shown to express and secrete a broad spectrum of proinflammatory and immunomodulating cytokines, but the role of these molecules in urticaria is largely unexplored. The data indicate that TNF-α and IL-3 are upregulated in lesional and nonlesional skin of chronic urticaria patients. The increased cytokine immunoreactivity of TNF-α and IL-3 in endothelial cells and keratinocytes are novel findings. The involvement of IL-8 in urticaria remains to be elucidated. The upregulation of inflammatory molecules in the skin of chronic urticaria patients may represent a low level priming of the cutaneous inflammatory and immunologic response apparatus, allowing for the maintenance of the disease even when the disease-eliciting factor (*eg*, activation of mast cells) is no longer apparent [20].

Mastocytosis is a condition characterized by mast cell hyperplasia. Clinical manifestations result principally from the reactions of mast cell–derived mediators [21]. Mastocytosis can be divided into presentations in which the skin is the only organ obviously involved (urticaria pigmentosa is one form; *see* Fig. 9-9) and systemic mastocytosis, either with or without skin involvement. Most patients with systemic mastocytosis experience a chronic, indolent course with episodic exacerbations. Antihistamines are the mainstay of treatment [22]. (*Adapted from* Fox and Russell [2].)

Types, Diagnostic Tests for, and Treatment of Physical Urticaria and/or Angioedema

Type	Diagnostic test	Treatment
Cold dependent	Ice cube test	H_1 antihistamines
Idiopathic (cutaneous only, or systemic)		Cyproheptadine HCl
Associated with abnormal serum proteins	Cryoproteins	Doxepin
Cold agglutinins		
Cryoglobulin		
Cryofibrinogen		
Donath-Landsteiner antibody		
Cold-induced cholinergic urticaria		
Cold-dependent dermatographism		
Delayed cold urticaria		
Familial cold urticaria		
Heat-induced disorder	Exercise	H_1 antihistamines
Cholinergic	Methacholine skin test	Hydroxyzine
Local heat urticaria		Danazol
Dermatographism	Stroking skin results in linear wheal	H_1 antihistamines
Idiopathic		
Following cutaneous allergic reaction		
Delayed form		
Mastocytosis/urticaria pigmentosa		
Delayed pressure angioedema	15-lb weight for 15 min	Corticosteroids
Idiopathic		
Associated with chronic idiopathic urticaria/angioedema		
Solar urticaria	Phototesting	Sunblock
		H_1 antihistamines
		Hydroxychloroquine

Type	Wavelength (nm)
I	290–320 (UVB) passively transferred (IgE)
II	320–400 (UVA)
III	400–700 (visible)
IV	290–900 passively transferred (IgE)
V	280–500
VI	400–500 (protoporphyrin IX)

Type	Diagnostic test	Treatment
Differential diagnosis SLE/photoallergic drug reaction		
PABA sunscreen blocks 280–320 (UVB)		
Window glass blocks		
Vibratory	Vortex for 4 min	H_1 antihistamines
		Diphenhydramine
		H_1 antihistamines
Aquagenic urticaria	Water compresses	H_1 antihistamines
Urticaria pigmentosa	Stroke skin	PUVA
	Darier's sign	
	"String of pearls"	

■ Figure 9-7.

Types, diagnostic tests for, and treatment of physical urticaria and/or angioedema. UVA—ultraviolet A; UVB—ultraviolet B; SLE—systemic lupus erythematosus; PABA—para-aminobenzoic acid; PUVA—psoralen ultraviolet light.

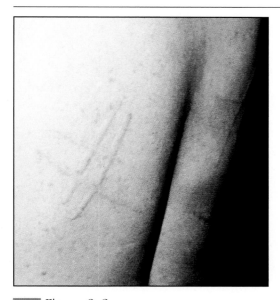

■ Figure 9-8.
Dermatographia. Dermatographia is displayed by stroking the back, resulting in long linear wheals and flares.

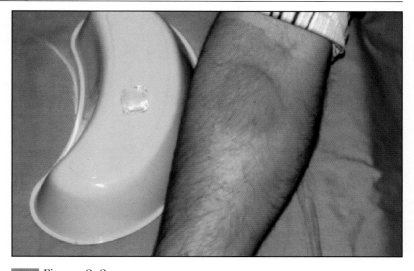

■ Figure 9-9.
Positive ice cube test in a patient with idiopathic cold-induced urticaria. This photograph was taken 5 minutes after the ice cube was removed.

■ Figure 9-10.
Solar urticaria. Solar urticaria is noted in this woman who had been wearing a tank top. These hives appear within minutes of sun exposure.

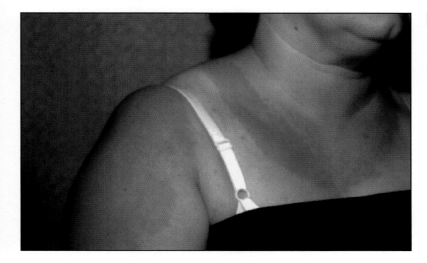

Mastocytosis

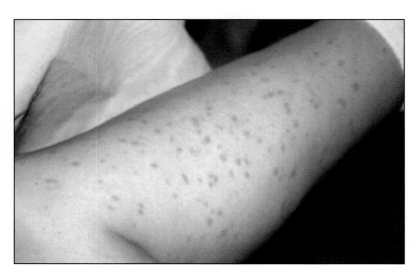

■ Figure 9-11.
Urticaria pigmentosa. This 24-year-old female patient first noted the appearance of multiple brown macules as a teenager. Stroking through these macules results in a "string of pearls" appearance of hives (a positive Darier's sign).

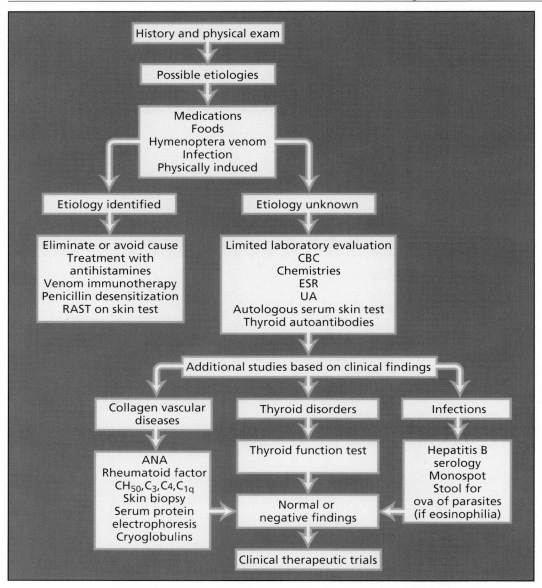

Figure 9-12.

Algorithmic approach to the workup of chronic urticaria. The possibility of an adverse or allergic reaction to venom, food, or a drug is always considered in the patient presenting with acute or recurrent episodes of urticaria and angioedema. If a comprehensive clinical evaluation is indeterminate, a cost-effective laboratory work-up is needed [23]. Because most episodes of acute urticaria are self-limiting or associated with an obvious allergic reaction, no further evaluation is necessary, with these exceptions: venom immunotherapy is required and penicillin desensitization is mandatory. Basic laboratory studies are needed to further evaluate the patient with unrelenting urticaria and/or angioedema (*see* Fig. 9-14). After a complete cognitive review of the clinical information and laboratory data, other immunologic studies may be ordered, although these tests are rarely indicated in an otherwise healthy individual with only cutaneous manifestations of urticaria and/or angioedema (as is the case with chronic idiopathic urticaria with or without angioedema) [24]. An evaluation for an occult malignancy or infection is not appropriate in most cases. Hidden food and food additive sensitivities are frequently considered as a cause of hives by the patient, but rarely can such a relationship between food and urticaria be established. A detailed food diary or elimination diet of a specific food or food additive can evaluate such possibilities. A hypoallergenic diet, such as a lamb and rice type diet, is sometimes required to determine if food is contributing. The double-blind, provocative oral challenge with a suspected food or food additive establishes a causal relationship, if one exists. A skin biopsy is not recommended in the evaluation of most cases of urticaria and angioedema, except in the cases of cutaneous vasculitis or refractory chronic urticaria or angioedema [25]. CBC—complete blood count; ESR—erythrocyte sedimentation rate; CH_{50}—total hemolytic complement; RAST—radioallergosorbent test.

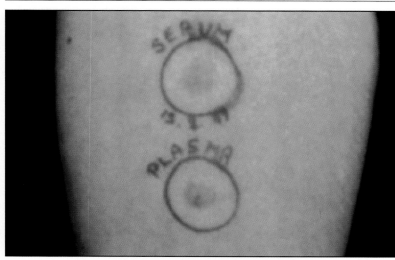

Figure 9-13.

A positive autologous serum or plasma skin test demonstrating the wheal and flare induced by the anti-IgE receptor antibody in a patient with chronic urticaria.

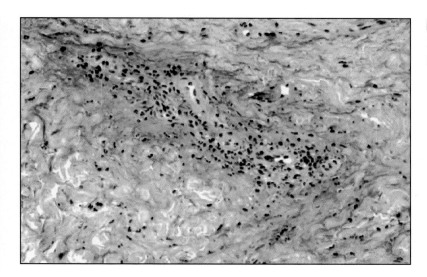

Figure 9-14.

Histopathology of chronic urticaria. Dermal edema and mild perivascular mixed cellular infiltration is characteristic.

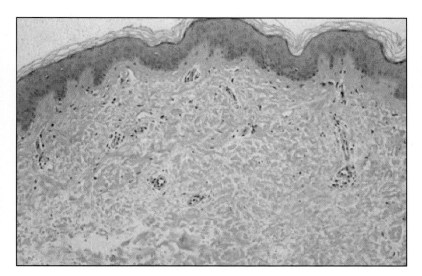

Figure 9-15.

Cutaneous vasculitis. This condition can involve dermal and deeper vessels of the skin. This biopsy specimen shows the intense neutrophilic infiltration, leukocytoclasis, and destructive changes of the superficial dermal postcapillary venules.

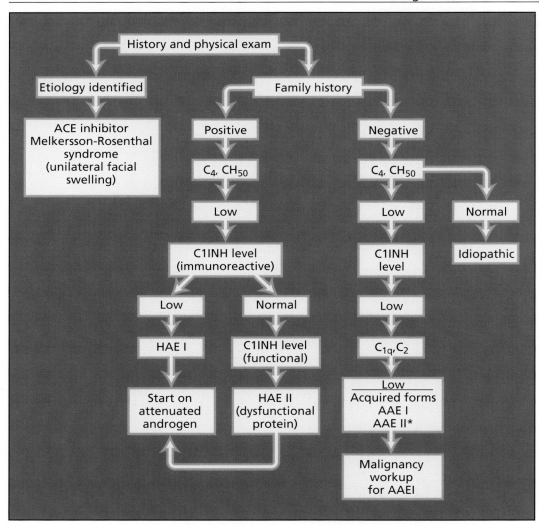

Figure 9-16.

Algorithmic approach to the workup of patients with angioedema without associated urticaria. The *asterisk* indicates that the autoantibody test is not commercially available. AAEI and II are less responsive to attenuated androgens than HAE. AAE I—acquired angioedema; AAE II—acquired angioedema II; ACE—angiotensin-converting enzyme; CH_{50}—total hemolytic complement; C1INH—C1 esterase inhibitor; HAE I—hereditary angioedema I; HAE II—hereditary angioedema II.

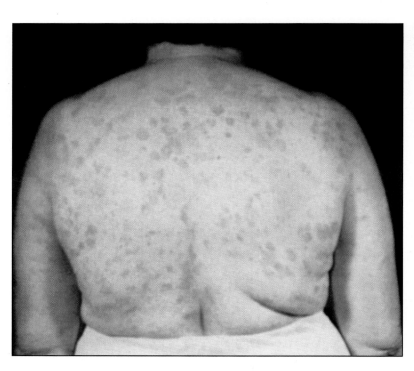

Figure 9-17.

An older woman with severe generalized chronic urticaria and non–life-threatening angioedema. The patient has not responded to antihistamines, and she has vitiligo and hypothyroidism.

Treatment

Investigation of Chronic Idiopathic Urticaria and/or Angioedema

In all patients	In certain patients
History and physical exam	Stool for ova and parasites
Provocative challenges for physical urticarias	Antinuclear factor
CBC	CH_{50}
ESR	Hepatitis B virus surface antigen and antibody
Urinalysis	Allergy skin testing or RAST
Blood chemistry profile	Serum protein electrophoresis
Autologous serum skin test	Cryoproteins
Thyroid autoantibodies	Skin biopsy

Figure 9-18.

Investigation of chronic idiopathic urticaria or angioedema. The rational therapy of urticaria is identification and then avoidance of the causative agents such as foods or medications, or of the specific conditions that induce physical urticarias. However, the precipitating cause is not always recognized immediately, or some other substance or activity is wrongly assigned.

With chronic urticaria and angioedema, avoidance of potentiating factors such as alcoholic beverages, heat, emotional stress, aspirin, and exertion is advocated. The treatment of this condition is generally considered palliative rather than curative [2]. Long-term treatment is the rule for patients with chronic urticaria and angioedema; therefore, careful selection of therapy is mandatory to maximize the benefit without resulting in severe drug side effects (*see* Fig. 9-15) [26]. Because most chronic urticaria is idiopathic, the physician should dispel patients' unrealistic expectations that there is a cause and reassure them that the prognosis is good and spontaneous remission is anticipated. CBC—complete blood count; ESR—erythrocyte sedimentation rate; CH_{50}—total hemolytic complement; RAST—radioallergosorbent test.

Chronic Idiopathic Urticaria and Angioedema Treatment Plan

Begin daily H_1 antihistamine
Hydroxyline or other classical/new
May use combinations (sedating and nonsedating)
Incomplete relief with above
Add daily H_2 antihistamine or doxepin
Add leukotriene modifier
For severe, refractory cases
Add corticosteroid for remission
Alternate day, tapering schedule
Other reported therapies in open clinical trials—limited cases
To steroid-dependent group (urticarial vasculitis, neutrophilic
    urticaria)
  Nifedipine
  Dapsone
  Hydroxychloroquine
  Azulfidine
  Stanozolol
  Methotrexate
  Cyclosporin/tacrolimus

Figure 9-19.

Chronic idiopathic urticaria and angioedema treatment plan. The acute phase treatment requires H_1 antihistamines. When the urticarial reaction is severe or accompanied by signs or symptoms of anaphylaxis, subcutaneous epinephrine, parenteral antihistamines, both H_1 and H_2 antagonists, and systemic corticosteroids are indicated.

H₁ Antihistamines Examples

Class	Generic name	Trade name	Doses (divided daily)
Piperazines	Hydroxyzine	Atarax (Pfizer)	40–200 mg
Piperidines	Cyproheptadine	Periactin (Merck)	8–32 mg
	Azatadine	Optimine (Schering)	2–4 mg
Ethanolamines	Diphenhydramine	Benadryl (Warner-Lambert)	25–200 mg
	Clemastine	Tavist (Novartis Consumer)	2.6–5.3 mg
Ethylenediamines	Tripelennamine	PBZ (Geigy)	75–200 mg
Propylamines	Chlorpheniramine	Chlor-Trimeton (Schering)	16–64 mg
Phenothialines	Methdilazine	Tacaryl (Westwood Squibb)	8–32 mg
Newer, less sedating	Fexofenadine hydrochloride	Allegra (Hoechst Marion Roussel)	60 mg to 180 BID
	Loratadine	Claritin (Schering)	10 mg to BID
	Cetirizine	Zyrtec (Pfizer)	10 mg to BID

Figure 9-20.

Antihistamines. **Antihistamines** are the mainstay of symptomatic management, mainly for pruritus. The diversity of mediators produced and the variety of inflammatory cells involved in urticarial reactions explain why antihistamines do not completely eliminate all the signs and symptoms of chronic urticaria. Sedation is common with most of the classic H₁ antagonists. The patient's tolerance for this side effect and others, such as dry mouth, urinary retention, and blurred vision will dictate the maximum antihistamine dose.

The limiting nature of the side effects of the classic antihistamines may not allow optimal control of the hives. There are six groups of classic H₁ antihistamines (*see* Fig. 9-16). The newer, less sedating antihistamines, fexofenadine, loratidine, and cetirizine are not necessarily more effective, but compliance improves when drugs are easy to take (daily and twice daily) and no symptomatic adverse effects are experienced. In general, when one antihistamine is ineffective or tachyphylaxis develops, the physician may select another antihistamine from a separate pharmacologic group. Hydroxyzine is traditionally first-line treatment for chronic idiopathic urticaria, and it remains the standard to which all other antihistamines are compared. When choosing two antihistamines for the patient with the more difficult chronic urticaria, choose from different groups.

The combination of hydroxyzine and cyproheptadine is particularly ineffective [27]. A popular combination is a nonsedating antihistamine in the morning and a sedating antihistamine, such as hydroxyzine, at bedtime. Patients with chronic urticaria should not be managed with "as needed" antihistamines exclusively, as this therapeutic rationale does not approach the problem from a preventive standpoint. Once an effective dose schedule is established with an antihistamine, the total dose can be gradually reduced according to the schedule until the lowest effective dose is found or the drug is withdrawn.

H₂ antihistamines may be necessary. The patient with inadequate control or on an H₁ or combination of H₁ agents at the highest tolerated or recommended dose should be prescribed an H₂ antihistamine. Cimetidine, 300 mg four times daily, or ranitidine, 150 mg twice daily, can be combined with an H₁ antihistamine. H₂ receptors make up about 10% to 15% of the total number of histamine receptors in the cutaneous vasculature [28]. The H₂ antihistamine should be discontinued after 3 to 4 weeks if there is no definitive clinical benefit.

Doxepin, a heterocyclic variant of amitryptaline, is approximately 800 times more potent than diphenhydramine in vitro on a molar basis, and doxepin is six times more potent than cimetidine. Clinical efficacy for doxepin in the management of chronic idiopathic urticaria has been established in doses ranging from 30 to 150 mg/d [29,30]. Doxepin is now considered a first-line treatment for chronic urticaria and/or angioedema. A concentrated syrup of doxepin (10 mg/L) allows for flexibility in dosing for the sedated patient.

Leukotriene modifiers, particularly the leukotriene receptor antagonists (*eg*, zafirlukast, montelukast) should be considered as add-on therapy with an antihistamine for patients with chronic urticaria and/or angioedema. Case reports indicate their value in conjunction with antihistamines. Leukotrienes (LTs) B4, C4, D4, and E4 are involved in the formation of the wheal and flare response in allergic reactions. A trial with one of these drugs for a period of 1 month is warranted in the chronic urticaria and/or angioedema patient who requires more than antihistamines for control of chronic urticaria. For those chronic urticaria and/or angioedema patients who respond to a LT-modifying drug, the agent should be continued until the patient is in clinical remission.

Corticosteroids are very effective in suppressing most signs and symptoms of all categories of urticaria. The physical urticarias (excluding delayed pressure urticaria/angioedema) are the

exception. Corticosteroids should be judiciously prescribed only in severe chronic urticaria and for uncontrolled exacerbations of urticaria and angioedema [13]. Their exact pharmacologic action is not completely understood. The patient should be tapered off the corticosteroids, with complete withdrawal of the drug prior to the onset of significant side effects (*see* Fig. 9-16). An alternate-day regimen of corticosteroids, prednisone 20 to 60 mg or equivalent dose of methylprednisolone, is used in the management of the patient with steroid-dependent chronic urticaria to maintain a clinical remission. Several months of therapy may be required. Corticosteroid-sparing agents and alternative drugs have been reported in the management of severe chronic urticaria [2,31]. Corticosteroid-sparing drugs have been reported in several case studies and include stanozolol, an attenuated androgen, and sulfasalazine, which is used in chronic inflammatory bowel disease. Methotrexate and cyclosporine are potent anti-inflammatory drugs reported to be effective in severe chronic urticaria and/or angioedema patients, but the side effects with these drugs must be carefully monitored. In particular, side effects with cyclosporine were unacceptable, despite the dramatic improvement observed with 6 mg/kg/d. Recent experiences with cyclosporine, 3.0 to 4.5 mg/d, are encouraging. Two thirds of patients on a 3-month trial had good to excellent results, with nearly one third in total remission [32]. A similar drug to cyclosporin, tacrolimus, which is used topically for atopic dermatitis, may be another choice for refractory chronic urticaria. Psoralen with ultraviolet A light (PUVA) treatments have anti-inflammatory effects in the skin. Plasmapheresis and intravenous γ-globulin infusions have been reported to help some patients who are identified to have the IgG autoantibody to the IgE high-affinity receptor α subunit.

Other drugs, including dapsone and hydroxychloroquine are effective treatment for urticarial vasculitis, *eg*, HUVS and SLE. Clinicians have prescribed these agents on a trial basis in steroid-dependent chronic urticaria and/or angioedema patients to reduce the requirements of corticosteroids or as a substitute for corticosteroids. The beneficial results are highly individualized. These results parallel similar reports with these drugs in steroid-dependent asthma. The anti-inflammatory properties of these drugs in the skin are important in suppressing chronic urticaria and/or angioedema. Prescribing such treatment without adequate knowledge of side effects and effectiveness places the patient at considerable risk from an off-label use of the drug. BID—twice daily; QD—every day.

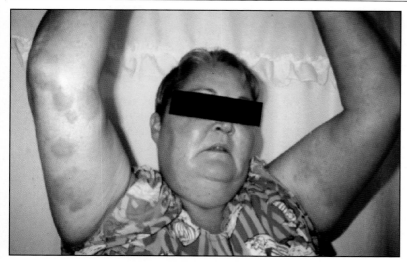

Figure 9-21.

Patient with severe chronic urticaria and angioedema for 7 months. Note her cushingoid appearance and the significant outbreak of urticaria while taking 50 mg of prednisone daily. She responded to cyclosporine and the prednisone was withdrawn.

References

1. Warin RP, Champion RH: *Urticaria*. London: WB Saunders; 1974.

2. Fox RW, Russell D: Drug therapy of chronic urticaria and angioedema. In *Pharmacologic Management of the Difficult to Treat Allergic Patient*. Edited by Kemp J. Philadelphia: WB Saunders; 1991: 45–63.

3. Casale TB, Sampson HA, Hanifin J: Guide to physical urticarias. *J Allergy Clin Immunol* 1988, 82:758–763.

4. Kaplan AP: Urticaria and angioedema. In *Allergy: Principles and Practice*, edn 5. Edited by Middleton E, Reed CE, Ellis F, *et al*. St. Louis: Mosby; 1998, 1553–1580.

5. Sanchez NP, Winkleman R, Schroeter AL: The clinical and histopathologic spectrum of urticaria vasculitis: study of 40 cases. *J Am Acad Dermatol* 1982, 7:599–605.

6. Rumbyrt JS, Katz JL, Schocket AL: Resolution of chronic urticaria in patients with thyroid autoimmunity. *J Allergy Clin Immunol* 1995, 96: 901–905.

7. Greaves MW: Chronic urticaria *N Engl J Med* 1995, 332:1767–1773.

8. Frank MM, Gelfand JA, Atkinson JP: Hereditary angioedema: the clinical syndrome and its management. *Ann Intern Med* 1976, 84:580–507.

9. Sheffer AL, Fearon DT, Austen KF: Clinical and biochemical effects of stanozolol therapy for hereditary angioedema. *J Allergy Clin Immunol* 1981, 68:181–187.

10. Paul E, Greilich KD, Dominante G: Epidemiology of urticaria. *Monogr Allergy* 1987, 21:87–115.

11. Kaplan AP: Urticaria and angioedema. In *Allergy*. Edited by Kaplan AP. New York: Churchill Livingstone; 1985:439–471.

12. Quaranta JH, Rohr AS, Rachelefsky GS: The natural history and response to therapy of chronic urticaria and angioedema. *Ann Allergy* 1989, 62:421–429.

13. Elias J, Boss E, Kaplan AP: Studies of the cellular infiltrate of chronic idiopathic urticaria: prominence of T lymphocytes, monocytes, and mast cells. *J Allergy Clin Immunol* 1986, 78:914–918.

14. Hide M: The pathogenesis of chronic idiopathic urticaria: new evidence suggests an autoimmune basis and implications for treatment. *Clin Exp Allergy* 1994, 24:624–627.

15. Grattan CEH, Wallington TB, Warin RP: A serological mediator in chronic idiopathic urticaria: a clinical, immunological, and histological evaluation. *Br J Dermatol* 1986, 114:583–590.

16. Grattan CEH, Boon AP, Eady RAJ, Winkelman RK: The pathology of the autologous serum skin test response in chronic urticaria resembles IgE-mediated late phase reaction. *Int Arch Allergy Immunol* 1990, 93:198–204.

17. Hide M, Francis DM, Grattan CEH, *et al*.: Autoantibodies against the high-affinity IgE receptor as a cause of histamine release in chronic urticaria. *N Engl J Med* 1993, 328:1599–1604.

18. Tong LJ, Balakrishran G, Kochan JP, *et al*.: Assessment of autoimmunity in patients with chronic urticaria. *J Allergy Clin Immunol* 1997, 99:461–465.

19. Sabroe RA, Poon E, Orchard GE: Cutaneous inflammatory cell infiltrate in chronic idiopathic urticaria: comparison of patients with and without anti-IgE RI or anti-IgE autoantibodies. *J Allergy Clin Immunol* 1999, 103:484–493.

20. Hermes B, Prochaska AK, Haas N: Upregulation of TNF-alpha and Il-3 expression in lesional and uninvolved skin in different types of urticaria. *J Allergy Clin Immunol* 1999, 103:307–314.

21. Metcalfe DD: Classification and diagnosis of mastocytosis: current status. *J Invest Dermatol* 1991, 96:2S–4S.

22. Metcalfe DD: The treatment of mastocytosis: an overview. *J Invest Dermatol* 1991, 96:55S–59S.

23. Charlesworth EN (ed.): Urticaria. In *Immunol Allergy Clin North Am*, vol 15. Philadelphia: WB Saunders; 1995.

24. Kanwar AJ, Greaves MW: An approach to the patient with chronic urticaria. *Hosp Pract* 1996, 3:171–189.

25. Winkleman RK, Reizner GT: Diffuse dermal neutrophilia in urticaria. *Hum Pathol* 1988, 19:389–393.

26. Tharp MD: Chronic urticaria: pathophysiology and treatment approaches. *J Allerg Clin Immunol* 1996, 98:S325–S330.

27. Harvey RP, Wegs J, Schocket AL: A controlled trial of therapy and chronic urticaria. *J Allergy Clin Immunol* 1981, 68:262–266.

28. Harvey RP, Schocket AL: The effect of H1 and H2 blockade on cutaneous histamine response in man. *J Allergy Clin Immunol* 1980, 65:136–139.

29. Goldgobel AB: Efficacy of doxepin in the treatment of chronic idiopathic urticaria. *J Allergy Clin Immunol* 1986, 78:867–871.

30. Greene SL, Reed CE, Schroeter AL: Double-blind crossover study comparing doxepin with diphenhydramine for the treatment of chronic urticaria. *J Am Acad Dermatol* 1985, 12:669–664.

31. Czarnetzki BM: Chronic urticaria. In *Current Therapy in Allergy, Immunology, and Rheumatology*, edn 4. Edited by Lichtenstein LM, Fauci AS. St. Louis: Mosby; 1992:49–52.

32. Greaves M: Chronic urticaria. *J Allergy Clin Immunol* 2000, 105:664–672.

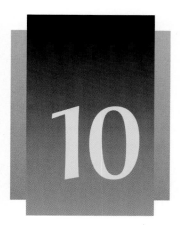

Atopic Dermatitis

Stacie M. Jones and Jay M. Kincannon

Atopic dermatitis is a chronic inflammatory disease of the skin characterized by intense pruritus, diffuse dryness, and chronically relapsing dermatitis. Individuals with a personal or family history of atopy are principally affected. The true prevalence of atopic dermatitis is unknown, but current estimates suggest that up to 10% of pediatric patients are affected. Sixty percent of affected individuals manifest characteristic lesions during the first year of life, and 90% of individuals will be affected by age 5 years. It is rare for symptoms to begin during adulthood.

The clinical course is variable and unpredictable; some children have mild disease with spontaneous remission by age 2 to 3 years, but others have a more persistent disease course with chronic, unremitting rash throughout childhood and into adulthood. The distribution of atopic dermatitis lesions varies with age (*see* Fig. 10-1). Infants and young children typically manifest rash on the face, trunk, and extensor surface of the extremities, with the pattern progressing to involve primarily the flexor surface of the extremities in older children. Adults often resolve their disease but continue to have evidence of "hand or foot eczema" that affects the palms and soles, respectively.

A strong correlation exists between atopic dermatitis and other atopic conditions such as asthma, food allergies, and allergic rhinitis. As many as 50% to 80% of children with atopic dermatitis develop allergic respiratory disease later in life. Evidence for the role of allergens in atopic dermatitis has long been recognized by practicing allergists. Investigators have demonstrated elevated levels of IgE antibody in 40% to 80% of patients with atopic dermatitis. The role of food allergy as a cause of atopic dermatitis, especially in infants and young children, has been repeatedly demonstrated. Aeroallergen sensitivity is most common in older children with atopic dermatitis and often complicates the disease course. Additionally, allergic sensitization to microorganisms (*eg,* *Staphylococcus aureus*) has been noted to be a cause of worsening or unremitting atopic dermatitis. In addition to allergens, the course of the disease can be influenced by environmental triggers (*eg,* irritant exposure, type of clothing, excessive heat, climate changes), psychosocial factors (*eg,* emotional upset and stress), and choice of occupation.

The rash of atopic dermatitis typically begins as an erythematous, papulovesicular eruption that progresses to a scaly, lichenified maculopapular dermatitis. Weeping and crusting lesions may occur and indicate the presence of bacterial superinfection. In addition, patients with atopic dermatitis have impaired cell-mediated immunity and are susceptible to severe viral infections with common organisms, such as herpes simplex and varicella.

Treatment of patients with atopic dermatitis is directed to control the chronically recurring condition and provide symptomatic relief (*see* Fig. 10-12). Environmental control (*eg,* cotton clothing) for reduction of specific allergen triggers and to minimize irritant contact with skin should be in place. Complete dietary restriction of specific food allergens should be instituted after the diagnosis of food allergy is confirmed. Skin care should focus on hydration, moisturization, reduction of itching, and control of inflammation. The use of daily soaking baths or wraps with the use of mild soaps (*eg*, Dove or Cetaphil) followed by the application of a moisturizing ointment (*eg*, petrolatum) several times a day can be very beneficial. Application of a topical steroid ointment twice daily to skin lesions helps to reduce the local inflammatory response. Topical tacrolimus ointment is a new nonsteroidal alternative

to steroid therapy that holds promise for both children and adults. Antipruritic agents should be used in liberal, scheduled dosing to reduce scratching. Lastly, oral antibiotic therapy is warranted in patients with open excoriations or oozing, crusting lesions to control bacterial superinfection. Alternate therapies such as oral steroid use, ultraviolet light therapy, and others should be reserved for patients who have severe cases and who are under the care of a specialist. The presence of atopic dermatitis is a relative contraindication for allergen immunotherapy because of the risk of disease exacerbation and progression.

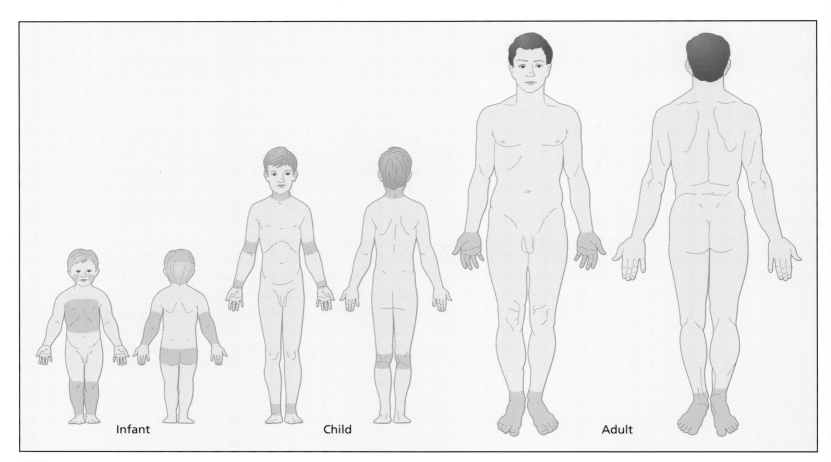

Infant   Child   Adult

■ Figure 10-1.

Age-related distribution of atopic dermatitis. Rash in infants is typically seen on the face, trunk, and extensor surfaces of the extremities. The rash moves to include both the extensor and flexor surfaces of the extremities in early childhood with progression

primarily to flexor surfaces in later childhood and adolescence. Atopic dermatitis rash in adults may be seen in any distribution but is most commonly limited to the palms and soles.

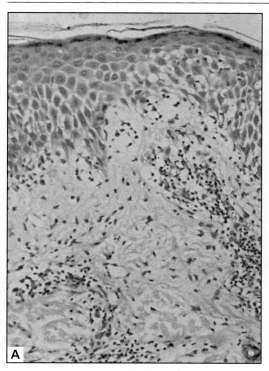 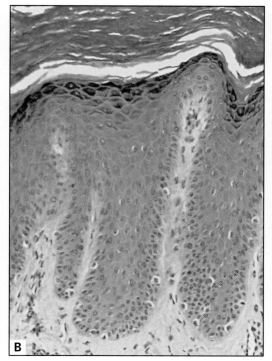 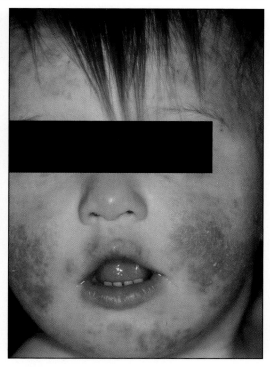

Figure 10-2.

Histopathology of atopic dermatitis. **A,** Acute atopic dermatitis lesion characterized by hyperkeratosis and hyperplasia of the epidermis with prominent spongiosis (edema) and mononuclear cell infiltrate, including monocytes, lymphocytes, eosinophils, mast cells, and Langerhans' cells. **B,** Chronic atopic dermatitis lesion characterized by marked hyperkeratosis of the epidermis with elongation of the rete ridges; parakeratosis and papillomatosis of the dermis with minimal spongiosis; and marked inflammatory cell infiltrate consisting of monocytes, macrophages, and lymphocytes. Langerhans' cells may be seen, but eosinophils are rare.

Figure 10-3.

Atopic dermatitis in an infant. This infant demonstrates the typical maculopapular, erythematous rash commonly seen on the face. This 5-month-old infant presented with a history of persistent rash starting at age 2 months. Subsequent allergy testing was positive to milk, and the infant improved after dietary restriction of milk protein and a formula change to a milk protein hydrolysate formula.

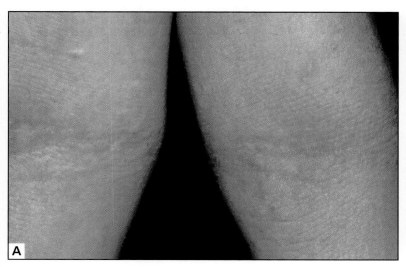 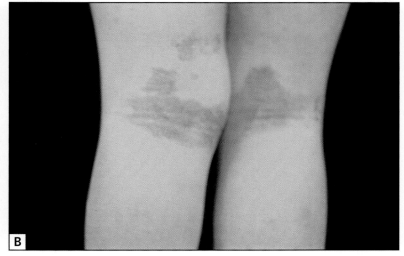

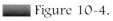**Figure 10-4.**

Atopic dermatitis in a child. Typical antecubital (**A**) and popliteal (**B**) lesions seen in atopic dermatitis of childhood. Treatment with hydration, a moisturizing ointment, and a topical anti-inflammatory ointment is warranted for symptomatic improvement of the disease.

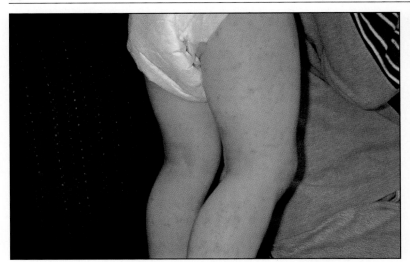

■ Figure 10-5.
Intense pruritus as a hallmark of atopic dermatitis. This young child has numerous linear excoriations typical of severe pruritus and secondary scratching. The liberal use of scheduled antihistamines and adequate skin hydration are essential to control itching and minimize traumatic injury with entry of microorganisms into the abraded skin.

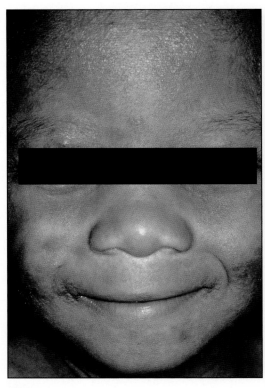

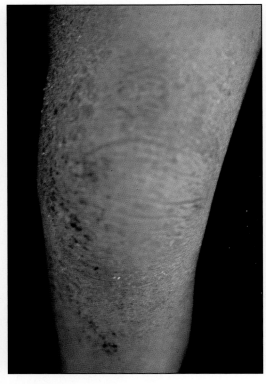

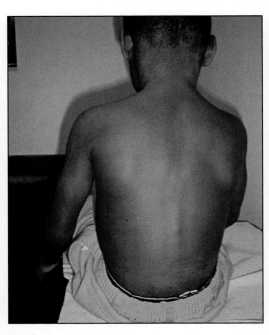

■ Figure 10-8.
Atopic features and ichthyosis. These characterize many patients with chronic disease. This 8-year-old boy has had atopic dermatitis since age 3 months. He had allergy to eggs during infancy and early childhood that yielded to multiple aeroallergen sensitivities by age 5 years. Note the chronic, hyperpigmented skin lesions and ichthyosis of the neck that signify long-standing disease.

■ Figure 10-6.
Atopic facies associated with atopic dermatitis. In this child, note the presence of allergic shiners, Dennie-Morgan lines, and central facial clearing in addition to his widespread facial and scalp dermatitis. These features indicate atopic disease.

■ Figure 10-7.
Lichenification in chronic atopic dermatitis. Long-standing atopic dermatitis with poor skin hydration and ongoing inflammatory disease results in the hyperpigmented, thickened skin known as lichenification.

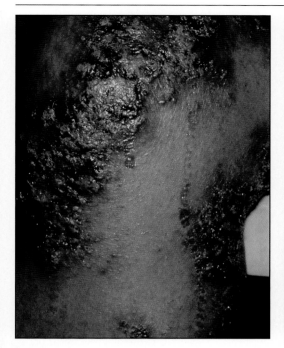

Figure 10-9.

Acute atopic dermatitis with secondary infection. In this patient, the acute atopic dermatitis lesions were complicated by superinfection with *Staphylococcus aureus*. Treatment requires both topical anti-inflammatory medications and systemic antibiotics. *S. aureus* infection of atopic dermatitis skin may further complicate the clinical course through a heightened allergic response (*ie*, production of toxin-specific IgE and "superantigen" function driving the T-cell immunologic response) to one or more of the *Staphylococcal* exotoxins, further emphasizing the need for systemic antibiotics at the first sign of infection.

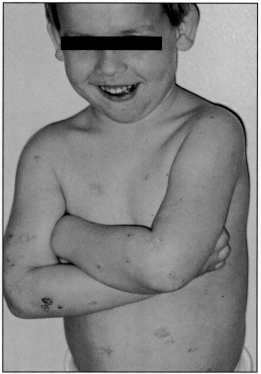

Figure 10-10.

Nummular eczema. This common disease variant of atopic dermatitis is characterized by well-circumscribed, circular lesions that occur primarily on the extensor surfaces of the extremities and on the trunk. Lesions are typically less pruritic than those of classical atopic dermatitis and are not usually associated with atopy. Nummular eczema can also be very recalcitrant to standard therapy.

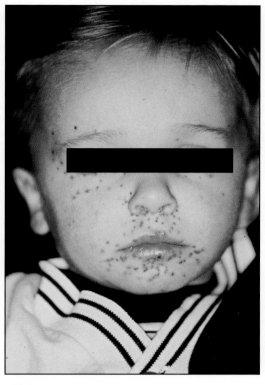

Figure 10-11.

Eczema herpeticum. Because of reduced cell-mediated immunity, children and adults with atopic dermatitis have increased susceptibility to viral skin infections such as herpes simplex and varicella. The occurrence of disseminated herpes simplex on the face of this patient is a medical emergency that requires aggressive antiviral therapy and attention by an ophthalmologist to ensure preservation of the patient's eyesight.

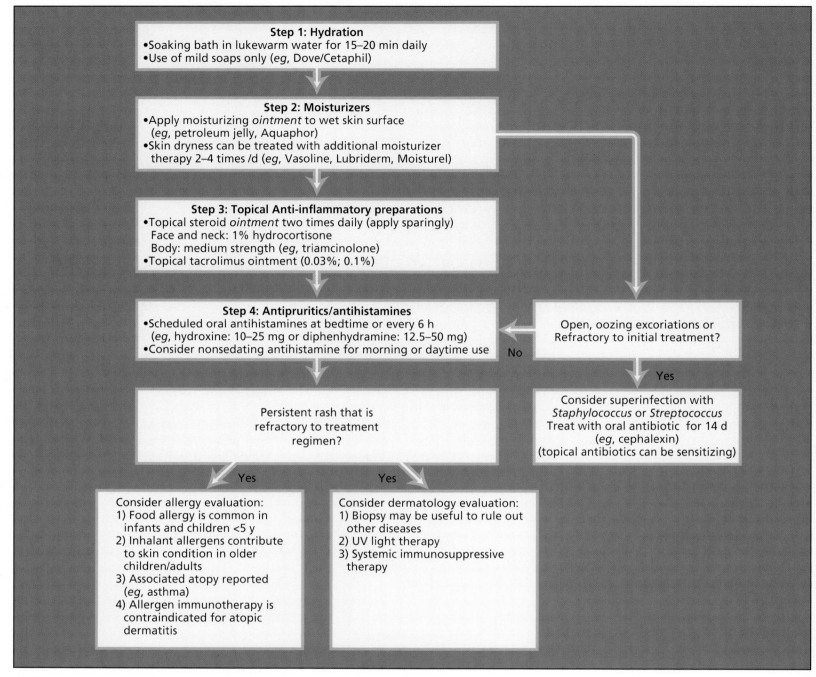

Step 1: Hydration
•Soaking bath in lukewarm water for 15–20 min daily
•Use of mild soaps only (*eg*, Dove/Cetaphil)

Step 2: Moisturizers
•Apply moisturizing *ointment* to wet skin surface
  (*eg*, petroleum jelly, Aquaphor)
•Skin dryness can be treated with additional moisturizer
  therapy 2–4 times /d (*eg*, Vasoline, Lubriderm, Moisturel)

Step 3: Topical Anti-inflammatory preparations
•Topical steroid *ointment* two times daily (apply sparingly)
  Face and neck: 1% hydrocortisone
  Body: medium strength (*eg*, triamcinolone)
•Topical tacrolimus ointment (0.03%; 0.1%)

Step 4: Antipruritics/antihistamines
•Scheduled oral antihistamines at bedtime or every 6 h
  (*eg*, hydroxine: 10–25 mg or diphenhydramine: 12.5–50 mg)
•Consider nonsedating antihistamine for morning or daytime use

Open, oozing excoriations or
Refractory to initial treatment?

No

Yes

Persistent rash that is
refractory to treatment
regimen?

Consider superinfection with
Staphylococcus or *Streptococcus*
Treat with oral antibiotic for 14 d
(*eg*, cephalexin)
(topical antibiotics can be sensitizing)

Yes   Yes

Consider allergy evaluation:
1) Food allergy is common in
   infants and children <5 y
2) Inhalant allergens contribute
   to skin condition in older
   children/adults
3) Associated atopy reported
   (*eg*, asthma)
4) Allergen immunotherapy is
   contraindicated for atopic
   dermatitis

Consider dermatology evaluation:
1) Biopsy may be useful to rule out
   other diseases
2) UV light therapy
3) Systemic immunosuppressive
   therapy

Figure 10-12.

Treatment algorithm for atopic dermatitis. Treatment of a patient with atopic dermatitis should focus on four basic steps: 1) hydration, 2) moisturization, 3) anti-inflammatory therapy (*eg*, topical steroids), and 4) antipruritic therapy. Tacrolimus ointment is a new nonsteroidal therapy that has shown promising disease-modifying action for both pediatric and adult patients with atopic dermatitis.

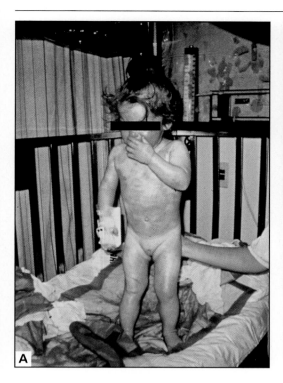 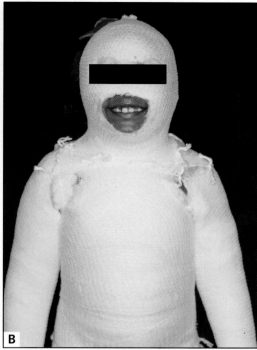

■ Figure 10-13.
Treatment for severe, refractory atopic dermatitis. Patients with erythroderma and severe atopic dermatitis require hospitalization for intravenous antibiotics and aggressive skin care, including total body wraps applied in a wet-to-dry fashion with topical steroids twice daily. **A,** Toddler with severe atopic dermatitis and erythroderma with evidence of superinfection. **B,** Older child with severe atopic dermatitis in full body wraps.

Recommended Reading

Boguniewicz M, Fiedler V, Raimer S, *et al.*: A randomized, vehicle controlled trial of tacrolimus ointment for treatment of atopic dermatitis in children. *J Allergy Clin Immunol* 1998, 102:637–643.

Burks AW, James JM, Hiegel A, *et al.*: Atopic dermatitis and food hypersensitivity reactions. *J Pediatr* 1998, 132:132–136.

Hanafin JM: Atopic dermatitis. *J Allergy Clin Immunol* 1984, 73:211–222.

Jones SM, Burks AW: Atopic dermatitis. In *Allergic Disease: Diagnosis and Treatment*, edn 2. Edited by Lieberman P, Anderson J. Totowa, NJ: Humana Press; 2000:231–260.

Leung DYM: Atopic dermatitis: new insights and opportunities for therapeutic intervention. *J Allergy Clin Immunol* 2000, 105:860–876.

Rajka G: *Essential Aspects of Atopic Dermatitis*. Berlin: Springer-Verlag; 1989:1–261.

Contact Dermatitis

Jere D. Guin

Contact dermatitis is a form of eczema that is caused by exposure to external agents. It tends to be recognizable as different from other forms of eczema by the pattern, which is something of an artifice. Contact with certain objects (*eg*, surgical and examination gloves, earrings, perfumes and colognes, jewelry, shoes, transdermal patches) is so typical in shape and location that the cause is often recognized by the patient. Unfortunately, some allergic causes are not obvious, and some patterns can be caused by more than one antigen, making it necessary to try to reproduce the eruption in a controlled environment by patch testing. This is not feasible with irritants, which have to be uncovered by the patient's history and physical findings.

Contact reactions comprise irritant and allergic contact dermatitis; protein contact dermatitis; immunologic, nonimmunologic, and uncertain forms of contact urticaria; and photoallergic and phototoxic eruptions. Allergic contact dermatitis is a delayed hypersensitivity reaction that typically appears 2 to 3 days after adequate exposure. On some skin areas that absorb well, such as the face, the eruption may appear the same day, but this is not usual. The pattern often reveals the probable source because it often coincides with the location of where a medication was applied or where an object was worn. For example, glove dermatitis tends to involve the hands to the wrist where the gloves contact the skin.

Irritant contact dermatitis is a nonallergic eczema caused by an external contactant. A typical example is soap or detergent dermatitis. This may also be superimposed on other forms of eczema such as atopic eczema. It may be indistinguishable from allergic contact dermatitis, but there are suggestive signs that help separate the two entities. Whereas allergic contact dermatitis tends to be delayed in onset, irritant reactions typically occur within a few minutes. However, delayed and cumulative irritant reactions are exceptions. Allergic reactions occur from very low concentrations, but irritant responses tend to be dose responsive. Allergic patch test reactions tend to become vesicular with weeping, oozing, and scaling that spread from the site and frequently become worse after first appearing. Irritant responses may look similar but often seem chapped. They also tend to be more localized to the original site of contact and tend to improve with time. Of course, allergic reactions only occur in sensitive persons, so they require prior exposure. Irritant responses tend to occur in everyone with adequate exposure.

Protein contact dermatitis is an allergic eczematous response to an IgE-mediated allergen probably bound to Langerhans cells. This is seen especially as hand eczema in some food handlers and health care workers. The eczema tends to appear within hours rather than days, but it is more delayed than the (immediate) urticarial reaction to scratch or prick tests.

Phototoxic reactions occur when light-absorbing agents cause a nonallergic injury from light exposure. In photoallergic reactions, a chemical is altered by light to produce the actual allergen. Photoallergens tend to also be light-absorbing chemicals, so there may also be a phototoxic element present.

The cause of allergic contact dermatitis is suspected from the pattern of the eruption and confirmed by comparing the patch test results with the opportunity for exposure from the patient's history. This determines the relevance. One can see patch test responses that are caused by preexisting allergies and are unrelated to the present episode, so it is necessary to compare the location and morphology of the eruption with the history and test results.

The patient's history can be helpful. People who tend to break out when wearing "cheap earrings" are likely to be sensitive to nickel. Health care workers who state: "I can wear vinyl gloves, but I break out when wearing rubber gloves" are probably allergic to rubber or rubber chemicals. A list of all products applied, especially when ingredients are known, also gives the physician some idea of the potential sensitizers that may be involved.

The morphology can be critically important. The "streaks" of poison ivy dermatitis are actually a hand-transfer pattern that clues the physician to look for an opportunity for exposure in the patient's history. Handprint patterns combined with obvious contact dermatitis around another site suggest the possibility of allergy to a therapeutic agent. A glovelike pattern on the hands and wrists is often seen in health care workers with glove dermatitis, and eczema of the plantar surface or on the dorsum of the feet tends to make one suspect shoe dermatitis. A common pattern seen today involves the shoulders, back, rib cage, and periaxillary region but spares the axillae and inner arm. This suggests clothing dermatitis. The pattern of eyelid dermatitis is more complex because it can be caused by many things and sometimes by more than one at any one time.

Lastly, managing the patient requires careful selection of the patch test materials likely to be associated with the eruption presented clinically and by the patient's history. Testing should be done to therapeutic agent used previously and agents one contemplates using. The patient should avoid contact with the suspected contactants and should apply therapeutic agents without the opportunity for hand transfer of contaminant agents. A good approach is to use a topical agent applied with vinyl glove, both of which the patient has been proved to be patch test negative. After the testing is completed, the patient should avoid the materials that give positive test results and should reinstitute exposure one at a time to those to which he or she is patch test negative.

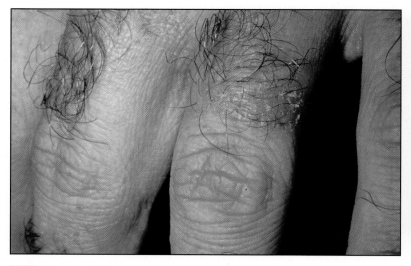

Figure 11-1.
Reaction to a ring in an individual who is allergic to gold. Allergy to gold is very common, but it seldom occurs where the jewelry is worn because, unlike nickel, gold is not easily solubilized in sweat. Abrasives that remove gold may cause black dermographism, which is often accompanied by contact dermatitis in allergic persons.

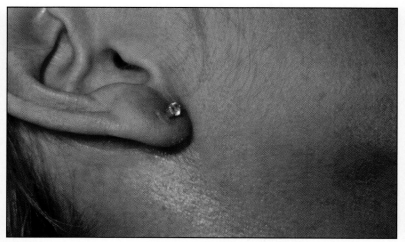

Figure 11-2.
A reaction in and around where ears are pierced strongly suggests allergy to earrings. Nickel is the most common allergen, but this person reacted to gold.

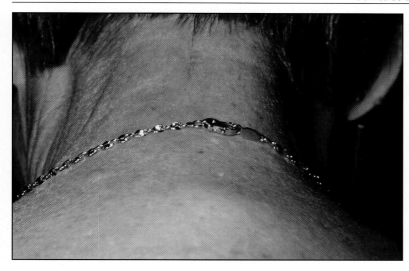

■ Figure 11-3.

Jewelry reaction in a patient allergic to gold.

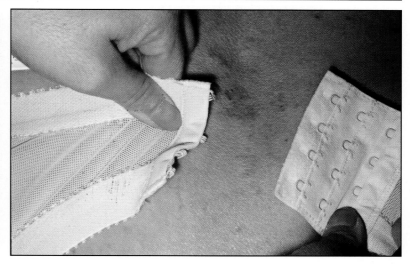

■ Figure 11-4.

Cobalt sensitivity is often similar to nickel sensitivity in its pattern. This cobalt-sensitive patient broke out directly under the hooks in her bra.

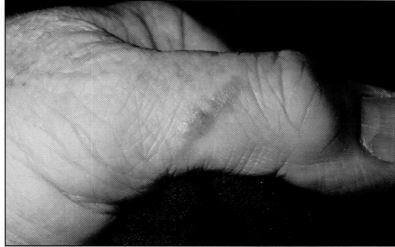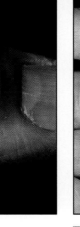

■ Figure 11-5.

A streak of vesicles or bullae strongly suggests poison ivy dermatitis in areas where the plant grows. The "streak" results from application of the antigen by a finger, which, because of a thick stratum corneum, itself does not break out.

■ Figure 11-6.

Hand eczema in a patient who packs cashews in a food processing plant. The allergen here is similar to that of poison ivy but differs in being an alk(en)yl resorcinol rather than an alk(en)yl catechol. The two plants are members of the same family and commonly cross-react. This patient was known to be extremely sensitive to poison ivy.

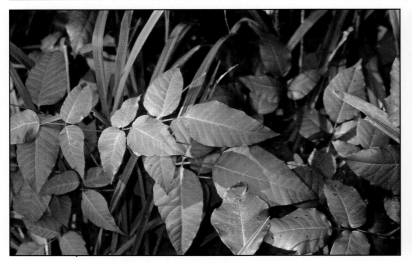

■ Figure 11-7.

Poison ivy (*Toxicodendron radicans* subsp. *radicans*). This clone was grown from plant containers from a nursery in Florida. The morphology of the leaflets is typical of poison ivy plants seen in some parts of Florida.

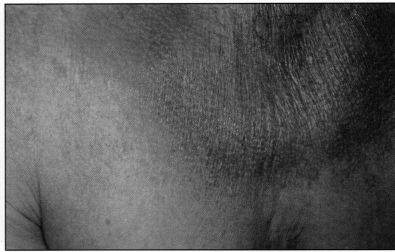

■ Figure 11-8.

Periaxillary dermatitis from sawdust in a sawmill worker. Patch testing was strongly positive to 10% sawdust in petrolatum. The location was apparently where the sawdust-contaminated clothing was wet from axillary sweat.

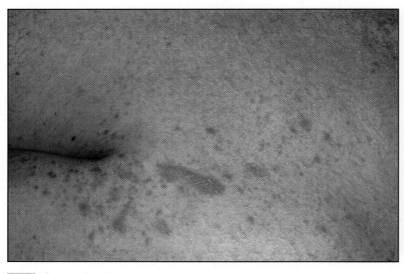

■ Figure 11-9.

Compositae dermatitis in a farmer. This man was allergic to bitter-weed *Helenium amarum*, which contains sesquiterpene lactones. Typically, these patients break out on exposed sites that sometimes closely resemble photosensitivity reactions. They are also common-ly photosensitive as well as *Compositae* allergic.

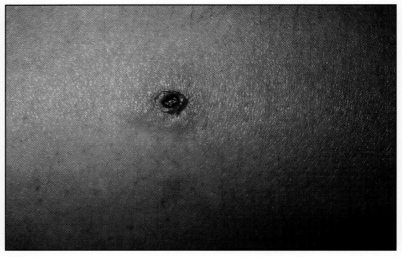

■ Figure 11-10.

Black spot poison ivy dermatitis. Here the antigen was left on in quantity, and it polymerized, leaving a black deposit. The reaction around the black stain is both irritant and allergic.

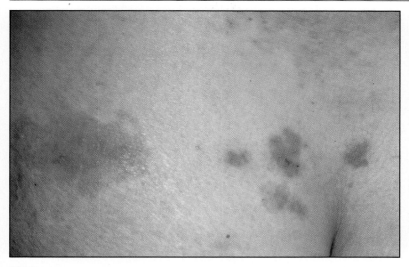

Figure 11-11.

A handprint contact reaction to English ivy (*Hedera helix*) in a retail florist. This plant is from the family *Araliaceae*, and persons allergic to it also tend to react to *Schefflera* spp., as this patient did.

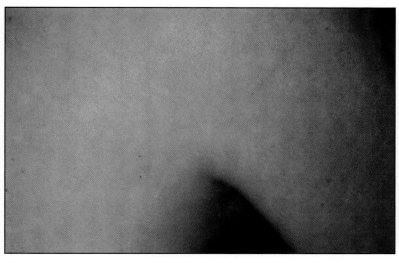

Figure 11-12.

Clothing dermatitis caused by allergy to a fabric finish. The eruption typically involves pressure areas over the trunk such as the shoulders, periaxillary areas, and rib cage, with prominent sparing of the axillae. Many such patients are allergic to formaldehyde; this patient was not.

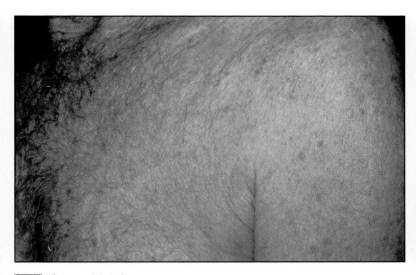

Figure 11-13.

Clothing (textile) dermatitis caused by a textile finish. Whereas the area around the axilla is more prominently affected, the axilla is spared. The patient had a ++ (erythema raised with vesiculation) reaction to the finish and a + (erythema, flat or slightly raised, without vesiculation) response to formaldehyde.

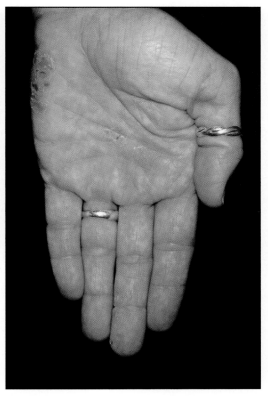

Figure 11-14.

Hand eczema in a massage therapist caused by allergy to the lotion she used in her work. Patch testing produced a +++ (bullous) reaction to formaldehyde and ++ (erythema raised with vesiculation) reactions to the lotion and two formaldehyde-releasing preservatives.

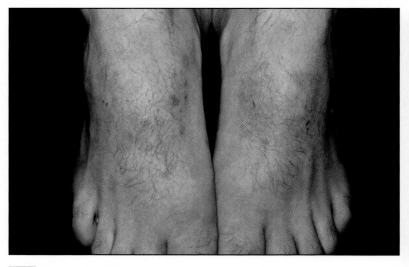

■ Figure 11-15.

Shoe dermatitis caused by allergy to dichromate and exposure to chrome-tanned leather.

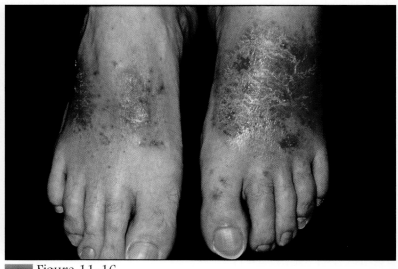

■ Figure 11-16.

Shoe dermatitis. This patient was patch test positive to several pairs of his shoes but also to several topical corticosteroids as well as preservatives in lotions that he had applied to the eruption without removing the cause.

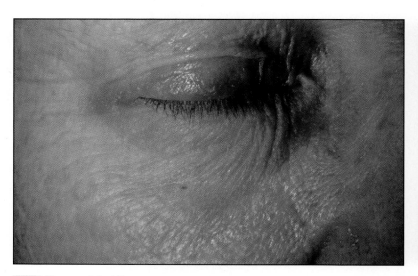

■ Figure 11-17.

Eyelid dermatitis caused by allergy to thimerosal and benzalkonium in eye drops prescribed for glaucoma.

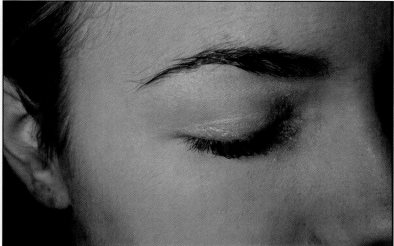

■ Figure 11-18.

Eyelid dermatitis (spontaneous flare-up) from exposure to nickel at a patch test site. The patient's results were clear when tested, strongly suggesting that nickel was the cause of her recent eyelid dermatitis. Nickel can be transferred from fingernails that have been filed by a metal nail file, a metal eyelash curler, or other sources. This patient's exposure was to nickel in her clarinet keys.

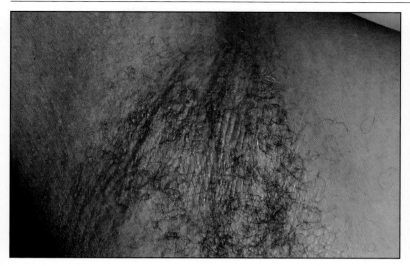

Figure 11-19.
Deodorant reaction caused by sensitivity to the fragrance in the product.

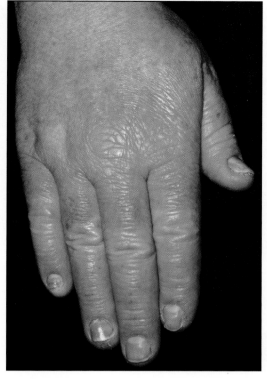

Figure 11-20.
Protein contact dermatitis to latex in a nurse, complicated by allergy to methylisothiazolinone or methylchloroisothiazolinone in a generic "baby wipe."

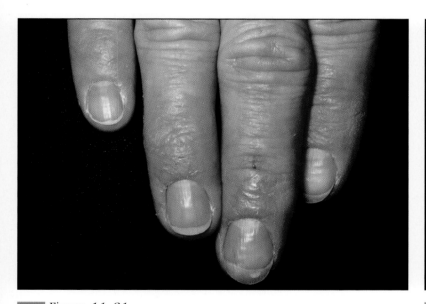

Figure 11-21.
Glutaraldehyde allergy complicating glove dermatitis. This is commonly seen in dental assistants and operating room nurses who handle cold sterilization solutions, which can penetrate their gloves.

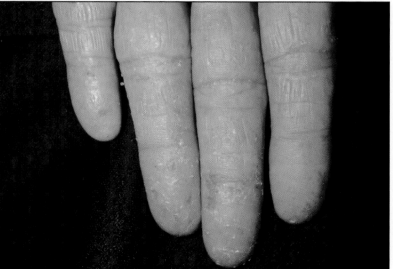

Figure 11-22.
"Dyshidrotic" eczema (pompholyx) from systemic contact dermatitis to nickel. This patient improved after avoiding nickel in her diet and taking disulfiram to chelate nickel.

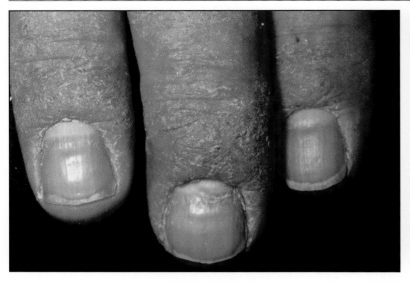

Figure 11-23.

Hand eczema in a metal worker from biocides in coolant.

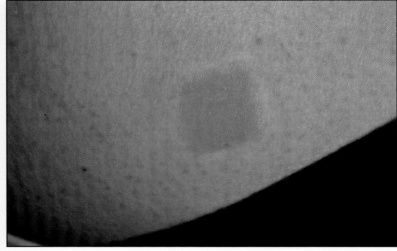

Figure 11-24.

Contact dermatitis to a clonidine patch used in the treatment of rosacea.

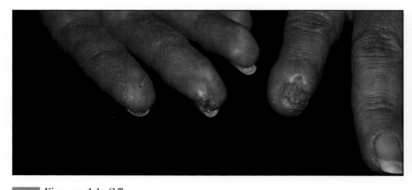

Figure 11-25.

Oncholysis and paronychia from allergy to cyanoacrylate adhesive used with artificial nail tips.

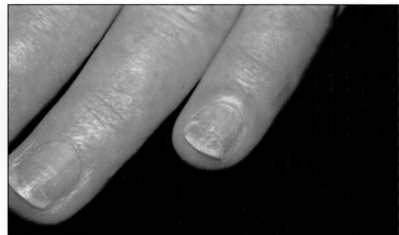

Figure 11-26.

Reaction to artificial nails. In this case, the reaction occurred to methacrylates, mainly 2-hydroxyethyl methacrylate. The eruption is identical to that from cyanoacrylates; many such patients are allergic to both.

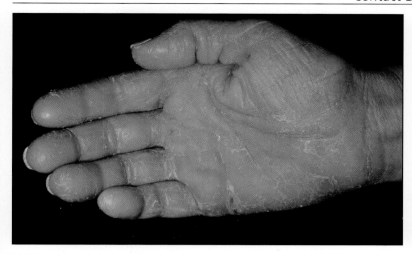

Figure 11-27.

Occupational hand eczema from an anaerobic sealant containing methacrylates.

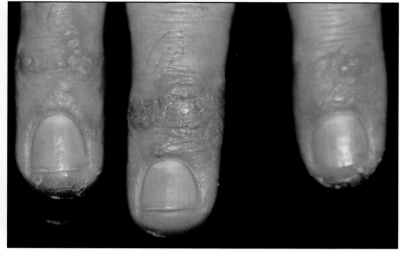

Figure 11-28.

Occupational contact dermatitis to epoxy resin used in taxidermy. This patient also became allergic to nitrile gloves used in a vain attempt to protect his hands. His mistake was in not removing the gloves within a few minutes, before the adhesive had time to penetrate the gloves.

Figure 11-29.

Occupational contact dermatitis in a hairdresser allergic to glyceryl monothioglycolate in acid permanents. This chemical also rapidly penetrates gloves, especially latex gloves. It also tends to remain in the customer's hair, serving as a chronic source of contact allergy for allergic customers and hairdressers.

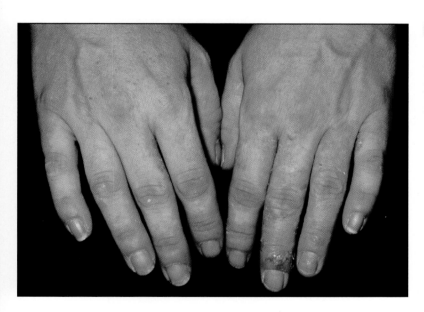

Allergic Eye Disorders

Leonard Bielory

The eye is a common target of inflammatory disorders that can either be triggered from external agents or from systemic immunologic hypersensitivity reactions. Due to the prominent vascularity of the eye embedded in a transparent medium, inflammatory reactions are immediately noticed by the patient. The eye and its surrounding tissues are also involved in a variety of other immunologically mediated disorders. When such reactions occur, they are not infrequently seen first by the primary care physician, who then is in the position to correlate ocular and systemic findings and to coordinate therapy so as to treat underlying disease (if present) rather than only local eye symptoms.

Ocular allergy is a common ocular problem that presents to the primary care health provider. It includes a spectrum of clinical disorders that involve different levels of activity that can be better appreciated through various clinical and immunopathologic methods. In seasonal allergic conjunctivitis there are minimal pathologic changes, such as an increase in mast cell activation, minimal presence of migratory inflammatory cells, and early signs of cellular mediators at the molecular level. In perennial allergic conjunctivitis, these markers are more pronounced with the increased duration of allergenic stimulation. In the more chronic forms of allergic conjunctivitis that range from vernal keratoconjunctivitis in children to atopic keratoconjunctivitis in adults, there is a persistent state of mast cell, eosinophil, and lymphocyte activation; noted switching from connective tissue to mucosal type mast cells; increased involvement of corneal pathology; and follicular development and fibrosis. The differential diagnosis of ocular inflammatory disorders includes a variety of other disorders that are presented in this chapter to assist healthcare providers in maximizing the care of their patients.

Atopic Disorders of the Eye

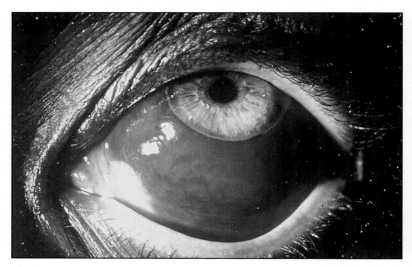

Figure 12-1.

Subconjunctival hemorrhage. Atopic disorders of the eye (or "the red eye") can be confused with a variety of conditions from the simple rupture of a blood vessel leading to a subconjunctival hemorrhage to the more serious sight-threatening conditions that are associated with intraocular inflammatory conditions. However, the most common hypersensitivity responses of the eye with highest morbidity are those associated with mast cell and IgE-mediated reactions.

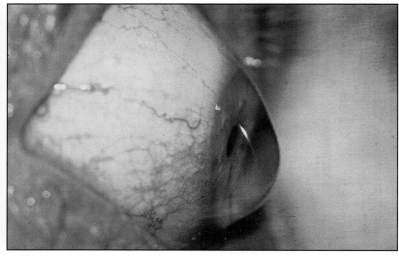

Figure 12-2.

Atopic keratoconjunctivitis. This condition is a common form of chronic allergic conjunctivitis that is underdiagnosed in the population of patients with eczema and asthma. This form of allergic conjunctivitis commonly affects older patients in the fourth and fifth decades of life. It is more commonly associated with blepharoconjunctivitis, cataract, corneal disease such as keratoconus and ocular herpes simplex as compared to the other chronic forms of ocular allergy.

Trantas' dots are a feature of the chronic forms of conjunctivitis such as vernal and atopic keratoconjunctivitis. These are small, white, elevated epithelial lesions seen at the corneal limbus. They can be associated with a grayish corneal infiltrate and superficial vascularization.

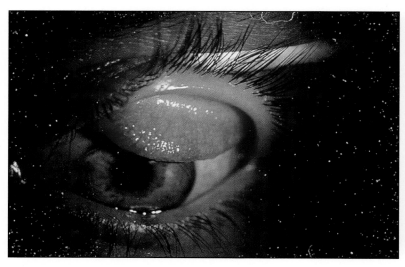

Figure 12-3.

Giant papillary conjunctivitis. This chronic form of allergic conjunctivitis has been directly linked to the continued use of contact lenses [2] and other forms of mechanical irritants on the surface of the eye. The allergic component is related to the typical allergic symptoms that become progressively worse during spring pollen season.

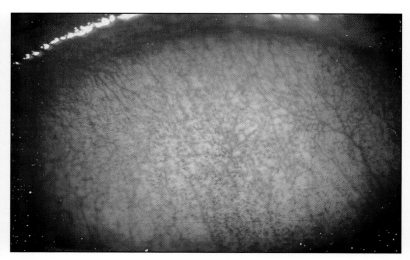

Figure 12-4.

Papillary hypertrophy. Upper tarsal papillary hypertrophy has been described in 5% to 10% of soft and 3% to 4% of hard contact lens wearers.

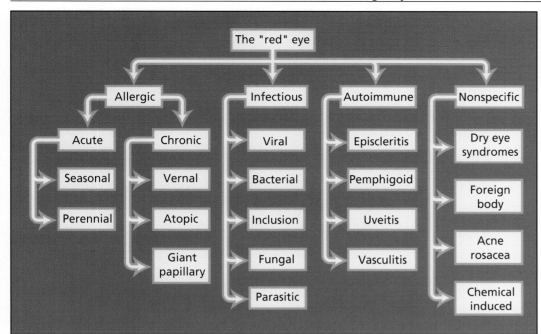

■ Figure 12-5.

Differential diagnoses of the red eye. The differential diagnoses of ocular allergic disorders includes a variety of other causes including allergic, infectious, autoimmune, and mechanical or nonspecific that activate the hypersensitivity responses of the extraocular and intraocular immunologically active tissues. These include acute and chronic allergic conditions (*eg*, giant papillary conjunctivitis, vernal conjunctivitis, atopic conjunctivitis, superior limbic conjunctivitis, follicular conjunctivitis); infectious causes (*eg*, chlamydial disease, molluscum contagiosum, Parinaud's oculoglandular syndrome); and miscellaneous disorders including keratoconjunctivitis sicca, acne rosacea, ocular pemphigoid, and blepharoconjunctivitis.

Immunologic Involvement of the Eye

Tissue	Disease
Lids	Blepharitis
	Contact dermatitis
Conjunctiva	Allergic conjunctivitis
	Atopic conjunctivitis
	Vernal conjunctivitis
	Giant papillary/conjunctivitis
	Pemphigus/pemphigoid
Sclera	Episcleritis
	Scleritis
Cornea	Corneal allograft rejection
	Amyloid deposition
Iris	Iritis
	Cyclitis
	Pars planitis
Vitreous	Vitreitis
Retina	Retinitis
Choroid	Choroiditis
Optic nerve	Optic neuritis
	Vasculitis (*eg*, temporal arteritis)
Extraocular muscles	Myasthenia gravis
	Orbital pseudotumor
	Vasculitis

■ Figure 12-6.

Ocular tissue and immunologic involvement [3]. Immunologic involvement of the eye can affect various tissues. Acute periorbital edema is a common manifestation of immediate hypersensitivity; it may occur following the systemic or local contact of an allergen to the rich mast cell supply found in this region. It usually produces symmetrical bilateral lid edema that may also be accompanied by conjunctival chemosis and urticarial cutaneous eruptions.

■ Figure 12-7.

Acute conjunctival chemosis. This condition commonly occurs in the absence of lid swelling due to the local deposition of allergen such as pollen or contact lens cleaning enzymes (*eg*, papain). Chemosis commonly is bilateral. The bulbar conjunctival surface typically gives a gelatinous appearance and is associated with hyperemia.

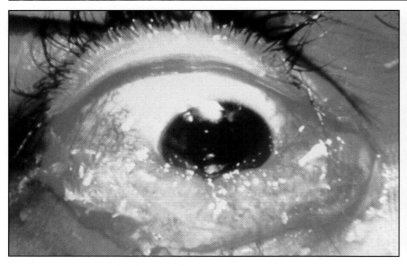

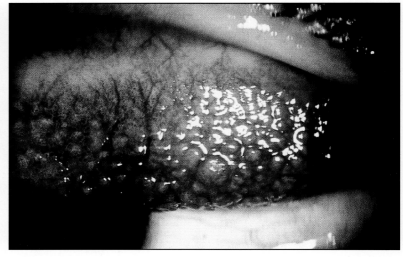

■ Figure 12-8.

Allergic conjunctivitis. Allergic conjunctivitis can occur as an acute or a severe form depending on the concentration of allergen on the conjunctiva. This patient who was allergic to cats had been petting a cat that touched his eye. There is marked edema of the lower conjunctival surface. This is often described by patients as "fried egg" in appearance, because the bulbar conjunctiva "bubbles up" like the white of an egg as it is being fried.

Allergic conjunctivitis is caused by the direct exposure of the ocular mucosal surfaces to the environmental airborne allergens such as the ubiquitous pollens. The allergen interaction at the interface of the conjunctiva triggers the estimated 50 million mast cells in this region. The prevalence of allergic conjunctivitis is more than 20% of the general population. Although the morbidity is high as measured by a variety of quality measurements, allergic conjunctivitis is seldom followed by permanent visual impairment [1]. (*From* Lieberman and Crawford [3]; with permission.)

■ Figure 12-9.

Cobblestoning. Vernal keratoconjunctivitis is a severe form of chronic allergic conjunctivitis that has a marked seasonal incidence—its frequent onset in the spring has led to the term *vernal catarrh*. It commonly starts in early childhood and "burns out" by the third decade of life. It can develop in a more limited form with just the limbus becoming involved. Vernal conjunctivitis is commonly associated with eczema on the forehead and cheeks. There is commonly an upper lip ptosis reflecting the chronic cellular infiltrate into the upper conjunctiva. Typically the upper palpebral conjunctival surface consists of giant papilla (*ie*, "cobblestoning"). Histologically, the papilla have a loose stroma in which collections of lymphocytes, plasma cells, and eosinophils are found. These papillae persist during the quiescent periods and become inflamed with edema and migration of inflammatory cells into the lesions. Mucus accumulation commonly occurs in the crevices between the papilla where the mucus-producing goblet cells are found. The changes in the lower tarsal conjunctiva are usually less striking, although similar to those found in the upper tarsal plates. Collections of mucus commonly accumulate in the lower fornix.

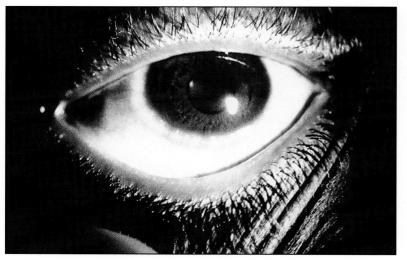

■ Figure 12-10.

Limbal vernal conjunctivitis. This condition may also occur in the absence of tarsal involvement. These lesions may also occur in the absence of tarsal involvement. They are heavily infiltrated with inflammatory cells and appear as grayish, gelatinous swellings at the limbus (at corneal scleral junction). The blood vessels are prominent and there is a paucity of mucus.

Nonatopic Disorders of the Eye

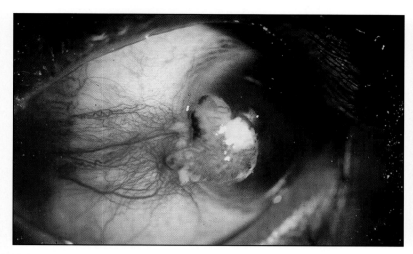

Figure 12-11.

Basal cell carcinoma. Cicatricial pemphigoid and tumors of the conjunctival surface (*eg*, basal cell carcinoma) are commonly associated with a localized erythematous reaction that may present with pruritis.

Focal scarring on the conjunctival surface may lead to symblepharon formation that are simply adhesions of one portion of the conjunctival surface to another. These are also found in cicatricial pemphigoid.

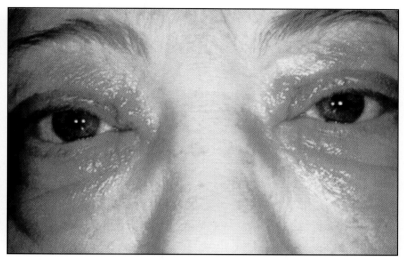

Figure 12-12.

Contact dermatoconjunctivitis. This delayed-type hypersensitivity reaction is a common problem associated with cosmetic preparations, contact lens solutions, topical drops, and ointments. The conjunctiva and eyelids are commonly involved. Patients commonly complain of irritation of the eye, discharge, and itchiness. The eyelid is erythematous and slightly swollen. In more severe reactions, the swelling and erythema are more marked and the skin may take on a weeping eczematous appearance.

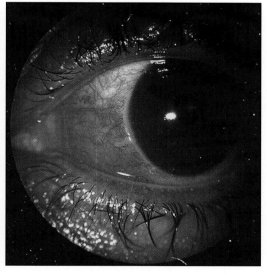

Figure 12-13.

Scleritis. There are four clinical categories of scleritis: nodular anterior, diffuse anterior, necrotizing anterior (*ie*, scleromalacia perforans), and posterior scleritis. The majority of patients with necrotizing scleritis have an underlying systemic immunologic disorder such as vasculitis, rheumatoid arthritis, systemic lupus erythematosus, Wegener's granulomatosis, polyarteritis nodosa, and Crohn's disease.

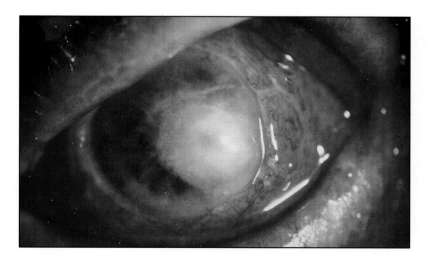

Figure 12-14.

Scleromalacia perforans is characterized by the progressive thinning of the sclera in the absence of symptoms due to the occlusion of the deep arteriolar vascular bed. It is nearly always associated with a chronic vasculitis such as rheumatoid arthritis.

Ophthalmologic Procedures in the Evaluation of Atopic Disorders of the Eye

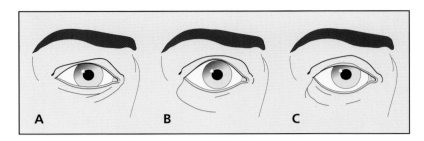

Figure 12-15.

Examination of the external eye. The position of the eyelid is important to note the position of the eyelid in respect to the pupil. **A,** The normal eye has the lid just touching the iris, but not the pupil. **B,** The exophthalmic eye has the eyelid not touching the iris at all, displaying the white of the sclera between the eyelid and the iris. **C,** In ptosis, the eyelid closely approximates the pupil, covering most of the upper iris.

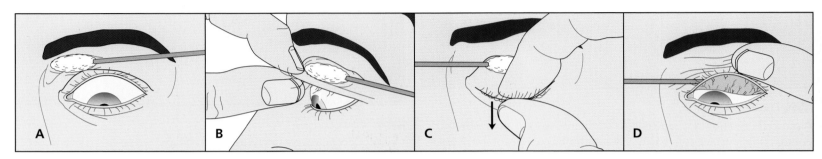

Figure 12-16.

Examination of the conjunctiva. The technique for evaluation of the bulbar and palpebral portion of the upper and lower conjunctiva requires the eversion of both lower lids and then the eversion of both upper lids. The eversion of the upper lid is performed by the placement of a cotton-tipped swab above the eyelid (*A*) and then, while the patient is asked to look downward, the upper eyelash is gently grasped (**B**). The upper eyelid is gently pulled down while placing pressure on the upper portion of the eyelid with the cotton swab (**C**), and then it is lifted over the surface of the swab **D**). This procedure is helpful when looking for papillary and follicular development in patients with more chronic forms of conjunctivitis.

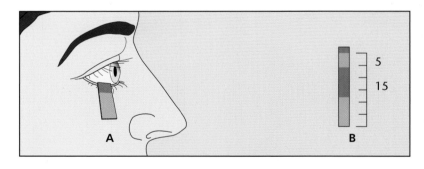

Figure 12-17.

The Schirmer technique. The Schirmer test measures the amount of tear secretion generated and absorbed by a special form of filter paper that is placed in the inferior cul-de-sac of an unanesthetized eye at the junction of the lateral one third and the medial two thirds of the eyelids (**A**). Normal tear secretion wets more than 10 mm of the filter paper at 5 minutes (**B**). The leading edge of the tear can be more easily discerned by using a filter with a dye marker incorporated into it.

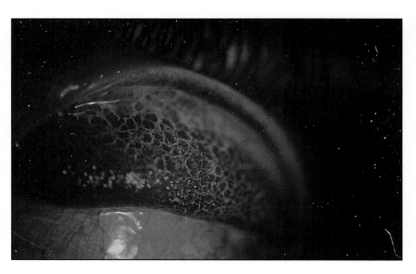

Figure 12-18.

Fluorescein examination. Fluorescein is an excellent tool to examine the subtle anatomic changes of the conjunctival surface. Instead of a smooth homogenous distribution in a normal patient, cobblestoning or follicular hypertrophy can be easily detected with the islands of "cobblestones" visible in a sea of cobalt blue fluorescein.

References

1. Donshik PC, Ehlers WH: The contact lens patient and the ocular allergies. *Int Ophthalmol Clin* 1991, 31:138–145.
2. Bielory L: Allergic and immunologic disorders: part I. Immunology of the eye. *J Allergy Clin Immunol* 2000, 106:805–816.
3. Lieberman PL, Crawford LV, eds.: Anaphylaxis and anaphylactic reactions. In *Management of the Allergic Patient: A Text for the Primary Care Physician*. New York: Appleton-Century-Crofts; 1982:300–309.

Recommended Reading

Bielory L: Allergic and immunologic disorders of the eye: part II. Ocular allergy. *J Allergy Clin Immunol* 2000, 106 (6 Pt 2):1019–1032.

Dinowitz M, Rescigno R, Bielory L: Ocular allergic diseases: differential diagnosis, examination techniques and testing. In *Diagnostic Testing of Allergic Disease*. Edited by Kemp S, Lockey D. New York: Marcel Dekker, Inc.; 2000:127–150.

Rhinitis

Stanley Fineman

hinitis is one of the most common illnesses seen in the medical office. Approximately 80 million people in the United States suffer with rhinitis. Although most patients have similar symptoms, there are some differentiating features in those with allergic trigger factors. An understanding of the differential diagnosis can help the practitioner differentiate between those patients with allergic rhinitis, which makes up 50% of the total, and those with nonallergic rhinitis [1].

Although rhinitis is not a life-threatening condition, it is associated with significant morbidity and reduction in quality of life. Allergic rhinitis has been reported to be responsible for over 800,000 missed work days and over 800,000 missed school days annually [2]. Quality of life parameters are significantly reduced in patients with allergic rhinitis [3]. The approach to therapy begins with avoidance of allergens and continues with medications. Antihistamines are usually considered first-line treatment, but other therapies, such as topical corticosteroids, are frequently needed. Allergen immunotherapy can be beneficial, particularly in allergic patients.

Mechanisms

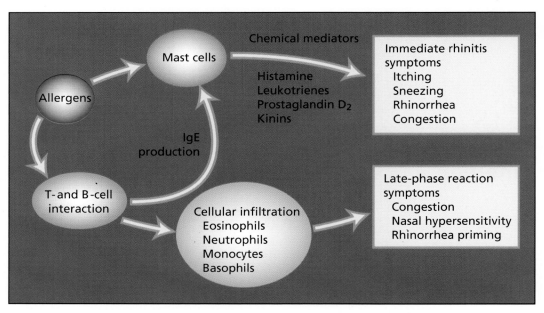

that may be preformed (*ie*, histamine and trypsin) or may be rapidly synthesized (*ie*, leukotrienes and prostaglandins). These chemical mediators produce the immediate symptoms of rhinitis including itching, sneezing, rhinorrhea, and congestion. The late-phase reaction occurs about 4 to 8 hours after allergen exposure and is associated with a cellular infiltration of the nasal mucosa with eosinophils, granulocytes, monocytes, and basophils. In a late-phase reaction, many of the same mediators are responsible for the late-phase reaction symptoms including histamine, leukotrienes, and kinins. Prostaglandin D_2 is not found in the late-phase allergic response in the nose. The late-phase symptoms include nasal congestion, rhinorrhea, increased nasal sensitivity, and priming. "Priming" refers to the phenomenon of increased sensitivity to specific allergen. There is also an increase in nonspecific sensitivity to irritants such as cigarette smoke.

Figure 13-1.

Mechanisms of allergic rhinitis. The pathophysiologic mechanism for allergic rhinitis is a biphasic reaction. The immediate phase is triggered with the interaction of allergen with IgE-sensitized mast cells in the nasal mucosa. These mast cells release chemical mediators

Etiology and Epidemiology

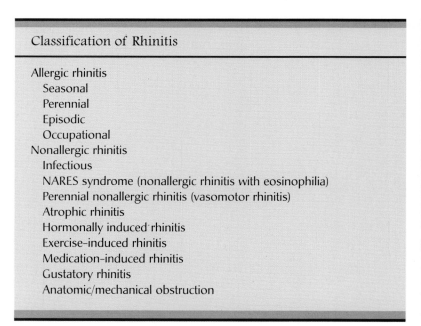

Classification of Rhinitis

Allergic rhinitis
    Seasonal
    Perennial
    Episodic
    Occupational
Nonallergic rhinitis
    Infectious
    NARES syndrome (nonallergic rhinitis with eosinophilia)
    Perennial nonallergic rhinitis (vasomotor rhinitis)
    Atrophic rhinitis
    Hormonally induced rhinitis
    Exercise-induced rhinitis
    Medication-induced rhinitis
    Gustatory rhinitis
    Anatomic/mechanical obstruction

Figure 13-2.

Causes of rhinitis. Allergic rhinitis is a common cause of rhinitis; however, in approximately 50% of patients there is no an allergenic trigger. (*Adapted from* Dykewicz *et al.* [1].)

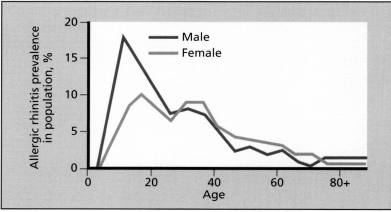

Figure 13-3.

Prevalence of allergic rhinitis. Rhinitis is one of the most common illnesses seen in outpatient practice. In the United States this condition affects approximately 40 million people. The prevalence peaks in early adolescence, then decreases with age.

Diagnosis

Differential Diagnosis Between Allergic and Nonallergic Rhinitis

Manifestation	Allergic rhinitis	Nonallergic rhinitis
Age of onset	Usually before 20	Usually after 30
Exacerbating factors	Allergen exposure	Irritant exposure, weather changes
Nature of symptoms		
Pruritus	Common	Rare
Congestion	Common	Common
Rhinorrhea	Common	Occasional
Sneezing	Frequent	Occasional
Eye symptoms	Frequent	Rare
Postnasal drainage	Not prominent	Prominent
Other related manifestations (*eg*, allergic conjunctivitis, atopic dermatitis)	Often present	Absent
Family history	Usually present	Usually absent
Physical appearance	Variable, classically described as pale, boggy, swollen—may appear normal	Variable, erythematous
Ancillary studies	Allergy skin tests always positive	Allergy skin tests negative
Nasal eosinophilia	Usually present	Present 15%–20% of the time (nonallergic rhinitis with eosinophilia)

Figure 13-4.

Differential diagnosis between allergic and nonallergic rhinitis.

Examination of the Nasal Cavity

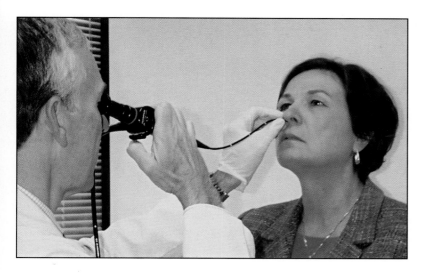

Figure 13-5.

A nasopharyngoscopic examination. Nasopharyngoscopy can be a useful tool to visualize pathology in the nasopharynx.

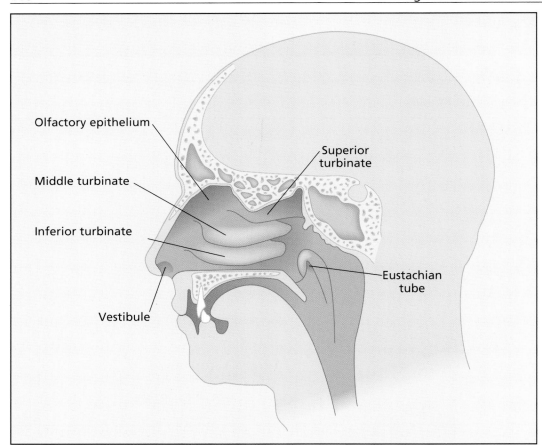

Figure 13-6.
Sagittal view of the inside of the nasal cavity.

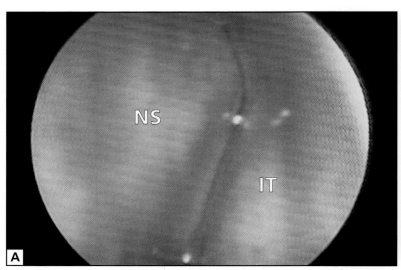

A

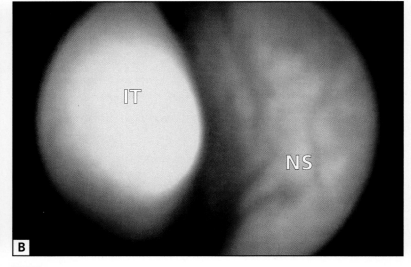

B

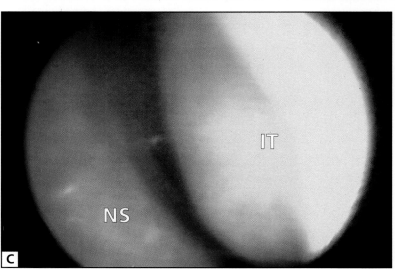

C

Figure 13-7.
Endoscopic view of the nasal mucous membrane. **A,** Swollen turbinate tightly bound to nasal septum, totally occluding all air space. **B,** Right side of another patient showing a white turbinate compared with the normal color of the septum. **C,** Left side of a third patient showing a white inferior turbinate contrasting to normal color of the septum. IT—inferior turbinate; NS—nasal septum.

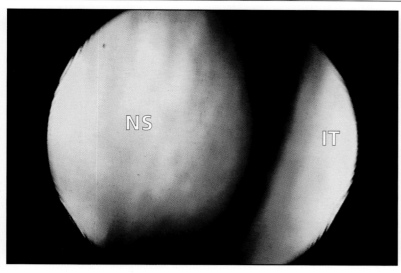

Figure 13-8.

Endoscopic view of deviated nasal septum into the left side of the patient's nose. IT—inferior turbinate; NS—nasal septum.

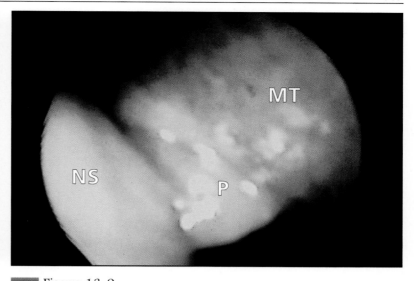

Figure 13-9.

Endoscopic view of a small nasal polyp seen between the turbinate and septum on the patient's left side. Polyps are usually gray in color and are movable, without pain perception. MT—middle turbinate; NS—nasal septum; P—polyp.

Physical Findings

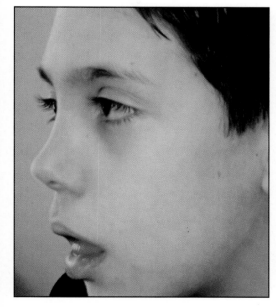

Figure 13-10.

The allergic appearance. The typical "allergic facies" has darkening of the infraorbital skin (allergic shiners) related to chronic nasal congestion. Mouth breathing and a "gaping mouth" are typically seen in children with allergic rhinitis.

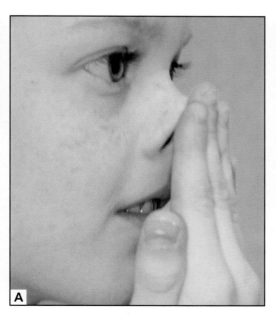 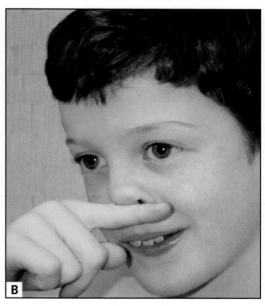

Figure 13-11.

The "allergic salute." Patients frequently have nasal pruritus, which causes repeated wiggling of the nose ("bunny nose"), or wiping and pushing of the nose ("allergic salute") as shown in *panels A and B.*

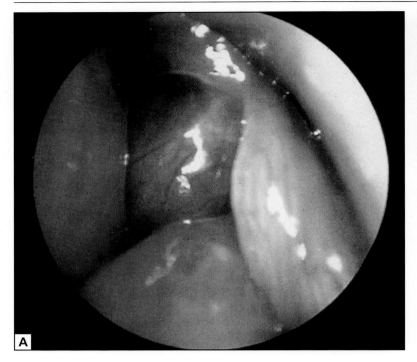

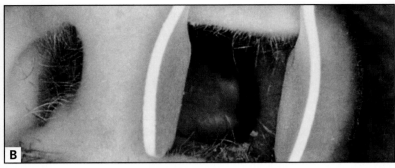

■ Figure 13-12.

Obstruction of the nose. Mechanical or anatomical obstruction can produce symptoms of rhinitis. A careful examination of the nose is crucial to rule out nasal polyps (**A**) and nasal septal deviation (**B**).

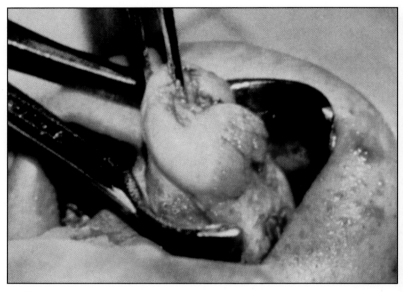

■ Figure 13-13.

Surgical removal of nasal polyp in an aspirin-sensitive asthmatic patient. (*From* Lieberman and Crawford [2]; with permission.)

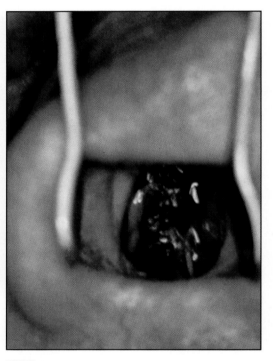

■ Figure 13-14.

Nasal tumor. Pigmentation of any polypoid structure or a polyp that bleeds should arouse suspicion of a nasal carcinoma or a malignant granuloma. These are usually unilateral, as opposed to polyps, which are usually bilateral. Both are associated with sinusitis. In nasal polyps, the sinusitis usually involves several sinuses; in nasal tumors, there is usually unilateral involvement of the maxillary or ethmoid sinus on the same side as the tumor. Although bleeding is a hallmark of nasal tumors, polyps are not usually associated with bleeding. (*From* Bull [3]; with permission.)

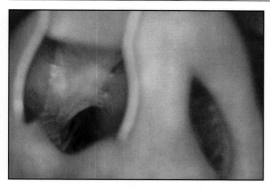

Figure 13-15.

Synechia formed between the turbinates and the septum following nasal trauma. Such synechia can occur as complications of septoplasties. They are usually visible on anterior nasal examination. (*From* Bull [3]; with permission.)

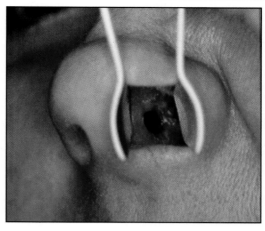

Figure 13-16.

Nasal septal perforation. Septal perforations produce alterations in nasal air flow, and thus patients often perceive nasal obstruction [4]. Many perforations fail to produce any symptoms whatsoever. However, patients often notice nasal bleeding occurring at the edges of the perforation. Perforations can be caused by the use of nasal sprays or cocaine. (*From* Bull [3]; with permission.)

Therapy

Environmental Control Measures Used to Reduce Allergen Exposure

House dust mite
Enclose mattress, box springs, pillows in allergen-proof casings
Wash bed linen on "hot cycle," 130° F
Reduce indoor humidity to <50%
Consider use of benzyl benzoate (acaricide) or tannic acid (to denature antigen)
Pollens
Avoid fresh-cut grass, do not mow lawn
Utilize air conditioning
Pets
Should be removed from home whenever possible
Cat allergen can be reduced by frequent bathing of cat (every 2 weeks)
Use of HEPA filter may be helpful

Figure 13-17.

Environmental control measures. Avoidance of the triggering allergens is an optimal way of controlling the symptoms of allergic rhinitis. HEPA—high-efficiency air filtration filter.

Comparison of Various Pharmacologic Approaches for the Treatment of Allergic Rhinitis Symptoms

	Sneezing	Itching	Congestion	Rhinorrhea	Eye Symptoms
Oral antihistamines	+++	+++	+ to –	++	++
Intranasal antihistamines	++	++	++	++	+ to –
Oral decongestants	–	–	++	–	–
Intranasal decongestants	–	–	+++	+ to –	–
Intranasal cromolyn	+	+	+	+	–
Intranasal corticosteroids	+++	++	+++	+++	+ to –
Intranasal anticholinergics	–	–	–	++	–

Figure 13-18.

Comparison of pharmacologic treatments of allergic rhinitis symptoms.

Characteristics of Representative First-Generation H_1 Antagonists Based on Chemical Classification

Chemical class	Examples	Comments
Ethanolamines	Diphenhydramine Clemastine Carbinoxamine	Significant antimuscarinic effects. Can be potent sedatives, but sedative potential varies, with clemastine producing the least amount. Can have some anti–motion-sickness activity
Alkylamines	Chlorpheniramine Brompheniramine Dexchlorpheniramine Tripolidine	Relatively moderate incidence of drowsiness. Moderate anticholinergic effect. No anti-emetic or anti–motion-sickness activity. Few gastrointestinal side effects
Ethylenediamines	Tripelennamine Pyrilamine Antazoline	Mild to moderate sedation. Slight anticholinergic effect. Some local anesthetic effect. As a group said to have frequent gastrointestinal side effects
Piperazines	Hydroxyzine Meclizine Cyclizine	Meclizine and cyclizine relatively low sedative activity with main use being for vertigo, anti-motion sickness, and antiemetic activity. Hydroxyzine has significant anticholinergic activity
Piperadines	Cyproheptadine Azatadine Phenindamine	Mild to moderate sedation. Little anticholinergic activity, antiemetic activity, and anti–motion sickness activity. Cyproheptadine has a potent antiserotonin effect
Phenothiazines	Methdilazine Promethazine Trimeprazine	Usually highly sedating. Main clinical use is as antiemetic

Figure 13-19.

Characteristics of representative first-generation H_1 antagonists based on chemical classification. The first-generation antihistamines are generally associated with more side effects, particularly sedation, anticholinergic and antiemetic activity, and antimuscarinic actions. These may be desirable in certain clinical situations, *eg*, motion sickness.

Characteristics of Second-Generation H₂ Antagonists

Name of drug	Formulations	Sedative potential	Associated with ventricular arrhythmias	Major route of metabolism secretion	Available with decongestant	Useful as rapid onset prn drugs
Fexophenodine (Allegra, Aventis Pharmaceuticals, Bridgewater Area, NJ)	30, 60, 180 mg	None	No	Mainly unmetabolized, 80% found in feces	Yes	Yes
Azelastine (Astelin, Wallace Laboratories, Cranbury, NJ)	Nasal spray: 137 μg/spray, 2 sprays	Reduced but possible	No	Liver	No	Yes
Cetirizine (Zyrtec, Pfizer, Parsippany, NJ)	5 or 10 mg; also available as a liquid (10 mg/10 mL)	Reduced but present	No	Kidney	No	Yes
Loratidine (Claritin, Schering-Plough, Kenilworth, NJ)	10 mg; or liquid, 10 mg/10mL; or dissolving RediTab	None, at recommended dose	No	Liver	Yes (pseudoephedrine); bid dosing	Yes

Figure 13-20.

Characteristics of second-generation H₂ antagonists. The second-generation antihistamines have been recommended as first-line therapy for patients with rhinitis [1]. The benefits of these preparations include relatively long duration of action and little or no sedation. bid—twice a day; prn—*pro re nata* (as circumstances require); qd—daily.

Topical Corticosteroid Preparations Used to Treat Rhinitis

Drug	Trade name	Type of delivery	Dose
Beclomethasone	Beconase (GlaxoSmithKline, Research Triangle Park, NC)	Fluorocarbon aerosol	1 spray = 42 μg 1–2 sprays each nostril bid to tid
	Beconase AQ (GlaxoSmithKline)	Liquid spray	
	Vancenase (Schering-Plough, Kenilworth, NJ)	Fluorocarbon aerosol	
	Vancenase AQ (Schering-Plough)	Liquid spray	
Triamcinolone	Nasacort (Aventis Pharmaceuticals, Bridgewater Area, NJ)	Fluorocarbon aerosol	1 spray = 55 μg 1–2 sprays each nostril qd to bid
	Nasacort AQ	Liquid spray	
Flunisolide	Nasalide (Roche Bioscience, Palo Alto, CA)	Liquid spray	1 spray = 25 μg 1 to 2 sprays each nostril bid
Mometasone	Nasonex (Schering-Plough)	Liquid spray	1 spray = 50 mg 2 sprays each nostril qd
Budesonide	Rhinocort (AstraZeneca, Wilmington, DE)	Fluorocarbon aerosol	1 spray = 32 μg 4 sprays each nostril qd
	Rhinocort Aqua (AstraZeneca)	Liquid spray	
Fluticasone	Flonase (GlaxoSmithKline)	Liquid spray	1 spray = 50 μg 1–2 sprays each nostril qd

Figure 13-21.

Topical corticosteroid preparations available to treat rhinitis.

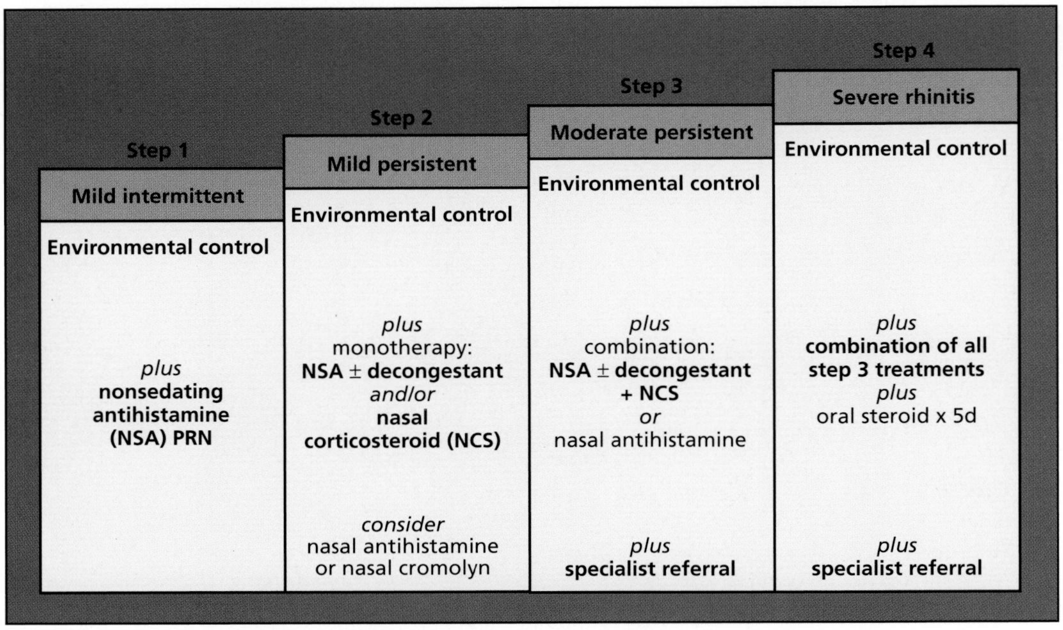

Figure 13-22.

Sample stepwise treatment for patients with rhinitis.

Criteria for Allergen Immunotherapy

Severity of rhinitis symptoms
Duration of rhinitis symptoms
Progression of rhinitis
Failure to respond to medical treatment
Presence of comorbid conditions, *eg*, sinusitis, asthma [1]

Figure 13-23.

Consideration for allergen immunotherapy in patients with allergic rhinitis. Allergen immunotherapy can be an efficacious therapy for allergic rhinitis. It has been shown to be effective in more than 20 placebo-controlled studies. The decision to use allergen immunotherapy should be based on the criteria listed in this table. The patients should demonstrate significant positive reactions to allergen, which correlate clinically with their symptoms.

Factors Involved in Considering Consultation with an Allergist-immunologist

Clarification of allergic trigger factors
Medical management is unsatisfactory at controlling symptoms
When allergen immunotherapy is a consideration
The patient's quality of life is detrimentally effected
Complications or a comorbid condition are also present
The duration of rhinitis symptoms is greater than 3 months
When patients require oral corticosteroids to control symptoms [1]

Figure 13-24.

Factors involved in considering consultation with an allergist-immunologist.

References

1. Economides A, Kaliner MA: Vasomotor rhinitis: making the diagnosis and determining therapy. *J Respir Dis* 1999, 20:463–464.

2. Malone DC, Lawson KA, Smith DH, *et al.*: A cost of illness study of allergic rhinitis in the United States. *J Allergy Clin Immunol* 1997, 99:22–27.

3. Meltzer EO, Nathan RA, Selner JC, Storms W: Quality of life and rhinitis symptoms: results of a nationwide survey with the SF-36 and RQLQ questionnaires. *J Allergy Clin Immunol* 1997, 99:S815–S819.

Recommended Reading

Baraniuk JN: Pathogenesis of allergic rhinitis. *J Allergy Clin Immunol* 1997, 99:S763–S772.

Busse WW: Role of antihistamines in allergic disease. *Ann Allergy* 1994, 72:371–375.

Dykewicz MS, Fineman SM, *et al.*: Joint task force practice parameters on diagnosis and management of rhinitis. *Ann Allergy Asthma Immunol* 1998, 81:463–518.

International Rhinitis Management Working Group: International consensus report on the diagnosis and management of rhinitis. *Allergy* 1994, 19:S5–34.

Spector SL: Overview of comorbid associations of allergic rhinitis. *J Allergy Clin Immunol* 1997, 99:S773–S780.

Sinusitis

Rande H. Lazar and Ron B. Mitchell

Sinusitis affects both adults and children and has become the most common chronic disease in the United States. New technologies such as CT scanning and rigid endoscopy have added to current understanding of the pathophysiology of this condition, and they have allowed better visualization of the paranasal sinuses and better access to them during surgery. The principal focus of interest in sinusitis is the so-called "ostiomeatal complex" — that part of the middle meatus where the ostia or openings of the frontal, anterior ethmoid, and maxillary sinuses become confluent and drain into the lateral nasal wall. If drainage of the sinuses is blocked by inflammation subsequent to infection or by some disease process, either medical or surgical therapy may be used to improve drainage.

Unimpaired drainage of the paranasal sinuses is essential for the resolution of sinusitis. The symptoms of sinusitis mimic those of an upper respiratory infection coupled with an inflammatory nasal event. These symptoms usually include headache, nasal congestion, facial pain, and postnasal discharge. Other symptoms include olfactory disturbance, halitosis and, in children, cough and irritability. It is important to differentiate between acute and chronic sinusitis. Acute sinusitis lasts for up to 12 weeks. After 12 weeks, the condition is classified as either subacute or chronic. Acute exacerbations of chronic sinusitis may also occur. Up to 50% of all acute sinus infections resolve spontaneously. In addition, acute sinusitis has a confirmed bacterial cause. Conversely, there is controversy surrounding the role of bacteria in chronic sinusitis. Most complications of sinusitis occur in association with acute sinusitis or in association with acute exacerbation of chronic sinusitis. These complications may range in severity from minor orbital cellulitis to potentially fatal intracranial abscess.

Many factors may contribute to the development of sinusitis. For example, anatomic problems can lead to poor drainage through the ostiomeatal complex. These problems may include septal deviation; concha bullosa characterized by an enlarged, air-filled middle turbinate; enlarged ethmoid bulla; and anatomic variants of the uncinate process. The cilia of cells in the mucosa of the paranasal sinuses propel mucus toward the ostiomeatal complex. It is this rhythmic ciliary beat, not the force of gravity, that produces fluid drainage of the sinuses. Ciliary function may be impaired by disease processes such as cystic fibrosis, primary ciliary dysfunction, or allergic disease. Immune deficiency may enhance the potential for sinus infection, even though drainage pathways and ciliary function may be normal. Primary immune deficiency is increasingly recognized as a cause of recurrent sinusitis and can include conditions such as IgG subclass deficiency, common variable immune deficiency, and C4 deficiency. Secondary immune deficiency can result from HIV infection or from immune suppression by either cytotoxic medication or high-dose steroids.

Imaging studies of the paranasal sinuses are used to supplement clinical diagnosis of sinusitis. Plain radiography of the sinuses is the most frequently used imaging modality. However, it does lack specificity and sensitivity versus coronal CT scans, particularly when the ethmoid sinuses are under study. Therefore, CT scans provide optimal radiologic visualization of the paranasal sinuses. Soft tissues in the region surrounding the ostiomeatal complex are readily identified in contrast to air in the nasal cavity, which allows changes in the mucosa of ostiomeatal complex to be monitored to an extent that is not possible with endoscopy. The ostiomeatal complex is displayed optimally in the coronal plane, along with relationship of the sinuses to the contents of the orbit and to the intracranial compartment. These images should be obtained for all patients who are candidates for surgery because they are useful in planning the surgical approach. To date, the use

of MRI has been restricted to the diagnosis of intracranial and intraorbital complications of sinusitis.

The management of sinusitis is medical and most commonly involves the use of antibiotics and inhaled nasal steroids. Antihistamines and nasal saline are often added to reduce allergic symptoms and to facilitate drainage. Surgery is reserved for patients in whom maximal medical therapy fails or who have complications of sinusitis. During the past 15 years there has been a fundamental change in emphasis in the surgical management of sinusitis. Functional endoscopic sinus surgery (FESS) has been used to facilitate drainage through the lateral nasal wall using minimally invasive techniques and thus reducing the need for radical procedures such as the Caldwell-Luc antrostomy.

The management of sinusitis, and particularly the increased use of endoscopic techniques and CT scanning, lends itself well to pictorial representation. This chapter illustrates the pathophysiology, causes, complications, and treatment of sinusitis.

Anatomy

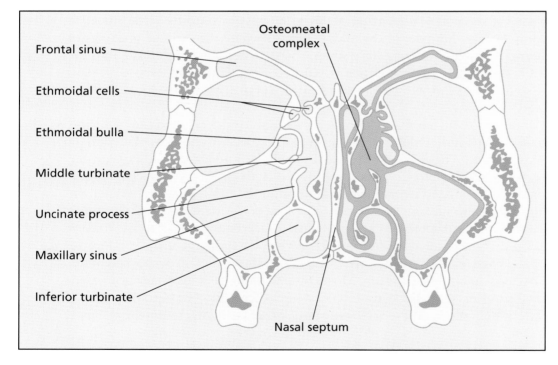

Figure 14-1.

The nose and sinuses. This coronal plane corresponds to a coronal CT scan (see Fig. 14-5).

Frontal sinus

Ethmoidal cells

Ethmoidal bulla

Middle turbinate

Uncinate process

Maxillary sinus

Inferior turbinate

Osteomeatal complex

Nasal septum

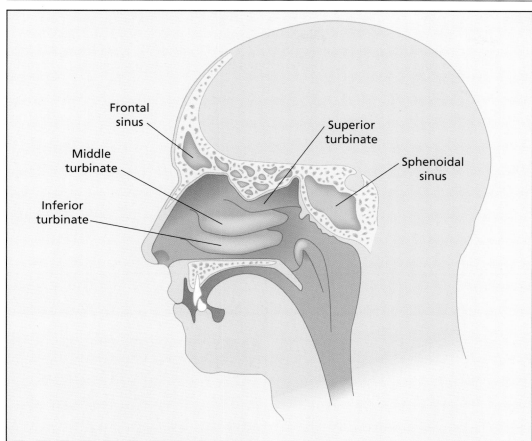

Figure 14-2.
The lateral nasal wall. This illustration shows the position of the inferior, middle, and superior turbinates. The relationship of the frontal and sphenoid sinuses is demonstrated.

Imaging

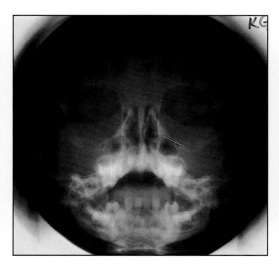

Figure 14-3.
Normal sinus radiograph (Waters' view). The extent of disease in the sinuses and particularly the anatomy of the ethmoid complex is poorly visualized.

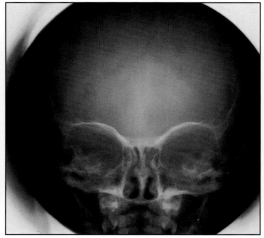

Figure 14-4.
Normal sinus radiograph (occipitofrontal view). This view is again poor at visualizing the ethmoid complex. The frontal sinus is normally well visualized but in this pediatric film the frontal sinuses are absent.

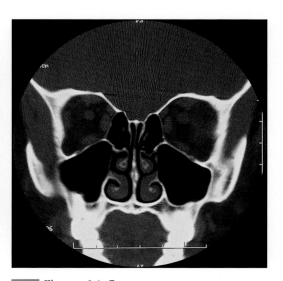

Figure 14-5.
Normal coronal CT scan of sinuses. CT is the modality of choice for the evaluation of sinusitis. It has replaced plain radiography for the evaluation of sinusitis because it gives better anatomic precision to the endoscopic sinus surgeon. CT also provides detailed information about mucosal changes and anatomical variants that cannot be visualized endoscopically.

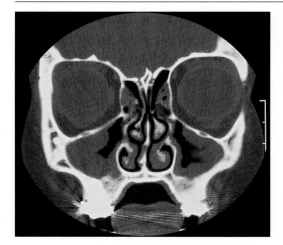

Figure 14-6.

Coronal CT scan of sinuses. The nasal septum, inferior and middle turbinates, maxillary and anterior ethmoid cells, and ostiomeatal complex are evident. Mucosal disease can be seen in both maxillary sinuses and anterior ethmoids. The osteomeatal complex is partially obstructed bilaterally.

Chronic Sinusitis

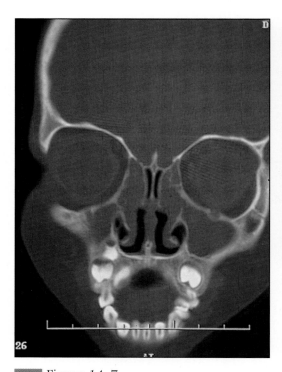

Figure 14-7.

Coronal CT scan of sinuses demonstrating pansinusitis. This scan is from a 6-year-old child with nasal obstruction and worsening pulmonary status. The child has cystic fibrosis. The scan shows complete obstruction of both osteomeatal complexes with extensive mucosal disease of bilateral maxillary and anterior ethmoidal sinuses. Note hypoplasia of the right maxillary sinus. Nasal polyposis in adults is more common and is associated with allergic disease and non-steroidal anti-inflammatory drug sensitivity. Children that present with nasal polyposis should be screened for cystic fibrosis.

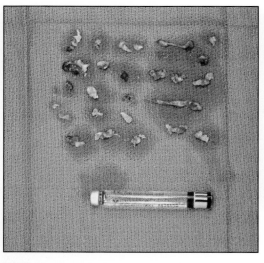

Figure 14-8.

Nasal polyposis. Nasal polyps are edematous lesions that typically arise from the ethmoidal sinuses and cause nasal obstruction to a variable degree. In some patients nasal polyposis can be extensive, causing widening of the ethmoid labyrinth, bone thinning, and mucocele formation. Nasal polyps usually have a respiratory epithelium with ciliated columnar cells and goblet cells.

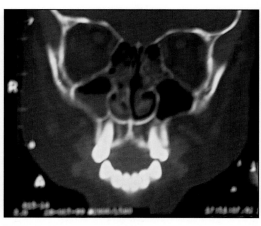

Figure 14-9.

Blockage of the osteomeatal complex. Bilateral blockage of the osteomeatal complex is apparent in this coronal CT scan. There is also fluid in the right maxillary sinus. The bony walls of the sinuses are well demonstrated. An excellent demonstration of soft tissue densities within the sinuses and nasal cavity is seen.

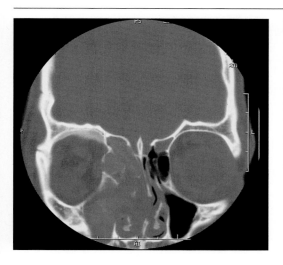

■ Figure 14-10.

Coronal CT scan showing a mass involving the nasal cavity and paranasal sinuses. The symptoms of a mass involving the nasal cavity and paranasal sinuses may be very similar to those of sinusitis secondary to inflammatory disease. If the lesion is unilateral it requires further investigation and biopsy. Although a CT scan gives an excellent anatomical display, it fails to predict the histologic nature of the process. A mass in the nasal cavity extending to the antrum is highly suggestive of an inverted papilloma. Some areas of calcification are often seen. More dense calcification is consistent with a chondroma or chondrosarcoma. The distinction between benign and malignant tumors is based on the extent of bony destruction. Malignant tumors characteristically produce aggressive bony destruction.

Endoscopic Sinus Surgery

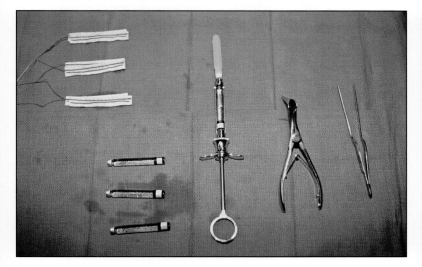

■ Figure 14-11.

Nasal preparation. The surgical intervention follows preoperative preparation of the nose to obtain optimal vasoconstriction and thus optimize visualization during surgery. Additionally it minimizes intra-operative bleeding. The surgical site is injected with 1% lidocaine with 1:100,000 epinephrine. This is followed by packing the nose with neurosurgical cottonoids soaked in 4% cocaine solution.

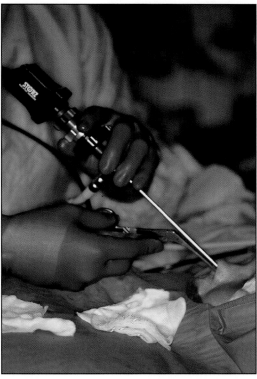

■ Figure 14-12.

Endoscopic examination of the nose. The most common instruments used are 4.0-mm-diameter scopes that are 0°, 30°, or 70°. The procedure can be performed in the office or in the operating room, under local or general anesthesia. The nasopharynx, middle meatus, and sphenoethmoidal recess are well visualized using this technique.

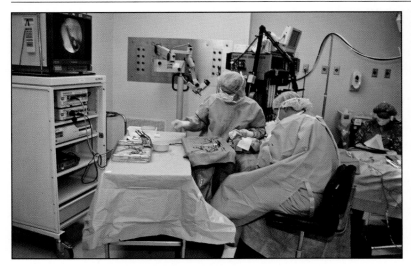

■ Figure 14-13.
Endoscopic sinus surgery. The examination is performed on a patient in the recumbent position. The monitor is used to aid visualization. The surgical approach is minimally invasive and aims to re-establish normal sinus physiology. Diseased tissue is removed while normal tissue is minimally traumatized.

Complications of Sinusitis

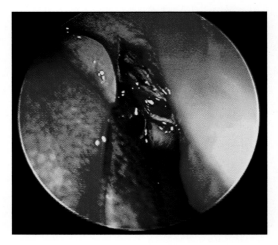

■ Figure 14-14.
Intraoperative diagnostic nasal endoscopy using a 4.0-mm-diameter telescope. The examination is performed after applying topical anesthesia in conjunction with a mild vasoconstrictor. The septum, the middle turbinate, and the lateral nasal wall are shown. The uncinate process is visualized in the lateral nasal wall.

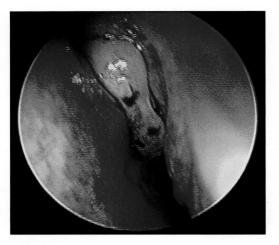

■ Figure 14-15.
Intraoperative diagnostic nasal endoscopy using a 4.0-mm-diameter telescope. The uncinate process has been partially removed to display the ethmoidal bulla. This represents the surgical approach to the anterior ethmoidal, maxillary, and frontal sinuses.

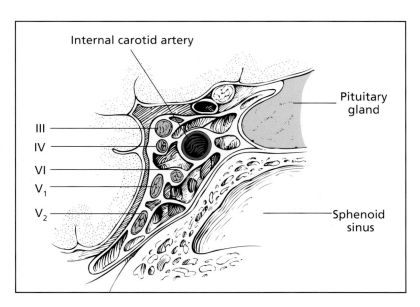

■ Figure 14-16.
The cavernous sinus in cross-section. Infection and occlusion of this sinus may follow sphenoid sinusitis or septic thrombophlebitis of the orbital veins. The neurovascular structures within the cavernous sinus may be involved in the inflammatory process, resulting in a number of clinical signs and symptoms. Spread of the inflammation into the internal carotid artery may lead to narrowing or occlusion of the artery, an event that may result in cavernous sinus thrombophlebitis, resulting in varying degrees of ocular motility deficits. Symptoms of involvement of cranial nerves V_1 and V_2 (*ie*, facial numbness or pain) are possible but are not frequently observed.

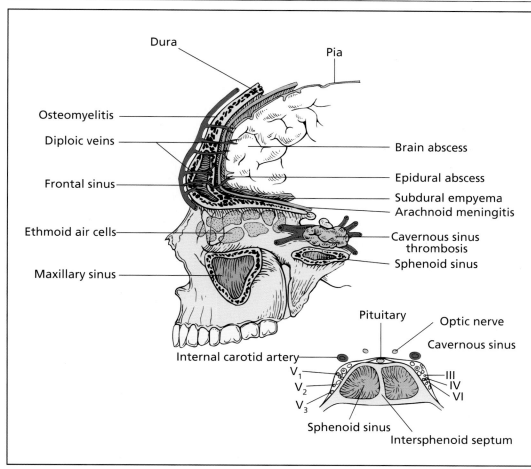

■ Figure 14-17.

Intracranial complications of sinusitis. The sagittal section shows the major routes for intracranial extension of infection, either directly or via the vascular supply. Note the proximity of the diploic veins to the frontal sinus and of the cavernous sinuses to the sphenoid sinus. The coronal section (*inset*) demonstrates the structures adjoining the sphenoid sinus. (*Adapted from* Vortel and Chow [1].)

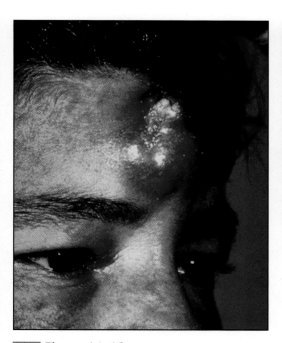

■ Figure 14-18.

Mucopyocele of the frontal sinus with perforation. Preoperative view.

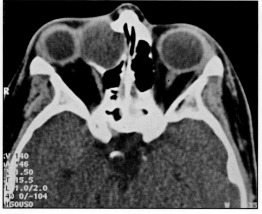

■ Figure 14-19.

Orbital complications of sinusitis. Most acute sinus infections are successfully treated with antibiotics. The close proximity of the sinuses and orbits, however, can lead to infection spreading to the orbit and thus lead to orbital cellulitis with pain, edema, and proptosis. This complication most commonly affects children. It can progress from mild orbital cellulitis to a subperiosteal abscess (seen in this axial CT scan) and to an orbital abscess. Cavernous sinus thrombosis is a serious and potentially fatal complication.

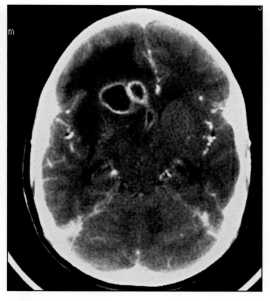

■Figure 14-20.

Intracranial complications of sinusitis. This axial CT scan demonstrates a frontal lobe abscess. Intracranial complications of sinusitis are less common than orbital complications, but the two can coexist. A subdural or intracerebral abscess may remain asymptomatic until it is of a significant size. The patient may present with increasing headaches, fever, seizures, and focal neurologic signs. Surgical intervention should be directed at treating both the complication and the underlying sinusitis.

Upper Respiratory and Head and Neck Infections

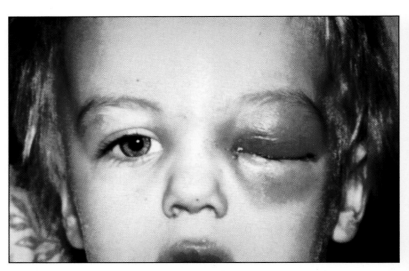

■ Figure 14-21.

Streptococcal bacterial cellulitis secondary to orbital trauma. A 2-year-old boy had nasal discharge, nasal congestion, and low-grade fever for about 10 days. The morning before presentation, he fell and sustained a 7-mm laceration just lateral to his left eye. Despite careful cleansing of the area, he developed dramatic periorbital swelling and erythema over the next 24 to 36 hours. His 9-year-old brother had had a "strep" throat the preceding week. Group A streptococcus was recovered from the culture of the wound. Bacterial cellulitis secondary to trauma is usually caused by *Staphylococcus aureus* or *Streptococcus pyogenes* (group A streptococcus). Parenteral therapy was initiated with good response.

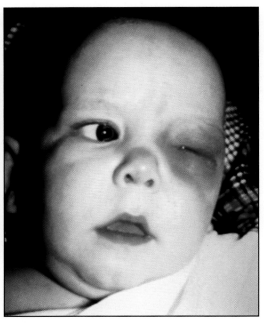

■ Figure 14-22.

Haemophilus influenzae type b bacteremic cellulitis. A 9-month-old boy had an upper respiratory tract infection for 3 days. On the morning of admission, he had a temperature of 40°C (104°F) and a small erythematous area under the medial portion of the lower lid. Within 6 hours, the erythema and swelling progressed to involve both upper and lower lids. The area was nontender. Eversion of the lids showed the globe to be normally placed with intact extraocular movements. The blood culture was positive for *H. influenzae* type b. Parenteral antibiotics were initiated and resolution was prompt. Within 24 hours, the erythema had receded partially, and the eye was approximately 25% open. In 48 hours, the eye was nearly completely open, and the cutaneous findings had resolved.

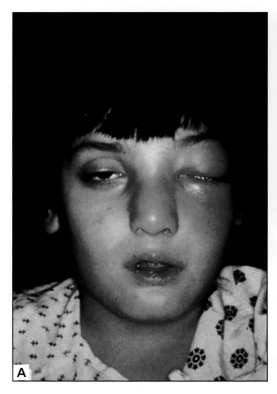

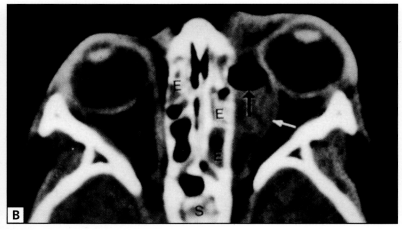

■ Figure 14-23.

Intra- and extraorbital suppurative complications of sinusitis. **A**, A 10-year-old boy had long-standing allergic symptoms, including chronic nasal discharge and congestion. For 3 days, he had left-sided facial pain and headache, with progressive swelling of his left eye. On physical examination, he was febrile to 38.4°C (101.2° F). When his lids were mechanically everted, his left globe was frozen and there was intense chemosis of the conjunctiva. **B**, An axial CT scan shows anterior and lateral displacement of his left eye. There is an air-fluid level (*black arrow*) in the area between the lateral border of the left ethmoid and the medial rectus of his left eye (*white arrow*). E—ethmoid air cells; S—sphenoid sinus.

References

1. Vortell JJ, Chow AW: Infections of the sinuses and parameningeal structures. In *Infectious Diseases*. Edited by Gorbach SL, Bartlett JG, Blacklow NR. Philadelphia: WB Saunders; 1992:432.

2. Wald ER: Rhinitis and acute and chronic sinusitis. In *Pediatric Otolaryngology*, edn 2. Edited by Bluestone CB, Stool SE. Philadelphia: WB Saunders; 1990:736.

Recommended Reading

Report of the Rhinosinusitis Task Force Committee Meeting: Alexandria, Virginia, August 17, 1996. *Otolaryngol Head Neck Surg* 1997, 117 (3 Pt 2):S1–S8.

15 Allergic Bronchopulmonary Aspergillosis

Gailen D. Marshall, Jr.

Allergic bronchopulmonary aspergillosis (ABPA) is a noninvasive, IgE-mediated hypersensitivity disease that occurs in 1% to 2% of all asthmatic patients and 10% of patients with cystic fibrosis. The typical clinical presentation includes varying combinations of pulmonary infiltrates, bronchospasm, eosinophilia, central bronchiectasis, and highly elevated serum IgE. ABPA is one of the clinical entities that make up the pulmonary infiltrates with eosinophilia (PIE) syndrome. Proper recognition of the specific PIE diagnosis is important for prognostic as well as therapeutic purposes. ABPA is the most common asthmatic presentation of PIE.

Aspergillus is a common genus of saprophytic molds found almost ubiquitously in warm climates. *Aspergillus* spp can cause a variety of clinical conditions distinct from ABPA. These include invasive aspergillosis, aspergilloma, hypersensitivity pneumonitis, chronic necrotizing pneumonia, and allergic fungal sinusitis (caused by a hypersensitivity reaction to *Aspergillus* that can aggravate concomitant asthma or ABPA). ABPA is not an invasive infectious disease and thus does not require or typically respond to antifungal therapy. Rather it is a hypersensitivity state caused by aberrant type I (IgE) mechanisms directed against *Aspergillus fumigatus* antigens.

The disease is significantly underdiagnosed, largely because it has not been regularly considered by clinicians. Eight major criteria are characteristic of ABPA. If all eight criteria are met, the diagnosis is obvious. The most common findings in ABPA are central bronchiectasis and elevated serum *Af* IgE/IgG, but the absence of either of these does not exclude the diagnosis if other criteria are met. Within the PIE syndromes, ABPA is the most common in those patients presenting with asthma. If a patient presents with wheezing, other diagnoses besides ABPA are more often considered. However, if there is evidence of purulent sputum or a need for recurrent systemic corticosteroids, ABPA should be considered. The clinical picture associated with ABPA can also be caused by other allergic bronchopulmonary mycoses.

The acute form of ABPA can be difficult to distinguish from an asthma exacerbation, whereas chronic ABPA can be mistaken for chronic obstructive pulmonary disease, particularly in an older patient with smoking history. Staging of ABPA is important for both prognostic as well as therapeutic strategies. The most characteristic radiologic findings in ABPA are pulmonary infiltrates and central bronchiectasis. Other radiographic findings seen in ABPA include perihilar infiltrates, tramlines (representing bronchial wall edema), and, occasionally, significant consolidation.

The specific therapeutic regimen for ABPA depends primarily on the stage of disease. Specific therapeutic goals should be set for each patient. These include 1) the rapid detection and treatment of pulmonary infiltrates (because these are believed to be the sites most at risk for development of bronchiectasis), 2) the management of associated lung diseases (asthma, fibrosis), and 3) the search for environmental sources of the fungus that can be controlled.

Pulmonary Infiltrates with Eosinophilia Syndrome

Diagnosis, Etiology, and Characteristics of the Pulmonary Infiltrates with Eosinophilia (PIE) Syndrome

Diagnosis	Asthma*	IgE†	Etiology	Characteristics
Löffler's syndrome	No	NV‡	Unknown	Transient PIE; no treatment needed
Eosinophilic pneumonia	No	V§	Infectious drug reaction	Treat infection; needs corticosteroids
Hypereosinophilic syndrome	No	NV	Unknown	Highest eosinophilia; multiple organs affected
Tropical eosinophilia	Yes	+¶	Filariasis	Treat with diethylcarbamazine
Allergic bronchopulmonary aspergillosis	Yes	++	*Aspergillus fumigatus*	Asthma with constitutional symptoms
Churg-Strauss syndrome	Yes	+	Unknown	Multisystem; use immunosuppressive treatment

*Asthma as a presenting component of the specific diagnosis.
†Serum IgE level measured at time of diagnosis.
‡Normal values (NV) typically < 400 ng/mL.
§Variable (V) can be normal or elevated.
Single plus sign indicates elevated levels (typically < 2000 ng/mL); *double plus sign* indicates highly elevated levels (often > 4000 ng/mL).

▬ Figure 15-1.

Diagnosis, etiology, and characteristics of diseases comprising the pulmonary infiltrates with eosinophilia syndrome (PIE). Within the PIE syndromes, allergic bronchopulmonary aspergillosis (ABPA) is the one most common, presenting with asthma. Löffler's syndrome and eosinophilic pneumonia do not commonly present with bronchospasm. Löffler's syndrome is typically transient and produces no significant symptomatology of its own, whereas eosinophilic pneumonia causes constitutional symptoms such as fever and productive sputum. Tropical eosinophilia should be suspected with a travel history to locations endemic for filaria (*Wuchereria bancrofti*). In a wheezing patient with eosinophilia and other systemic involvement (*ie*, renal, hepatic, neurologic, cutaneous), Churg-Strauss vasculitis should be considered. Clinical and laboratory findings typical of vasculitis (*ie*, extreme complement consumption) are commonly found. Hypereosinophilic syndrome should be considered when other causes have been eliminated and multiorgan eosinophilia is established.

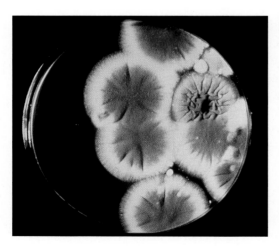

▬ Figure 15-2.

Aspergillus fumigatus. Aspergillus is a common genus of saprophytic molds commonly found in warm, moist areas such as moldy hay (barns), potting soil, compost piles, decaying vegetation (*eg*, forest floors), crawl spaces, and sewage treatment plants. The various species are highly thermotolerant, growing from 15°C to 53°C. These molds produce septated hyphae that measure 7 to 10 μm in diameter and characteristically branch at a 45°-angle. *A. fumigatus* is the most common of the species to cause disease in humans.

Diagnosis

Differential Diagnosis of Aspergillus-related Diseases

Invasive aspergillosis
Hypersensitivity pneumonitis
Chronic necrotizing pneumonia
Allergic fungal sinusitis

Figure 15-3.

Differential diagnosis of aspergillus-related diseases. For patients presenting with wheezing, other diagnoses besides allergic bronchopulmonary aspergillosis are more often considered. If evidence of purulent sputum exists or there is a need for recurrent systemic corticosteroids, ABPA must be considered. In children, cystic fibrosis may present with wheezing, sputum production, and bronchiectasis. Asthmatic bronchitis, sarcoidosis, pneumonia, chronic obstructive pulmonary disease or congestive heart failure can all present with various combinations of the above symptoms. Other diseases must be considered that present with eosinophilia (hypoadrenalism, collagen vascular diseases, neoplasms, parasitism) or highly elevated IgE (Job's syndrome, atopic dermatitis).

The clinical picture associated with ABPA can also be caused by other allergic bronchopulmonary mycoses, such as *Alternaria, Candida, Curvularia,* and *Drechslera.* This is important to note because tests for specific IgE and IgG for *Aspergillus fumigatus* would likely be negative. Proper diagnosis might be directed if evidence of specific fungi could be recovered in sputum from affected patients.

Diagnostic Criteria for Allergic Bronchopulmonary Aspergillosis

Asthma
Pulmonary infiltrates (via radiography)
Peripheral blood eosinophilia
Elevated serum IgE
Elevated IgE and IgG to *Aspergillus fumigatus*
Precipitating antibodies ("precipitins") to *A. fumigatus*
Positive allergy skin test to *A. fumigatus*
Central bronchiectasis (with normal tapering of distal bronchi) via tomograms or CT of the chest

Figure 15-4.

Diagnostic criteria for allergic bronchopulmonary aspergillosis (ABPA). This table shows the eight major criteria characteristic of ABPA. Pulmonary infiltrates may not be present if the patient has received systemic corticosteroids. Peripheral blood eosinophilia may also be affected by systemic corticosteroids. Serum IgE is usually highly elevated, on an order of 1000 ng/mL or higher).

Clinical Stages

Clinical Stages of Allergic Bronchopulmonary Aspergillosis

Stage	Clinical Characteristic	Systemic Steroids Needed	IgE Level	Comments
I	Acute	Yes (2 mo)	+++	Most responsive to systemic CS
II	Remission	No	+	May last indefinitely
III	Exacerbation	Yes	++ to +++	May also have constitutional symptoms
IV	Steroid dependent	Yes	++	Fail repeated attempts to taper CS
V	Fibrosis	Yes	?	Permanent obstruction; death from pneumonia or cor pulmonale

Figure 15-5.

Clinical stages of allergic bronchopulmonary aspergillosis (ABPA). Staging of ABPA is important for both prognostic as well as therapeutic strategies. The basic assumptions are that chronic disease follows uncontrolled acute episodes, and that irreversible pulmonary damage can be prevented by corticosteroid therapy.

Stage I is the acute phase, with little or no permanent damage. This stage is most likely to have most or all of the diagnostic criteria. Pulmonary infiltrates are very commonly observed along with significant peripheral blood eosinophilia. This stage is typically most responsive to short-term, high-dose corticosteroid therapy.

Stage II, remission, is defined as no subsequent chest infiltrates after tapering and discontinuing corticosteroids for at least 6 months. Total serum IgE levels often decrease substantially (although not always to normal) and remain low while in remission. Remission can be permanent, although exacerbations up to 7 years later have been reported.

Stage III, exacerbation, is characterized by new pulmonary infiltrates unexplainable from other diagnoses and a marked elevation in serum IgE (at least double, typically three- to 10-fold). The clinical picture is exacerbation of asthma symptoms with or without constitutional symptoms such as malaise, fever (usually < 38.5°C), myalgias, and sputum production.

Stage IV, steroid-dependent asthma from APBA, is recognized by exacerbations (asthma, new chest infiltrates, elevation in IgE) from either stage I or III patients when repeated attempts to taper systemic corticosteroids fail. Although the IgE level may remain low, *Aspergillus fumigates*–specific IgE and IgG levels are typically elevated.

Stage V is end-stage fibrotic lung disease from repeated inflammatory episodes of ABPA. These patients have defined ABPA as well as an irreversible obstructive-restrictive clinical picture, and have steroid-dependent asthma. With worsening end-stage lung disease despite corticosteroid therapy, death typically occurs from acute respiratory failure (*eg*, superimposed pneumonia) or cor pulmonale.

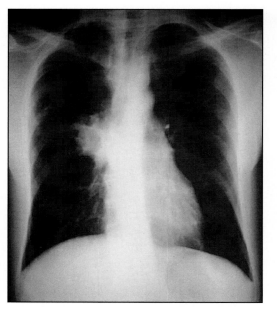

Figure 15-6.

Chest radiograph from a patient with pulmonary infiltrates with eosinophilia syndrome. The most common radiologic finding in allergic bronchopulmonary aspergillosis (ABPA) is pulmonary infiltrates. Plain films of the chest can be most useful, from the initial infiltrate recognition (see Fig. 15-3) to a baseline study to distinguish the development of fibrosis. Other findings such as mucoid impactions or new infiltrates can be an indicator of disease exacerbation or progression. A characteristic finding in APBA is the development of ring shadows, typically 1 to 2 cm in diameter, which reflect ecstatic central bronchi with peribronchial thickening seen *en face*. If seen tangentially, the dilated bronchus is called a parallel-line shadow. These findings are most common in the posterior segments of the upper lobe. Other radiographic findings seen in ABPA include perihilar infiltrates, tramlines (representing bronchial wall edema), and, occasionally, significant consolidation. Although none of these latter findings are specific for ABPA, their presence is associated with disease activity and may be useful markers for response to therapy.

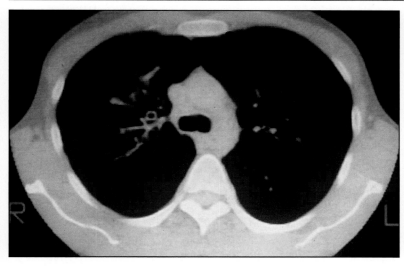

Figure 15-7.

Central bronchiectasis associated with allergic bronchopulmonary aspergillosis (ABPA). The most characteristic radiologic finding in ABPA is central bronchiectasis (CB). Those patients who have ABPA without CB (ABPA-S) may represent early disease that has not yet progressed to bronchiectasis or may truly be a disease variant. CB is most readily found by hilar tomography. CT scan may be useful but can, because of its axial orientation, give false negatives. Recent work suggests the potential for high-resolution CT in differentiating ABPA patterns from other pulmonary diseases caused by *Aspergillus*.

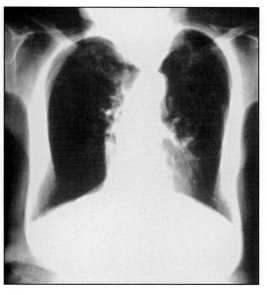

Figure 15-8.

Stage V fibrosis in allergic bronchopulmonary aspergillosis. Stage V (fibrosis) patients have a poorer prognosis. An initial FEV_1 (forced expiratory volume in 1 second) of 0.8 L or less is a very poor prognostic indicator. Daily corticosteroids are usually indicated. Some stage V patients remain stable on daily corticosteroids. Most do not and progress to parenchymal destruction with development of fibrosis, cor pulmonale, and pulmonary hypertension. These complications are managed until death.

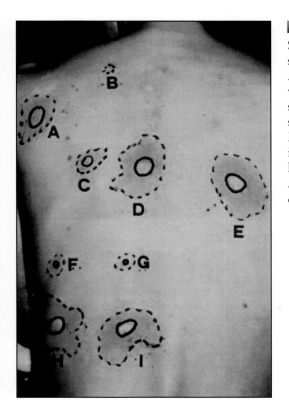

Figure 15-9.

Skin test responses in allergic bronchopulmonary aspergillosis (ABPA). This photograph shows skin test reactivity to recombinant *Aspergillus fumigatus* and human proteins in an ABPA patient. For intradermal skin tests, 100 µL of the protein solutions (10 to 1 µg/mL) was injected with a syringe. A 0.01% histamine dihydrochloride solution (*A*) and 0.9% saline solution (*B*) were used as positive and negative controls, respectively. The reactions show that 10-g fungal (*D*) and human (*E*) P2 protein or fungal (*H*) and human (*I*) MnSOD are able to elicit a wheal that is comparable to the size of the skin reaction induced by the positive histamine control. C shows the reaction to a challenge with 1 ng human P2 protein. The patient lacks IgE to rAsp f 3 (*F*) and rAsp f 11 (*G*), two additional *A. fumigatus* allergens. The absence of reactions to skin challenges with these allergens demonstrates the specificity of the test.

Treatment

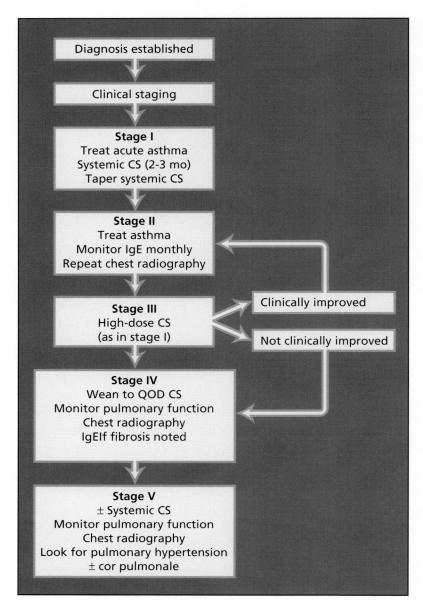

Diagnosis established

↓

Clinical staging

↓

Stage I
Treat acute asthma
Systemic CS (2-3 mo)
Taper systemic CS

↓

Stage II
Treat asthma
Monitor IgE monthly
Repeat chest radiography

↓

Stage III
High-dose CS
(as in stage I)

→ Clinically improved

→ Not clinically improved

Stage IV
Wean to QOD CS
Monitor pulmonary function
Chest radiography
IgEIf fibrosis noted

↓

Stage V
± Systemic CS
Monitor pulmonary function
Chest radiography
Look for pulmonary hypertension
± cor pulmonale

Figure 15-10.

Treatment paradigm for allergic bronchopulmonary aspergillosis (ABPA). The specific therapeutic regimen for ABPA patients depends primarily on the stage of disease. In 60% to 70% of patients with ABPA, asthma is the most persistent symptom. Thus, proper control of asthma symptoms is a major consideration for chronic control. In stages I and III, systemic corticosteroids (CS) are usually necessary. These should be given in relatively large amounts (0.5 mg/kg prednisone, up to 40 mg) daily for at least 2 weeks and converted to alternate-day regimens for at least 2 to 3 months. Serum IgE levels typically decrease as remission is achieved. Thus, a monthly monitoring of IgE for the first year is useful because pulmonary infiltrates may worsen in up to 30% of ABPA patients with little or no pulmonary symptoms. Sharp increases in IgE levels (at least doubling) are often associated with new pulmonary infiltrates long before development of clinical symptoms. After a 3-month trial, tapering and discontinuation of corticosteroids can be attempted, dictated by clinical symptomatology, IgE levels, and chest radiographs. The patient may remain in stage II (remission) indefinitely but should be followed up at frequent intervals for the first year with IgE determinations and clinical assessment. When exacerbation occurs (stage III), repeat therapy as in stage I can be attempted. If the patient progresses to stage IV, alternate-day corticosteroids should be administered repeatedly. Even in a stable stage IV patient on prednisone, exacerbations will occur. If symptoms are primarily asthmatic with no new chest infiltrates or sharp increases in serum IgE, other medications such as bronchodilators, cromolyn, and even anticholinergics may be used.

Recommended Reading

Cockrill BA, Hales CA: Allergic bronchopulmonary aspergillosis. *Ann Rev Med* 1999, 50:303—316.

Hinson KFW, Moon AJ, Plummer NS: Bronchopulmonary aspergillosis. *Thorax* 1952, 7:317–333.

Oermann CM, Panesar KS, Langston C, *et al.*: Pulmonary infiltrates with eosinophilia syndromes in children. *J Pediatr* 2000, 136:351–358.

Wark PA, Gibson PG: Allergic bronchopulmonary aspergillosis: new concept of pathogenesis and treatment. *Respirology* 2001, 6:1–7.

16 Hypersensitivity Pneumonitis

Michael C. Zacharisen and Jordan Fink

Hypersensitivity pneumonitis is a non-IgE, non-mast cell–mediated inflammatory lung disease that is characterized by both respiratory and systemic symptoms. Although this disease is also called extrinsic allergic alveolitis, the pathophysiology involves the pulmonary interstitium, small and medium airways, and the alveoli. Hypersensitivity pneumonitis is significantly less common than asthma and is more difficult to diagnose. The exact disease prevalence is unknown, but estimates range from 7% in dairy farmers up to 70% of exposed individuals in industrial settings [1]. This discrepancy may result from the case definition of hypersensitivity pneumonitis, exposure variables, and risk factors, which are poorly characterized.

Although respiratory disease does not readily lend itself to pictorial representation, the important diagnostic features of this disease can be illustrated with the use of radiographic and specific laboratory studies. The most important information that results in arriving at a correct diagnosis is obtained from a careful, detailed, and accurate environmental history that includes the home, workplace, and hobbies. The most prominent respiratory symptoms are dyspnea, or nonproductive cough, and, rarely, wheezing. Although symptoms of rhinitis, conjunctivitis, and dermatitis are not part of the disease manifestations, fever and influenza-like symptoms after exposure to the offending agent are classic symptoms of acute disease. This pattern of symptoms can be easily misinterpreted as an acute viral process. In contrast to asthma, a personal or family history of atopy does not predispose patients to this disease, and smoking may protect against the development of hypersensitivity pneumonitis. This probably relates to the toxic effect of smoke on alveolar macrophage function. The physical examination is typically normal between episodes in those with acute hypersensitivity pneumonitis. During an acute exacerbation, dry-end inspiratory rales are characteristic. Findings in patients with chronic hypersensitivity pneumonitis are similar to those of other chronic interstitial lung diseases and primarily include dyspnea on exertion. The subacute form of hypersensitivity pneumonitis is intermediate between the acute and chronic forms and typically presents with advancing respiratory symptoms over a period of months. After the diagnosis has been established, the currently recommended treatment approach is avoidance of the offending antigen and, if needed, use of oral corticosteroids. Early treatment is encouraged in an effort to prevent recurrent symptoms and more severe or chronic disease [2].

Antigens in Hypersensitivity Pneumonitis

Source	Antigen	Disease
	Bacteria	
"Moldy" hay, grain, compost	Thermophilic actinomycetes (*Micropolyspora faeni*, *T. vulgaris*)	Farmer's lung
Humidifier or air conditioner	Thermophilic actinomycetes, *Klebsiella* spp.	Ventilation pneumonitis
Ultrasonic cool mist humidifier	*Bacillus cereus, Klebsiella oxytoca, Cephalosporium acremonium*	Humidifier lung
"Moldy" sugarcane (bagasse)	*T. sacchari, T vulgaris*	Bagassosis
Humidifier or air conditioner	*T. candidus, T sacchari*	Ventilation pneumonitis
Compost	*T. vulgaris*	Residential composter's lung
Mushroom compost	*T. candidus, T viridis*	Mushroom worker's lung
Used metal working fluid	*Pseudomonas fluorescens, Acinetobacter lwoffii*	Machine operator's lung
	Fungi	
Moldy hay	*Penicillium brevicompactum*	Farmer's lung
Moldy basement shower	*Epicoccum nigrum*	Basement shower hypersensitivity pneumonitis
Moldy malt dust	*Aspergillus* spp.	Malt worker's lung
Moldy wood dust	*Alternaria* spp.	Woodworker's lung
Moldy cork dust	*Penicillium frequentans*	Suberosis
Cheese mold	*Pencillium caseii*	Cheese worker's lung
Moldy Japanese house dust	*Trichosporum cutaneum, Trichosporum ovoides*	Summer-type hypersensitivity pneumonitis
Moldy maple bark	*Cryptostroma corticale*	Maple bark stripper's disease
Moldy flooded basement	*Pezizia domiciliana*	El Niño lung
Moldy redwood dust	*Pullularia* spp.	Sequoiosis
Moldy humidifier water	*Cephalosporium acremonium, S. virdis, Cladosproiodes* spp., *Curvularia spiciferia, Helminthsproium sativum, Paecilomyces variotii, Pencillium mix, Aspergillus flavus, A glacus,* and *A. nidulans*	Humidifier lung
	Animal proteins	
Avian dust, droppings, feathers, and sera	Avian serum proteins (pigeon, duck, chicken, dove, turkey, parakeet, parrot, lovebird, goose)	Bird breeder's disease, pigeon breeders disease, duck fever, plucker's lung, turkey handler's lung
Rat urine–contaminated dust	Rat urine or serum proteins	Laboratory worker's lung
Gerbil excreta	Gerbil proteins	Gerbil lung
Animal pelts (*ie*, cat)	Animal fur dust	Furrier's lung
Oyster or mollusk shell dust	Oyster shell protein	Oyster shell lung
Infested wheat flour	*Sitophilus granarius*	Wheat weevil disease, Miller's lung
Cocoon fluff	Silkworm larvae	Sericulturist's lung disease
Pituitary snuff	Bovine and porcine antigens	Pituitary snuff user's lung
	Amoebae	
Contaminated humidifier	*Naegleria gruberi, Acanthamoeba castellani*	Ventilation pneumonitis
	Drugs	
Drug	Amiodarone, gold, β-adrenergic blocker, sulfasalazine, intravesicular BCG, nitrofurantoin, minocycline, procarbazine, methotrexate, chlorambucil, mesalamine, fluoxetine, HMG-CoA reductase inhibitors, cyclosporin, clozapine, intranasal heroin	Medication-induced hypersensitivity pneumonitis
	Chemicals	
Paint catalyst	Toluere di-isocyanate	Paint refinisher's disease
Paint catalyst	Diphenylmethane diisocyanate (MDI)	Bathtub refinisher's lung
Epoxy resin	Phthalic anhydride	Epoxy resin worker's lung
Plastics industry	Trimellitic anhydride	Plastic worker's lung
	Other	
Wet plaster or stucco	Esparto grass	Stipatosis
Veterinary feed	Soybean hull	
Wood dust or sawdust	Cabreuva wood, pine, cedar, oak, mahogany, and spruce pulp	Wood dust disease
Insecticide	Pyrethrum	Pyrethrum hypersensitivity
Nut industry in Spain	Tiger nut dust	pneumonitis

Figure 16-1. (*on previous page*)

Antigens in hypersensitivity pneumonitis. The number and diversity of antigens incriminated in producing hypersensitivity pneumonitis continue to increase. The antigens are usually derived from microorganisms, animal and plant products found in organic dust, low molecular weight chemicals used in industry, and medications. Thermophilic bacteria that thrive at temperatures above 60°C are the cause of farmer's lung, one of the earliest recognized triggers of hypersensitivity pneumonitis. Various fungi have also been implicated in many different occupations as well as in the home environment. Some antigens appear restricted to certain regions of the world such as Japanese summer-type hypersensitivity pneumonitis, which is caused by *Trichosporum* spp in the home. Despite the broad array of antigens, the clinical picture is strikingly similar. As the causative agents are identified, measures to control exposure to them has resulted in prevention of further outbreaks or cases, making them of historical interest only. BCG—bacillus Calmette-Guérin; HMG-CoA—3-hydroxy-3-methylglutaryl coenzyme A; TDI—toluene diisocyanate.

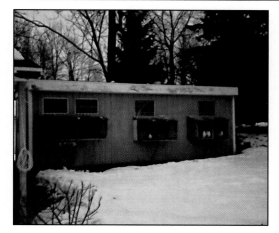

Figure 16-2.

Pigeon breeding as a cause of hypersensitivity pneumonitis. Pigeon breeding for the purpose of racing and showing is a popular hobby and sport. Pigeon coops can range in size from 6 × 6-foot lofts to large barns that hold hundreds to thousands of birds. The cleaning of the coops generates small respirable particles that contain feather blooms or dust and intestinal proteins from droppings [3]. Although intermittent exposure to cleaning the coop or during bird shows can result in recurrent, acute symptoms of hypersensitivity pneumonitis, keeping birds indoors causes chronic low-grade exposure that may result in chronic hypersensitivity pneumonitis as the presenting diagnosis. (*Courtesy of* Steve Yanke, Sheboygan Falls, WI.)

Clinical Findings in Patients with Hypersensitivity Pneumonitis

	Acute Form	**Chronic Form**
Symptoms	4 to 6 hours after exposure	Insidious over months
Dry cough	Common	Common
Dyspnea on exertion	Common	Common
Fever, chills	Common	Uncommon
Weight loss or anorexia	Uncommon	Common
Fatigue	Common	Common
Wheezing	Uncommon	Occasional
Pulmonary function	Normal between attacks	
Spirometry	Restriction	Restriction and obstruction
Diffusion capacity	Decreased	Decreased
Radiographic studies	Typically lacks adenopathy, pleural fluid	Bronchiectasis not characteristic
Chest radiography	Bilateral interstitial infiltrates, reticular–nodular	Diffuse interstitial fibrosis, honeycombing and fibrosis
Chest CT scan	Ground-glass appearance	Scattered small, round opacities; nodules
Laboratory studies		
CBC and differential	Leukocytosis	Normal
ESR	Elevated	Normal or elevated
Serum precipitins	Present	Present
Bronchoscopy studies	Cultures negative	Cultures negative
BAL T-cell markers	Lymphocytosis, CD8+ > CD4+	Lymphocytosis, CD8+ > CD4+
Pathologic studies	No vasculitis	No vasculitis
Open lung biopsy	"Foamy" macrophages, lymphocytic pneumonitis	Diffuse interstitial fibrosis, noncaseating granulomas

Figure 16-3.

Clinical findings in patients with hypersensitivity pneumonitis. The symptoms of acute hypersensitivity pneumonitis can easily be misconstrued as acute lower respiratory tract infections. The apparent response to empiric treatment with antibiotics frequently corresponds with avoidance of the antigen. Therefore, a high index of suspicion is required to arrive at the correct diagnosis in a timely fashion. The diagnosis is traditionally based on a constellation of clinical, laboratory, and pulmonary function findings in the setting of an exposure to an offending antigen [4]. Purposeful inhalation challenge is usually reserved for unusual cases and should be performed in a hospital setting where treatment can be immediately rendered in the event of a severe respiratory event. BAL—bronchoalveolar lavage; CBC—complete blood count; ESR—erythrocyte sedimentation rate.

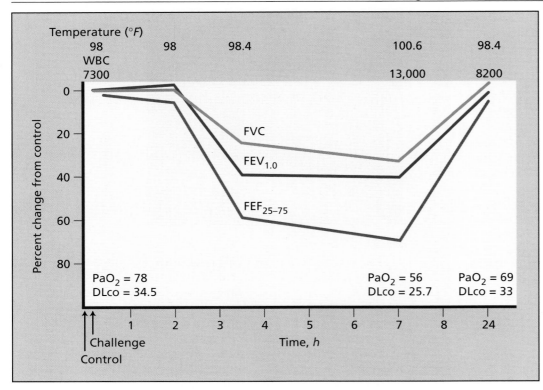

Figure 16-4.

Pulmonary function tests in hypersensitivity pneumonitis. This drawing illustrates the late-onset reaction after inhalation of pigeon antigen by a sensitized pigeon breeder. The finding is that of a restrictive ventilatory defect as seen by a decrease in both FVC (forced vital capacity) and the FEV_1 (forced expiratory volume in 1 second) occurring 6 to 8 hours after challenge. In this acute reaction, systemic findings include fever, elevation of total white blood cells (WBCs), and a decrease in lung diffusion capacity. Some individuals have a dual response in spirometry, with both an early and late phase decrease in FVC and FEV_1 measurements. The lung function changes spontaneously resolve over time with avoidance of the triggering antigen or can be more rapidly improved with treatment with oral corticosteroids.

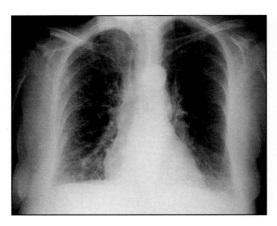

Figure 16-5.

Chest radiograph of patient with acute hypersensitivity pneumonitis. If hypersensitivity pneumonitis exacerbations are widely spaced, the chest radiograph is usually normal. During acute exacerbations, chest radiographic findings typically reveal soft, patchy bilateral lower lobe ill-defined parenchymal densities. This represents active alveolitis, which resolves over several days. After resolution of the acute phase or with subacute hypersensitivity pneumonitis, findings include nodulations and fine reticulations with general coarsening of the bronchovascular markings. End-stage hypersensitivity pneumonitis is characterized by fibrosis with honeycombing and parenchymal contraction. High-resolution CT of the chest is no better than conventional radiographs in the diagnosis of acute hypersensitivity pneumonitis. However, for subacute or chronic forms, the chest CT scan may better delineate centrilobular nodules and small, round ground-glass opacities and areas of emphysema [5]. Limited data are available to determine the usefulness of lung diffusion scans except in drug-induced pneumonitis. Traditional magnetic resonance imaging scans have been limited by the low proton density of lung tissue and loss of signal caused by motion. Techniques that use ultrashort gradient echoes that reduce cardiac and respiratory motion artifact may be useful in identifying reversible changes.

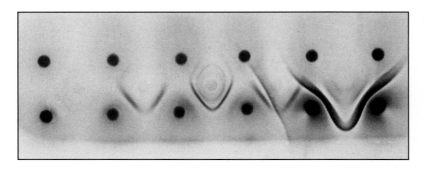

Figure 16-6.

Serum-precipitating antibodies as demonstrated by Ouchterlony double immunodiffusion gel system. An agar gel diffusion system is shown that demonstrates the presence of serum-precipitating antibodies specific to the offending antigen. Antigen is placed in the five central wells (light in color), and serum from the affected patient is placed in the top wells. Serum from unexposed normal control patients is placed in the bottom wells. The intensity of the stained bands represents the precipitating antigen–antibody complexes that have formed in various degrees. This immunologic finding confirms exposure to the specific antigen, but it does not confirm the disease itself because the demonstration of elevated levels of serum-precipitating antibody occurs in nearly all ill individuals and approximately 50% of similarly exposed but asymptomatic individuals. Not all antigens are available for all circumstances, thus requiring sampling of airborne mist, dust, liquids, or solids and the subsequent preparation of material to be used in testing. Skin testing is not routinely used because irritative and both false-positive and false-negative reactions can occur.

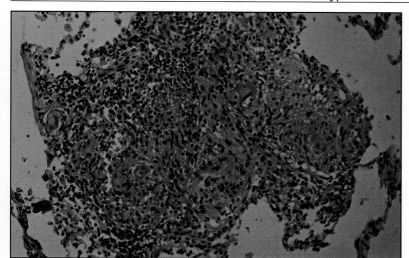

■ Figure 16-7.

Lung biopsy specimen of a patient with hypersensitivity pneumonitis. This low-power view from an open lung biopsy reveals noncaseating granulomas and a lymphocytic infiltrate. The majority of these cells are CD8+ lymphocytes, but CD4+ cell numbers are increased as well. Pathologic findings from patients with chronic hypersensitivity pneumonitis reveal luminal and mural alveolitis, granulomas, intra-alveolar buds, and interstitial fibrosis. The major cell type found is lymphocyte, but intra-alveolar macrophages with a "foamy" appearance are characteristic [6]. Compared with sarcoid lung disease, the granulomas are smaller and more loosely arranged and are located closer to the alveoli rather than to the bronchioles. Open-lung biopsy continues to be the preferred method because transbronchial biopsy may not provide adequate tissue samples for a specific diagnosis. Not all patients require biopsy to arrive at a diagnosis of hypersensitivity pneumonitis.

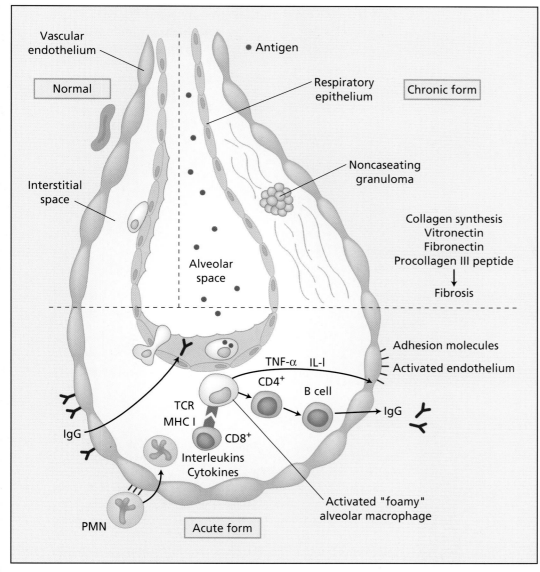

■ Figure 16-8.

Pathophysiology of hypersensitivity pneumonitis. This simplified schematic illustrates the proposed mechanism of hypersensitivity pneumonitis that takes place during the acute and chronic phases of the disease. The exact mechanism is unclear, particularly in humans. Animal studies have yielded significant information regarding mechanisms but may not exactly parallel human disease. After small organic particulate matter is inhaled into the peripheral airways, it combines with specific antibody, which is engulfed and processed by alveolar macrophages in the pulmonary interstitium. These macrophages become activated and express cell surface markers (including CD80 and CD86 and heat shock protein) and release proinflammatory cytokines (including interleukin (IL)-1 and tumor necrosis factor-α), as well as activating complement [7]. These mediators lead to endothelial activation with upregulation of adhesion molecules (intercellular adhesion molecule-1 and E-selectin), which attract and promote adhesion of neutrophils. The activated alveolar macrophage presents processed antigen to CD8+ T lymphocyte at the T-cell receptor in the context of major histocompatibility complex class I. The T cell, in turn, releases a host of mediators, including IL-2, -8, -10, -12, and -16. IL-8 acts a potent chemoattractant for neutrophils, which release superoxide anion, hydroxyl radicals, and toxic oxygen radicals. These products produce acute inflammation. CD4+ T cells also interact with activated alveolar macrophages. Further cell–cell interaction with B cells leads to the development of plasma cells that produce specific IgG. The effect of cytokines is inflammation with collagen synthesis and secretion of vitronectin, fibronectin, and procollagen III peptide.

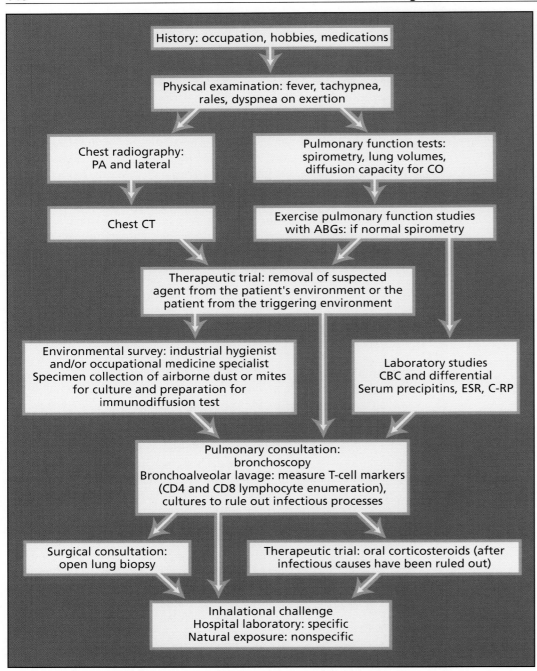

Figure 16-9.

Diagnostic algorithm for the evaluation of hypersensitivity pneumonitis. The evaluation process for a patient with possible hypersensitivity pneumonitis generally requires a multidisciplinary approach. The most important process is obtaining a thorough environmental history, documenting exposures in the workplace, hobbies, and home. The examination may show normal results or have findings of interstitial lung disease. Various radiologic studies are helpful, beginning with plain chest radiographs. Consultation with a pulmonologist who can perform bronchoscopy with bronchoalveolar lavage is helpful in ruling out other disorders as well as providing information regarding the cellular milieu within the alveoli. An industrial hygienist who is skilled in evaluating work environments and personal residences and who is familiar with heating, ventilation, and air conditioning systems can collect personal air samples as well as necessary fluid or soil specimens for microbial analysis for use in preparing antigen for gel diffusion experiments. ABG—arterial blood gas; CBC—complete blood count; C-RP—C-reactive protein; ESR—erythrocyte sedimentation rate.

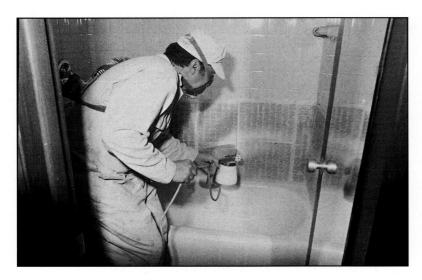

Figure 16-10.

A spray painter who is using a paint containing di-isocyanates as hardeners. This group of simple chemicals likely combines with a serum protein and haptenizes to become allergenic [8]. In addition to causing hypersensitivity pneumonitis, exposure to di-isocyanates can also lead to occupational asthma. Because avoidance measures are the key factor in preventing hypersensitivity pneumonitis, patients should be instructed to wear properly fitting face masks with appropriate filters for filtration. In addition to personal protection, proper room ventilation is required. Despite these precautions, patients occasionally require transfer to a different area or retraining for another occupation.

References

1. Lopez M, Salvaggio J: Epidemiology of hypersensitivity pneumonitis/allergic alveolitis. *Monogr Allergy* 1987, 21:70–86.

2. Fink JN, Zacharisen MC: Hypersensitivity pneumonitis. In *Allergy Principles and Practice*. Edited by Middleton E, Reed CE, Ellis EF, *et al*. St Louis: Mosby-Yearbook; 1998:994–1004.

3. Baldwin C, Todd A, Bourke S, *et al*.: Pigeon fancier's lung: identification of disease-associated carbohydrate epitopes on pigeon intestinal mucin. *Clin Exp Immunol* 1999, 117:230–236.

4. Richerson HB, Bernstein IL, Fink JN, *et al*.: Guidelines for the clinical evaluation of hypersensitivity pneumonitis. *J Allergy Clin Immunol* 1989, 84:839–844.

5. Muller NL, Miller RR: Computed tomography of chronic diffuse infiltrative lung disease: part 2. *Am Rev Respir Dis* 1990, 142:1440–1448.

6. Kawanami O, Basset F, Barrios R, *et al*.: Hypersensitivity pneumonitis in man: light- and electron-microscopic studies of 18 lung biopsies. *Am J Pathol* 1983, 110:275–289.

7. Israel-Assayag E, Dakhama A, Lavigne S, *et al*.: Expression of costimulatory molecules on alveolar macrophages in hypersensitivity pneumonitis. *Am J Respir Crit Care Med* 1999, 159:1830–1834.

8. Baur X: Hypersensitivity pneumonitis (extrinsic allergic alveolitis) induced by isocyanates. *J Allergy Clin Immunol* 1995, 95:1004–1010.

9. Salvaggio JE: Extrinsic allergic alveolitis (hypersensitivity pneumonitis): past, present, and future. *Clin Exp Allergy* 1997, 27:18–25.

Pulmonary Function Testing and Bronchial Provocation

Ronald L. Morton and Nemr S. Eid

Pulmonologists, allergists, and respiratory physiologists measure lung function through a series of tests called pulmonary function tests (PFTs). These tests determine the gas exchange properties of the lung, thereby allowing us to decide if disease (*ie*, obstructive or restrictive lung disease) is present. This chapter focuses on several key aspects of PFTs: the physiology behind the test, the clinical utility of spirometry, the use of bronchoprovocation challenge testing, and the application of infant PFTs in practice.

The first section demonstrates the normal physiology behind the use of PFTs. An understanding of normal lung physiology helps the clinician differentiate persons with normal airflows and lung volumes from those with intrinsic lung disease (*ie*, asthma, chronic obstructive pulmonary disease, interstitial lung disease [ILD]). The American Thoracic Society (ATS) established specific reference values for lung function testing [1]. In addition, physicians who perform lung function testing in children must meet certain standard quality performance measures [2]. Lung function tests can also help predict disease progression as well as disease prognosis; indeed, a retrospective cohort study [3] found PFTs followed longitudinally to be an independent predictor of long-term mortality. We refer the reader to several key reference texts [4,5] to gain a deeper understanding of the physiology behind the test.

The application of PFTs in the office setting facilitates physicians in evaluating patients with obstructive or restrictive lung disease. Through a series of case vignettes, this section emphasizes how PFTs can aid in the diagnosis of a patient with respiratory symptoms. One important—and, perhaps, underused—application for PFTs is their use in the evaluation and longitudinal follow-up of patients with asthma [6–8]. The measurement of lung volumes in the preoperative evaluation of patients with scoliosis [9] or pectus excavatum determines the degree of restriction and the response to surgical correction. Another important use of PFTs is in the determination of the degree of diffusion impairment in a patient who has undergone radiation therapy or chemotherapy [10].

Another practical way to measure the function of the lung is to determine the degree of airway reactivity after either a pharmacologic (*eg*, methacholine, adenosine monophosphate, histamine), physiologic (*eg*, cold air, allergens), or exercise challenge [11–15]. The section on bronchoprovocation challenge testing demonstrates the use of the methacholine challenge test in patients with suspected underlying asthma and normal initial spirometry. Our case illustrates a 5-year-old child with a chronic cough who had normal initial spirometry test results. However, his methacholine challenge test result was strongly positive, indicating underlying airway hyperreactivity.

Another new tool in the armamentarium of clinicians is the application of infant pulmonary function testing (IPFT) in the evaluation of infants with persistent or recurrent wheezing [16–22]. We illustrate the use of the flow-volume loop obtained at tidal breathing in a young infant with persistent wheezing. The flow-volume loop helps to differentiate the location (central vs peripheral airways) and degree of airway obstruction. One study [22] found a good correlation between the shape of the flow-volume loop obtained on IPFT and the findings on flexible bronchoscopy in an infant with persistent noisy breathing.

Physiologic Basis of Pulmonary Function Testing

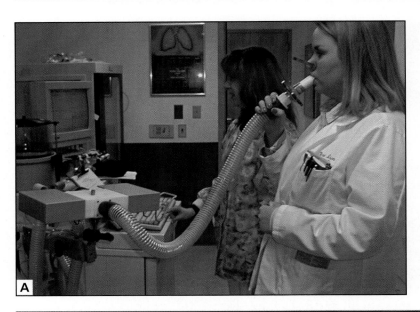

Figure 17-1.

Demonstration of spirometry. A forced vital capacity (FVC) is the volume of gas exhaled after a maximal inspiration. The forced expiratory volume in one second (FEV_1) measures the volume of airflow (L/s) after a full inspiration. The peak expiratory flow (PEF) is the greatest flow rate that can be obtained during a forced expiration starting from total lung capacity (TLC). **A,** The forced expiratory flow ($FEF_{25\%–75\%}$) is calculated from a forced expiration by measuring the slope of the line between 25% and 75% of vital capacity. From these measurements, the clinician determines whether a pattern of airflow obstruction or restriction is present. **B,** Normal spirometry. Airflows are measured before and after a bronchodilator challenge. Normal values for FVC and FEV_1 are greater than 80% predicted. A decrease in forced midrange expiratory flow measurements ($FEF_{25\%–75\%}$ and FEF_{75}) suggests small airway disease [1]. A reversible change after bronchodilator administration is noted in the small airways ($FEF_{25\%–75\%}$) in this patient. One study found that the $FEF_{25\%–75\%}$ may be useful in predicting the presence of bronchial hyperresponsiveness [8].

B. Normal Spirometry Results

Spirometry	Prebronchodilator		Postbronchodilator		Change, %
	Actual	Predicted, %	Actual	Predicted, %	
FVC, L	1.01	108	1.02	109	1
FEV_1, L	0.95	136	0.99	142	4
FEV_1/FVC, %	94.00	126	97.00	131	3
$FEF_{25\%–75\%}$, L/s	1.19	87	1.90	140	60

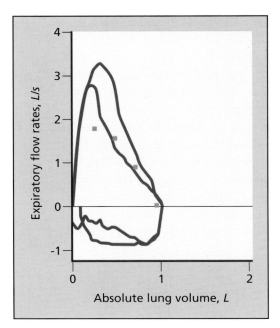

Figure 17-2.

Normal flow-volume loop. The flow-volume loop rises rapidly to a peak value during early expiration and then descends slowly throughout the remainder of expiration. The descending portion of the flow-volume loop is independent of effort over most of the lung volume. The flow-volume loop always follows a flow-volume envelope, which it does not penetrate. The unique behavior of the flow-volume curve is caused by the dynamic compression of the airways [4]. The shape of the flow volume is helpful in determining whether an intrathoracic or extrathoracic airway obstruction is present. If the inspiratory limb (*ie,* below the horizontal axis) is squared off or truncated, it suggests extrathoracic airflow obstruction, such as seen in vocal cord dysfunction [23].

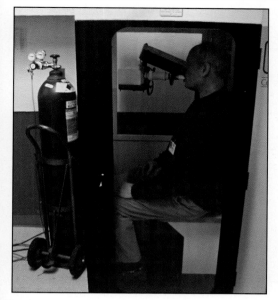

Figure 17-3.

Body plethysmography. The patient sits in an airtight box. At the end of a normal expiration, a shutter closes in the mouthpiece while the patient continues to make respiratory efforts. Functional residual capacity (FRC) is measured based on Boyle's law ($P_1V_1 = P_2V_2$). The body plethysmograph measures the total volume of gas in the lung, including any behind trapped airways.

Normal Lung Volumes

Spirometry	Pre-Drug Measured	Predicted, %	Predicted
MVV, *L/min*	108	87	124
Lung Volumes	**Pre-Drug Measured**	**Average Predicted, %**	
VC, *L*	3.74	96	3.88
TLC, *L*	4.97	94	5.31
FRC, *L*	2.54	111	2.29
ERV, *L*	1.31	108	1.21
RV, *L*	1.23	113	1.08
RV/TLC, *%*	25.00	> 121	20.00
IC, *L*	2.43	81	3.02
He equivalent, *min*	2.50		

Figure 17-4.

Normal lung volumes. The functional residual capacity (FRC) can also be measured using the helium dilution method, in which a known concentration of helium is allowed to equilibrate within the lungs ($C_1 \times V_1 = C_2 \times V_2$). The values for normal lung volumes are predicted between 80% to 120%. The ratio of residual volume (RV) to total lung capacity (TLC) corrects for lung volume, with the normal measured value ranging from 25% to 30%. MVV—maximal ventilatory volume; VC—vital capacity.

Comparison of Tests for Obstructive Pulmonary Disease Versus Restrictive Pulmonary Disease

Test	Obstructive Pulmonary Disease	Restrictive Pulmonary Disease
VC	↓	↓
FEV$_1$	↓	↓
FEV$_1$/FVC	↓	Normal
FRC	↑	↓
RV	↑	↓
TLC	↑	↓

Figure 17-5.

Interpretation of tests of ventilatory function. The specific patterns observed on tests of ventilatory function (airflows and lung volumes) helps to differentiate between obstructive (asthma, emphysema, chronic bronchitis) and restrictive (interstitial lung disease [ILD], kyphoscoliosis, muscular dystrophy) pulmonary disease. FEV$_1$—forced expiratory volume in 1 second; FRC—functional residual capacity; FVC—forced vital capacity; RV—residual volume; TLC—total lung capacity; VC—vital capacity.

Spirometry in the Clinical Setting

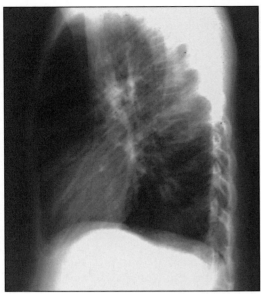

Figure 17-6.

Lateral chest radiograph demonstrating marked hyperinflation (flattening of the diaphragms and anterior cardiac air). An 8-year-old boy presented with a history of chronic cough. The cough was described as having a dry, hacking quality and was worse at night and after exercise. There was no family history of asthma.

Positive Response to Bronchodilators

Spirometry	Prebronchodilator		Postbronchodilator		
	Actual	Predicted, %	Actual	Predicted, %	Change, %
FEV, L	1.68	101	1.86	112	10
FEV, L	1.37	98	1.67	120	21
FEV_1/FVC, %	82.00		90.00		
$FEF_{25\%-75\%}$, L/s	1.30	62	1.84	87	41
TLC, L	3.08	144			
RV, L	1.26	265			
RV/TLC, %		183			

Figure 17-7.

Positive response to bronchodilators. The pulmonary function test of the boy in Figure 17-6 is shown. According to guidelines of the American Thoracic Society, a positive response to bronchodilators is defined as a 12% or greater improvement in forced expiratory volume in 1 second (FEV_1) [1]. A positive response to bronchodilators is observed in both the large (FEV_1) and small ($FEF_{25\%-75\%}$% [forced expiratory flow between 25% and 75% of vital capacity]) airways. Reversibility of airflow limitation with bronchodilators is a hallmark of asthma. The $FEF_{25\%-75\%}$ is decreased, which indicates small airway disease. FRC—functional residual capacity; FVC—forced vital capacity; RV—residual volume; TLC—total lung capacity.

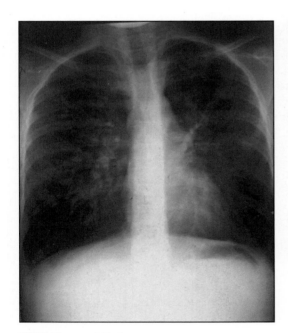

Figure 17-8.

The lungs of an 8-year-old girl with chronic cough. She had been treated for "allergy" and "bronchitis" with multiple medications and 3 years of immunotherapy. She had a chronic cough with green sputum production. Her height and weight were normal. Her chest examination revealed moist crackles over all lung fields.

Pulmonary Function with Severe Airflow Obstruction

Spirometry	Prebronchodilator		Postbronchodilator		
	Actual	Predicted, %	Actual	Predicted, %	Change, %
FVC, L	1.20	7.37	1.25	76.7	
FEV_1, L	0.72	53.3	0.72	53.3	0
FEV_1/FVC (%)	60.40		58.00		
$FEF_{25\%-75\%}$, L/s	0.33	15.6	0.36	16.7	
TLC, L	2.59	105.6			
RV, L	1.39	246.3			
RV/TLC, %	53.80				

Figure 17-9.

Pulmonary function test (PFT) result with severe airflow obstruction. This PFT result from the girl in Figure 17-8 illustrates severe airflow limitation in both the large and small airways. Both the forced expiratory volume in 1 second (FEV_1) and $FEF_{25\%-75\%}$% (forced expiratory flow between 25% and 75% of vital capacity) are decreased, and the residual volume (RV) is markedly elevated, indicating severe air trapping. The differential diagnosis for severe obstructive pulmonary disease includes severe asthma, cystic fibrosis, bronchopulmonary dysplasia (or chronic lung disease of infancy), and bronchiolitis obliterans. FVC—forced vital capacity; TLC—total lung capacity.

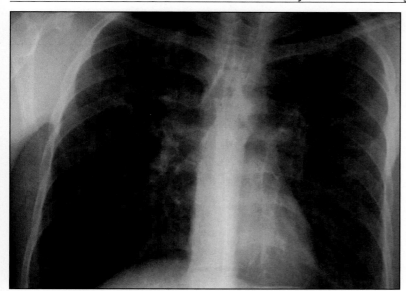

■ Figure 17-10.

Chest radiograph of an 18-year-old man with cystic fibrosis. The chest radiograph shows advanced lung disease with cystic changes, areas of bronchiectasis in the right upper lobe, and hyperinflation. Pulmonary function tests are used to follow the disease course and response to therapy during an acute exacerbation of the disease.

Pulmonary Function Tests in a Young Adult Patient with Advanced Cystic Fibrosis

Spirometry	Pre-drug Measured Value	Predicted, %	Predicted Values	Post-drug Measured*	Predicted, %	Change, %
FVC, L	0.76	24	3.15	0.83	26	18
FEV$_1$, L	0.59	24	2.53	0.68	27	14
FEF$_{25\%-75\%}$, L	0.55	17	3.19	0.65	20	17
FEF$_{max}$, L/s	1.17	20	5.93	1.40	24	19
FEF$_{50\%}$ (L/s)	0.94	22	4.38	0.70	16	-25
FEV$_1$/FVC, %	78.00	98	80.00	82.00	102	4

Spirometry	Pre-drug Measured	Predicted, %	Predicted, %
MVV, L/min	21	21	100

Lung Volumes	Pre-drug Measured	Average Predicted, %	Predicted, %
VC, L	0.76	24	3.15
TLC, L	2.10	50	4.22
FRC, L	1.50	73	2.06
ERV, L	0.16	16	0.99
RV, L	1.34	126	1.07
RV/TLC, %	64.00	253	25.00
IC, L	0.60	28	2.16
He equivalent, *min*	4.00		

■ Figure 17-11.

Pulmonary function test (PFT) results in a young adult patient with advanced cystic fibrosis. The PFTs show a severe mixed obstructive and restrictive pattern. The airflows (FVC [forced vital capacity] and FEV$_1$ [forced expiratory volume in 1 second]) are both decreased, with decreased lung volumes indicating severe restrictive disease. A significant response to bronchodilators is observed. ERV—expiratory reserve volume; FRC—functional residual capacity; IC—inspiratory capacity; RV—residual volume; TLC—total lung capacity; VC—vital capacity.

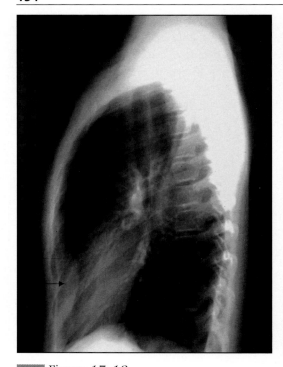

Figure 17-12.

Chest radiogram with pectus excavatum. This child presented to the pulmonary function laboratory for preoperative evaluation before repair of pectus excavatum. Pulmonary function test results are shown in Figure 17-13.

Mild Restrictive Pattern on Pulmonary Function Test

Spirometry	Pre-drug Measured*	Predicted, %	Predicted Value
FVC, L	2.90	74	3.90
FEV$_1$, L	2.64	72	3.67
FEF$_{25\%-75\%}$, L	3.19	79	4.03
FEF$_{max}$, L/s	5.51	69	8.01
FEF$_{50\%}$ (L/s)	3.33	72	4.63
FEV$_1$/FVC, %	91.00	97	94.00
Spirometry	**Pre-drug Measured**	**Predicted, %**	**Predicted, %**
MVV, L/min	93	7	120
Lung Volumes	**Pre-drug Measured**	**Average Predicted, %**	**Predicted, %**
VC, L	2.95	76	3.90
TLC, L	4.25	85	5.02
FRC, L	2.25	95	2.36
ERV, L	0.95	72	1.32
RV, L	1.30	125	1.04
RV/TLC, %	31.00	147	21.00
IC, L	2.00	75	2.66
He equivalent, min	2.00		

Figure 17-13.

Mild restrictive pattern on pulmonary function tests (PFTs). PFTs demonstrate a reduction in the vital capacity (VC) and FEV$_1$ (forced expiratory volume in 1 second) without a reduction of the ratio of FEV$_1$ to FVC (forced vital capacity). In restrictive lung disease, the expansion of the lung is impaired. This may involve diseases of the lung parenchyma (*eg* interstitial lung disease, pulmonary fibrosis), pleura (*eg*, pneumothorax, pleural effusion), chest wall (*eg*, scoliosis), or neuromuscular disease. FRC—functional residual capacity; RV—residual volume; TLC—total lung capacity.

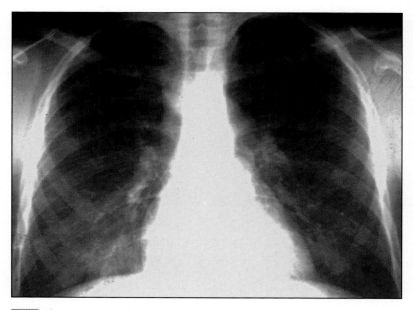

Figure 17-14.

Chest radiograph with increased interstitial markings. This 14-year-old boy with a history of pulmonary hemosiderosis was referred for further evaluation. Pulmonary hemosiderosis is a disease characterized by repeated bouts of bleeding in the lung parenchyma.

Pulmonary Function Test with a Decreased Diffusion Capacity

Spirometry	Actual	Predicted, %
FVC, L	2.44	81
FEV$_1$, L	2.26	88
FEF$_{25\%-75\%}$, L/s	3.18	90
TLC, L	2.83	73
RV, L	0.32	36
D$_L$CO, $mL/min/mm\ Hg$	9.64	43

Figure 17-15.

Pulmonary function test with a decreased diffusion capacity. The normal value for diffusing capacity of carbon monoxide at rest (D$_L$CO) is 25 mL/min/mm Hg. The D$_L$CO is corrected for blood volume to account for the association of the carbon monoxide with hemoglobin. D$_L$CO is decreased with decreased blood volume or increased thickness of the alveolar-capillary membrane. FEV$_1$—forced expiratory volume in 1 second; FVC—forced vital capacity; RV—residual volume; TLC—total lung capacity.

Bronchial Provocation Challenge Testing

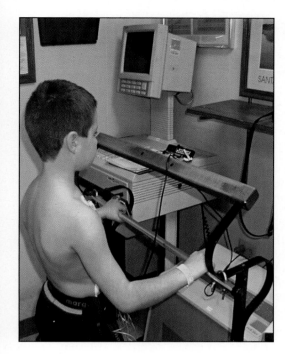

■ Figure 17-16.

Exercise challenge testing. The patient exercises on a treadmill until a target heart rate is achieved. Pulmonary function is assessed both 5 minutes (early response) and 30 minutes (late response) after exercise to determine the degree of airway responsiveness.

Pulmonary Function Tests Before and After Exercise

Spirometry	Pre-drug Measured	Predicted, %	Predicted Value	Post-drug Measured*	Exercise Predicted, %	Change, %
FVC, L	4.03	104	3.88	3.83	99	–4
FEV$_1$, L	3.20	83	3.86	2.70	70	–15
FEF$_{25\%-75\%}$, L	2.88	69	4.17	1.97	47	–31
FEF$_{max}$, L/s)	5.85	76	7.69	5.47	71	–6
FEF$_{50\%}$(L/s)	2.96	68	4.37	2.53	58	–14
FEV$_1$/FVC, %	79.00	80	99.00	70.00	71	–11

■ Figure 17-17.

Pulmonary function tests before and after exercise. An exercise challenge test is often performed if the patient reports shortness of air or dyspnea with exertion. A 15% or greater decrease in forced expiratory volume in 1 second (FEV$_1$) after exercise indicates a positive exercise challenge test result and increased airway hyperresponsiveness (*ie*, exercise-induced asthma). FEF—forced expiratory flow; FVC—forced vital capacity.

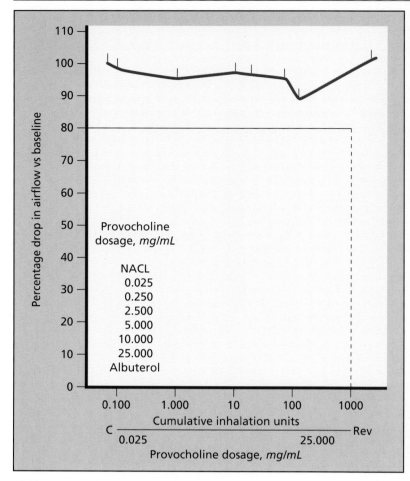

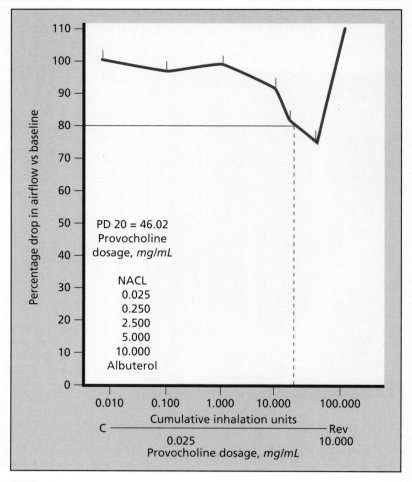

■ Figure 17-18.

Normal bronchoprovocation challenge test result. Sodium chloride is administered as a control before the challenge agent and used as a baseline. The *vertical axis* plots the percentage decrease in airflow FEV_1 (forced expiratory volume in 1 second) compared with baseline. The *horizontal axis* represents the cumulative inhalation units (CIU) as well as the actual drug dosages in micromoles (mg/mL). The CIU represents the cumulative dose administered throughout the test. The *hash marks* on the tracing plot the drop in FEV_1 compared with baseline at each provocative dose. The provocative doses used throughout the test are shown. The PC_{20} measures the provocative concentration that induces a 20% decrease in FEV_1.

■ Figure 17-19.

Methacholine challenge testing. The effect of an inhaled provocative agent (methacholine) on nonspecific airway responsiveness is tested. The PC_{20} is less than 8 mg/mL in patients with asthma and greater than 10 mg/mL in healthy individuals. The PC_{20} in this individual is between 5 and 10 mg/mL, indicating increased airway responsiveness. The Childhood Asthma Management Program (CAMP) demonstrated a positive correlation between increasing airway responsiveness and disease severity in children with mild to moderate asthma [11].

A. Normal Pulmonary Function Tests

Function	Predicted, %	Pre-drug Measured*	Predicted, %	Post-drug Measured*	Predicted, %	Change, %
FVC, L	1.33	1.26	94	1.34	100	6
FEV_1, L	1.18	1.05	89	1.13	96	8
FEV_1/FVC, L	0.86	0.83	97	0.84	98	1
PEFR	2.78	2.42	87	2.70	97	12
$FEF_{25\%-75\%}$ L	1.57	0.99	63	1.14	73	15
$FEF_{75\%-80\%}$ L/s		0.73		0.45		22
EXP test time, s		2.40		2.37		-1

Pre–: First-time testing, variable efforts, much coaching required
Post–: Maximum point effort, reproducible tests

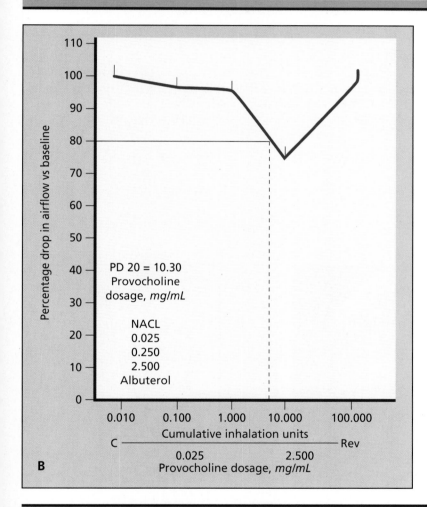

B

■ Figure 17-20.

A, Normal pulmonary function test. A 5-year-old child presented with a history of chronic cough. Methacholine challenge test was performed to determine the degree of airway hyper-responsiveness. **B,** Positive methacholine challenge test result for the patient in **A**. A 20% decrease in FEV_1 (forced expiratory volume in 1 second) at a provocative concentration (PC_{20}) of methacholine less than 2.5 mg/mL demonstrates increased airway hyperresponsiveness and underlying asthma. **C,** Pulmonary function tests in the same 5-year-old child. The patient presents during an acute exacerbation of his asthma with constant coughing. The pulmonary function tests show a severe obstructive pattern with a significant response to bronchodilators. He was admitted to the hospital. His FEV_1 improved to 69% predicted after 2 days of treatment with intravenous steroids and nebulized bronchodilators. FEF—forced expiratory flow; FVC—forced vital capacity; PEFR—peak expiratory flow rate.

C. Pulmonary Function Tests in a Child with Chronic Cough

Function	Predicted, %	Prebronchodilator Actual	Predicted, %	Postbronchodilator Actual	Predicted, %	Change, %
FEV, L	1.37	0.47	34	0.56	41	19
FEV, L	1.21	0.32	27	0.42	35	31
FEV_1/FVC, %	0.86	0.68	79	0.76	88	12
PEFR, L/s	2.87	0.71	25	0.85	30	20
$FEF_{25\%-75\%}$ L/s	1.60	0.21	13	0.35	22	67

Infant Pulmonary Function Tests

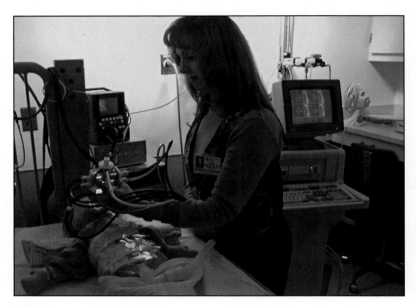

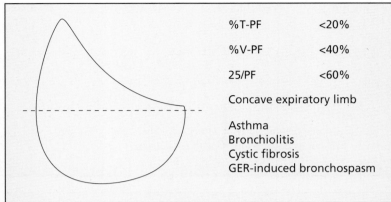

Figure 17-22.

Flow-volume loop with obstructive pattern. The ratio of the terminal to the peak expiratory flow at 25% of the previous expiration (FEF_{25}/PFEF) is measured at tidal breathing and with forced expiration. The normal values for FEF_{25}/PFEF are greater than 0.6.

Figure 17-21.

Infant pulmonary function testing. Airflow is measured at tidal breathing and a flow-volume curve is produced. Total pulmonary compliance and airway resistance are measured. The patient is wrapped in a Velcro jacket, and airflow is measured with forced exhalation using the "hugger technique" [19]. The normal shape of the flow-volume loop is oval.

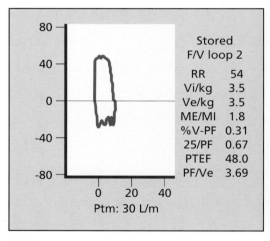

Figure 17-23.

Severe extrathoracic upper airway obstruction (UAO). The inspiratory limb of the flow-volume loop is truncated, suggesting an extrathoracic airway obstruction such as that seen with laryngomalacia, vocal cord paresis, laryngeal web or cyst, and subglottic stenosis or web. The mid-expiratory to mid-inspiratory flow (ME/MI) ratio is greater than 1.4.

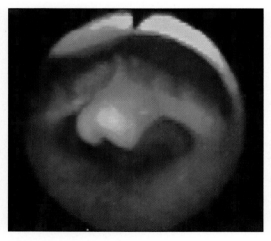

Figure 17-24.

Severe laryngomalacia. A flexible laryngoscopy was performed to evaluate the upper airway for other possible congenital airway lesions. A floppy epiglottis collapsing to the posterior pharynx is observed confirming the diagnosis of laryngomalacia. Treatment is supportive, and the condition improves by 12 to 24 months of age as the cartilage matures.

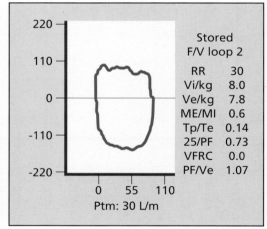

Figure 17-25.

Intrathoracic upper airway obstruction (UAO) versus nasal obstruction. Intrathoracic UAO results in expiratory wheezing or stridor. The flow-volume curve shows truncation of the expiratory limb, suggesting possible intrathoracic UAO. The mid-expiratory to mid-inspiratory flow (ME/MI) ratio is less than 0.65. The differential diagnosis includes tracheomalacia, intraluminal masses, vascular rings, or extrinsic compression. An upper gastrointestinal series aids in the diagnosis.

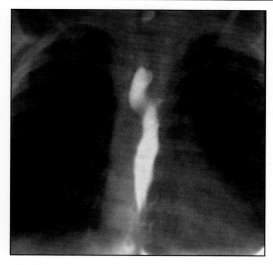

■ Figure 17-26.

Barium esophogram showing the anatomy of the esophagus and trachea. Posterior compression of the barium column suggests a vascular ring, which is confirmed on a magnetic resonance image of the chest. Treatment is surgical correction of the vascular ring.

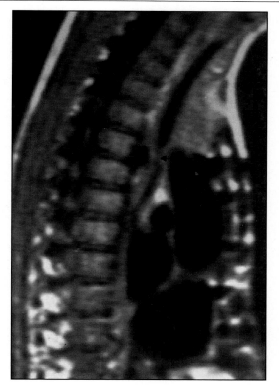

■ Figure 17-27.

Vascular ring encircling the trachea. A magnetic resonance image of the chest confirms a vascular ring that is causing compression of the trachea.

References

1. American Thoracic Society: Lung function testing: selection of reference values and interpretive strategies. *Am Rev Respir Dis* 1991, 144:1202–1218.

2. Enright PL, Linn WS, Avol EL, *et al.*: Quality of spirometry test performance in children and adolescents: experience in a large field study. *Chest* 2000, 118:665–671.

3. Schünemann HJ, Dorn J, Grant BJ, *et al.*: Pulmonary function is a long-term predictor of mortality in the general population: 29-year follow-up of the Buffalo health study. *Chest* 2000, 118:656–664.

4. West JB: *Respiratory Physiology: The Essentials*, edn 5. Edited by Coryell PA. Baltimore: Williams & Wilkins; 1995.

5. Cherniack RM. *Pulmonary Function Testing*, edn 2. Edited by Biello LA. Philadelphia: WB Saunders; 1992.

6. Voter KZ, McBride JT: Pulmonary function testing in childhood asthma. *Immunol Allerg Clin North Am* 1998, 18:133–147.

7. Eid N, Yandell B, Howell L, *et al.*: Can peak expiratory flow predict airflow obstruction in children with asthma? *Pediatrics* 2000, 105:354–358.

8. Alberts WM, Ferris MC, Brooks SM, Goldman AL: The $FEF_{25-75\%}$ and the clinical diagnosis of asthma. *Ann Allergy Asthma Immunol* 1994, 73:332–225.

9. Vedantam R, Lenke LG, Bridwell KH, *et al.*: A prospective evaluation of pulmonary function in patients with adolescent idiopathic scoliosis relative to the surgical approach used for spinal arthrodesis. *Spine* 2000, 25:82–90.

10. Fanfulla F, Pedrazzoli P, Da Prada GA, *et al.*: Pulmonary function and complications following chemotherapy and stem cell support in breast cancer. *Eur Respir J* 2000, 15:56–61.

11. Weiss ST, Van Natta ML, Zeiger RS for the Childhood Asthma Management Program Research Group: Relationship between increased airway responsiveness and asthma severity in the childhood asthma management program. *Am J Respir Crit Care Med* 2000, 162:50–56.

12. Ownby DR, Peterson EL, Johnson CJ: Factors related to methacholine airway responsiveness in children. *Am J Respir Crit Care Med* 2000, 161:1578–1583.

13. Xuan W, Peat JK, Toelle B, *et al.*: Lung function growth and its relation to airway hyperresponsiveness and recent wheeze. *Am J Respir Crit Care Med* 2000, 161:1820–1824.

14. Pratter MR, Bartier TC, Dubois J: Bronchodilator reversal of bronchospasm and symptoms incurred during methacholine bronchoprovocation challenge: documentation of safety and time course. *Chest* 1993, 104:1342–1345.

15. Avital A, Godfrey S, Springer C: Exercise, methacholine, and adenosine 5-monophosphate challenges in children with asthma: relation to severity of the disease. *Pediatr Pulmonol* 2000, 30:207–214.

16. Martinez FD, Wright AL, Taussig LM, *et al.*, and the Group Health Medical Associates: Asthma and wheezing in the first six years of life. *N Engl J Med* 1995, 332:133–138.

17. Martinez FD, Morgan WJ, Wright AL, *et al.*, and the Group Health Medical Associates Personnel: Diminished lung function as a predisposing factor for respiratory illness in infants. *N Engl J Med* 1988, 1112–1117.

18. Dezateux C, Stocks J, Fletcher ME: Impaired airway function and wheezing in infancy. *Am J Respir Crit Care Med* 1999, 159:403–410.

19. Sheikh S, Goldsmith LJ, Howell L, *et al.*: Comparison of lung function in infants exposed to maternal smoking and in infants with a family history of asthma. *Chest* 1999, 116:52–58.

20. Kavvadia V, Grenough A, Dimitriou G: Early prediction of chronic oxygen dependency by lung function test results. *Pediatr Pulmonol* 2000, 29:19–26.

21. Jones M, Castile R, Davis S, *et al.*: Forced expiratory flows and volumes in infants: normative data and lung growth. *Am J Respir Crit Care Med* 2000, 161:353–359.

22. Filippone M, Narne S, Pettenazzo A, *et al.*: Functional approach to infants and young children with noisy breathing. *Am J Respir Crit Care Med* 2000, 162:1795–1800.

23. Kapoor S, Kurtland G, Tunnessen WW: Recurrent, severe wheezing in a 17-year-old: seeking a new chord. *Contemporary Ped* 2000, 17:27–36.

18

Allergen Immunotherapy

Rosa Codina and Richard F. Lockey

Many studies suggest that exposure to indoor allergens is an important factor in the increased incidence and prevalence of allergic diseases in developed countries. The average person in these countries spends more than 90% of their time indoors and, in comparison to outdoor seasonal allergens, the concentration of most indoor allergens is greater and exposure more prolonged.

Many different allergens are present indoors. Evidence for a dose-response relationship between exposure and sensitization has been described for both dust mites and other allergens. Sensitization to allergens derived from the mites, *Dermatophagoides* spp, German cockroach (*Blattella germanica*), American cockroach (*Periplaneta americana*), rat (*Rattus norvegicus*), and mouse (*Mus musculus*) is commonly associated with asthma in North American cities [1]. However, cats and/or dogs are the most important sources of indoor allergens in northern Scandinavia and in US mountain states [2,3]. In Arizona and central Australia, *Alternaria*, an outdoor mold, is the primary allergen associated with asthma [4,5]. Sensitization to mite, cat, cockroach or *Alternaria* allergens has been associated with severe asthma in adults and children seen in various clinics or emergency departments in the United States [6].

Sensitization to grass and ragweed pollen allergens has also been associated with asthma exacerbations necessitating emergency treatment [7]. However, in population studies using multiple regression analysis, sensitization to grass, ragweed, or tree pollen has not been shown to be an independent risk factor for asthma [8]. Platts-Mills *et al.* [1] described in detail the characteristics of the main indoor allergens with the World Health Organization and International Unit of Immunology Societies.

Allergen immunotherapy is an effective treatment for allergic rhinoconjunctivitis and allergic asthma and is the only treatment available for venom hypersensitivity. Such therapy is indicated only for patients with demonstrated sensitivity to clinically relevant allergens. Knowledge of the aeroallergens in a given area and their cross-reactivity is necessary in the design of an immunotherapy protocol. Optimal doses of allergen immunotherapy are necessary for successful immunotherapy, and allergen immunotherapy is a relatively safe therapeutic modality with systemic reactions occurring in approximately 1/200 injections. Identification of patients at risk for systemic reactions is an essential component of patient evaluation. Adequate waiting time should be ensured for all patients undergoing immunotherapy.

Vaccines

Allergen Vaccines Used in the United States

Type of Vaccine	Scientific Name
Dust mites	*Dermatophagoides pteronyssinus*
	Dermatophagoides farinae
Epithelia	
Cat	*Felis domesticus*
Dog	*Canis familiaris*
Hymenoptera venoms	
Honey bee	*Apis mellifera*
Wasps	*Polistes* spp
Hornets	*Vespa* spp, *Dolichovespula* spp
Yellow jackets	*Vespula* spp
Fire ants	*Solenopsis* spp
Weeds	
Ragweed	*Ambrosia* spp
Plantain	*Plantago* spp
Mugwort	*Artemisia* spp
Pigweed	*Amaranthus* spp
Lambs quarter	*Chenopodium* spp
Grasses	
Rye	*Lolium* spp
Blue	*Poa* spp
Fescue	*Festuca* spp
Orchard	*Dactylis* spp
Sweet vernal	*Anthoxanthum* spp
Bermuda	*Cynodon* spp
Bahia	*Papalum* spp
Johnson	*Sorghum* spp
Trees	
Birch	*Betula* spp
Oak	*Quercus* spp
Cedar	*Juniperus* spp
Olive	*Olea* spp
Molds	*Alternaria* spp
	Cladosporium spp
	Aspergillus spp
	Penicillium spp
Foods	
Cod fish	*Gadus* spp
Shrimp	*Penaeus* spp
Peanut	*Arachis hypogaea*

Figure 18-1.

Allergen vaccines used in the United States. Allergen immunotherapy is now used to treat allergic rhinoconjunctivitis, allergic asthma, and insect hypersensitivity. The aim of such therapy is to decrease sensitivity to allergens by the gradual administration of increasing doses of allergen vaccines. The World Health Organization position paper, titled "Allergen Immunotherapy: Therapeutic Vaccines for Allergic Diseases" [9], was so named to indicate that allergen vaccines, which were previously referred to as allergen extracts, modify or downregulate the immune response that causes allergic diseases. The term *diagnostic allergen vaccine* replaces that of *allergen extract*. The new term refers to diagnostic testing with allergens and therapeutic allergen vaccine.

During the first half of the century, efficacy of allergen immunotherapy was based primarily on clinical observations. However, during the past 40 or more years, scientific investigations of allergens and of the immunologic complexities of the allergic reaction have improved the understanding of allergen immunotherapy with allergens derived from pollen, mammals, dust mites, molds, and insects. It is now clear that immunotherapy modifies the immune reaction that causes allergic diseases.

Mite and Insect Allergens

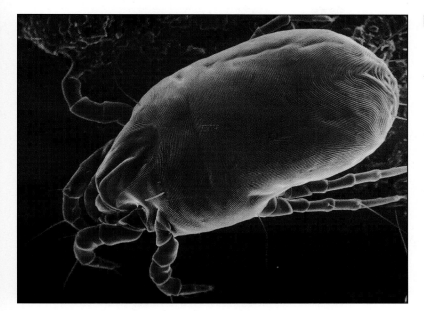

Figure 18-2.

Dermatophagoides farinae. The most common mites found in house dust are *Dermatophagoides farinae* and *Dermatophagoide pteronyssinus.* They belong to the family Pyrogliphydae and are known as "house dust mites." However, storage mites such as species of the family Glyciphagidae or predator mites from the family Cheyletidae are also present in house dust. All mites present in house dust are potential sensitizers and are thus considered as "domestic mites." For the production of allergen vaccines, mites are grown in pure mite cultures. Source materials are either pure mite bodies or whole mite cultures. Whole-mite cultures contain the different stages of the mite biologic cycle and fecal pellets, to which mite allergic subjects are exposed under natural conditions. However, they contain contaminants from the culture medium. Both types of allergen vaccines have similar clinical effects [10].

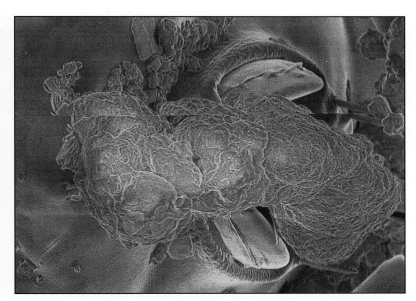

Figure 18-3.

Mite fecal pellet. Thirteen different groups of mite allergens have been identified. Mite allergens are present in mite bodies and fecal pellets. Mite fecal pellets are rich in group 1 (Der p1 + Der f1) allergens. With dust mites, a level of 2 µg/g of group 1 allergens per gram of dust and/or 100 mites per gram of dust is a risk factor for sensitization in genetically predisposed individuals. However, some investigators hypothesize that the threshold level for sensitization may be lower than 2 µg/g of dust of group 1 and that there is not a "safe," maximum level of exposure for some susceptible individuals. Ten µg/g of group 1 allergens per gram of dust and/or 500 mites per gram of dust are associated with asthma symptoms in dust mite–sensitive individuals. However, lower levels may also cause symptoms [1].

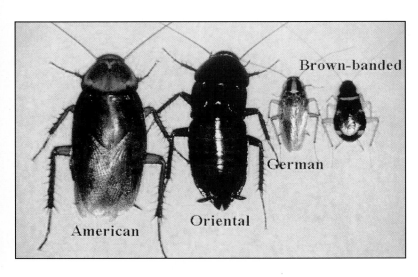

Figure 18-4.

Indoor cockroaches. More than 4000 different cockroach species exist worldwide, but only eight of these species have been found indoors. The German cockroach (*Blattella germanica*) and American cockroach (*Periplaneta americana*) are the most common species found in the United States. Other species found indoors are the oriental cockroach (*Blatta orientalis*) and the brown-banded cockroach (*Supella longipalpa*). Common allergens from cockroaches are Bla g1 and Bla g2 from *B. germanica* and Per a 1 from *P. americana.* Threshold levels of cockroach allergens to cause sensitization and symptoms are controversial. However, 2 U Bla g2 (≈ 80 ng) per gram of dust and 8 U Bla g2 (≈ 320 ng) per gram of dust have been associated with sensitization and symptoms, respectively [1]. (*Courtesy of* Dr. Clyde Ogg, University of Nebraska).

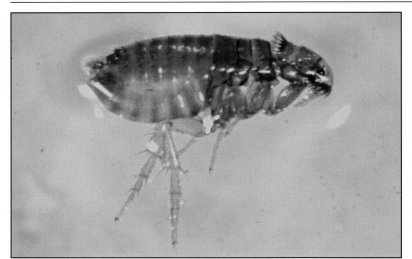

■ Figure 18-5.

Cat flea. There are at least 2400 known flea species, but fewer than 20 of these bite humans. Cat and dog fleas are found in homes, and it has been suggested that cat flea (*Ctenocephalides felis felis*) allergens may contribute to the allergenicity of house dust in areas with a heavy flea infestation [11]. Therefore, they could be important indoor allergens in households with mammalian pets. (*Courtesy of* the US Department of Agriculture.)

Mammal Allergens

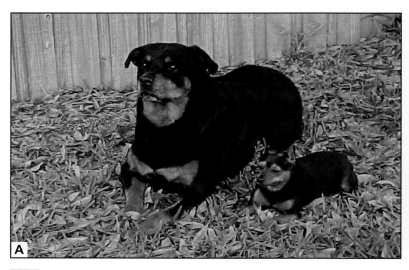

A

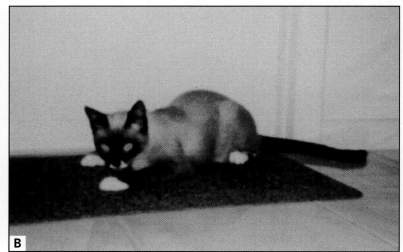

B

■ Figure 18-6.

Dogs (**A**) and cat (**B**). These animals are not only common pets, they are also known sources of indoor allergens. Other mammals, such as rats, mice, and ferrets are mainly associated with occupational allergy, but they are also kept as pets and their allergens are present in house dust. In fact, probably all mammals contain allergens, and exposure, however it occurs, is the key factor for sensitization and the development of allergies.

The most important allergens from dogs (*Canis familiaris*), Can f1, and from cats (*Felis domesticus*), Fel d1, are present in serum, hair, dander, pelt, and saliva. Albumin is another dog and cat allergen that is responsible for cross-reactivity among different mammal species. Although the presence of dog and cat breed-specific allergens has been extensively discussed, there is no evidence that supports this and all breeds of dogs or cats should be considered equivalent sensitizers. However, the production of Fel d1 is under hormonal control, and its synthesis is higher in male cats than in female cats. The threshold levels of cat allergens to cause sensitization and symptoms are controversial. However, 2 µg Fel d1per gram of dust and 8 µg Fel d1 per gram of dust have been associated with sensitization and symptoms, respectively [1]. Threshold levels of dog allergens to cause sensitization and symptoms are unknown, but they are probably similar to cat allergen. Dander is the optimal source material, and allergen vaccines are prepared from a mixture of at least five different breeds of either animal; the same combination of breeds should be used from batch to batch of allergen vaccine [10].

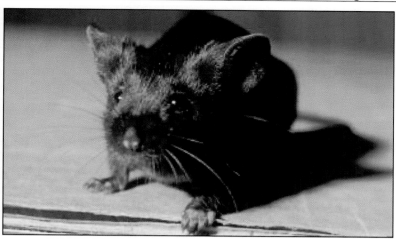

■ Figure 18-7.

Mouse. Rodent allergens are occupational sensitizers. However, rat (*Rattus norvegicus*) and mouse (*Mus musculus*) allergens are associated with asthma in inner cities, and because rodents are also domestic pets, they should be considered potential sources of indoor allergens. Rodents have permanent proteinuria, and several urinary proteins are inhaled by humans. From the mouse, two major allergens have been identified, Mus m1, which is prealbumin and Mus m2, a glycoprotein. The major allergens from rat are Rat n1 and Rat n2, and a third allergen, Rat n3 with a MW of 200 K, has been described. Two major allergens, Cav p1 and Cav p2, have been described in guinea pig (*Cavia porcellus*); they are present in urine and pelt. The major allergen from rabbit (*Oryctolagus cuniculus*), Ory c1, is present in saliva and fur, and in urine in low concentrations [12]. (*Courtesy of* Eric Jukes, from the London and Southern Counties Mouse and Rat Club.)

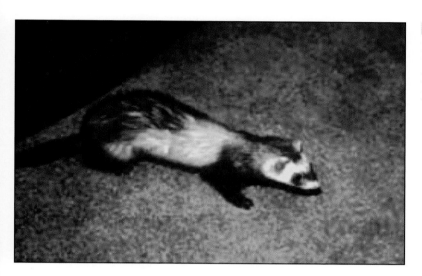

■ Figure 18-8.

Ferret. Sensitization to mammals from the carnivora order has been described as a cause of occupational sensitization [13,14]. However, ferrets (*Mustela putorius furo*) are also kept in homes as pets and may cause sensitization in pet ferret owners [15].

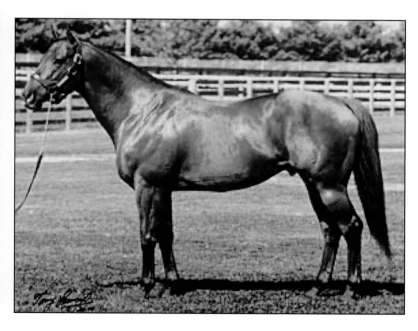

■ Figure 18-9.

Horse. Cows (*Bos domesticus*) and horses (*Equus caballus*) are common causes of occupational sensitization in rural populations. The major allergens from cow are Bos d1, Bos d2, Bos d3; from horse, Equ c1, Equ c2, Equ c3 [12].

Fire Ant and Hymenoptera Allergens

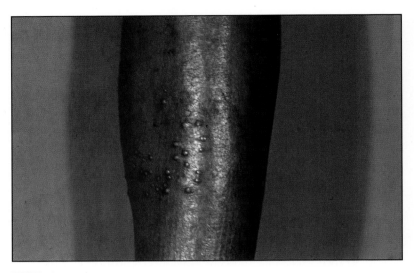

Figure 18-10.

Fire ant pustula. Fire ants belong to the genus *Solenopsis*. *Solenopsis invicta* and *Solenopsis richteri* were introduced to the United States from South America, and they are referred as "imported" fire ants. These two species are more aggressive than the native fire ants, *Solenopsis xyloni* and *Solenopsis aurea*. Fire ant stings are common in the southeastern United States. Fire ant venoms contain alkaloids with hemolytic, bactericidal, insecticidal, and cytotoxic properties; thus the sting causes a sterile pustula at the sting site. Fire ant whole-body vaccine contains 31 antigenic components, 21 of which are also present in fire ant venom. Whole-body vaccines are also used for skin testing. The efficacy of fire ant whole-body vaccine for immunotherapy has not been yet proved in double-blind control studies [17].Hymenoptera venoms are known sources of potent allergens.

Although many Hymenoptera insects are capable of stinging, only species from the families Apidae (bees), Vespidae (wasps, hornets, and yellowjackets), and Formicidae (ants) sting people frequently. All Hymenoptera venoms contain the allergens hyaluronidase and phospholipase, which have enzymatic activity; Apidae, Vespidae, and Formicidae contain unique allergens as well as homologous allergens with some degree of cross-reactivity. Hymenoptera-allergic subjects often are sensitive to several venom allergens, which can be caused by exposure to different insects or to cross-reactivity among different venoms. Such information influences the choice of venoms for immunotherapy [16].

Outdoor Allergens

Outdoor Allergen Cross-Reactivity

Trees
    Cedar, juniper, cypress
    Birch, alder, hazelnut
    Oak species
    Walnut, pecan, hickory
    Olive, ash, privet
Weeds
    Ragweed spp
    Sages, mugworts
    Chenopodium, amaranth
Grasses
    Timothy, June, rye, orchard, fescue, Bermuda, blue, salt

Figure 18-11.

Outdoor allergen cross-reactivity. In 1990, Curtis reported that injections of certain pollen extracts appear to benefit subjects with rhinitis and/or asthma.

Immunologic Mechanisms

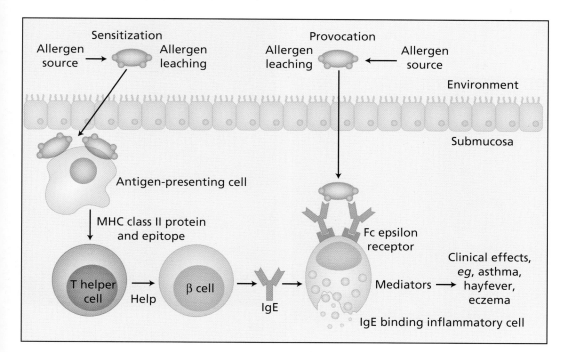

Figure 18-12.

Immunologic mechanisms involved in allergic disease. Allergic inflammation is characterized by IgE-dependent activation of mast cells, basophils, and eosinophils. It is also characterized by imbalance in the CD4+ T helper-1 and T helper-2 cells. These two types of CD4+ cells promote inflammatory responses with different characteristics that oppose each other. Allergic inflammation is associated with upregulated production of T helper-2 cytokines, such as interleukin (IL)-4, IL-5, and IL-13. Il-4 and IL-13 mediate IgE heavy chain isotype switching, whereas IL-5 is a selective growth factor for terminal differentiation and activation of eosinophils and their retention in tissues.

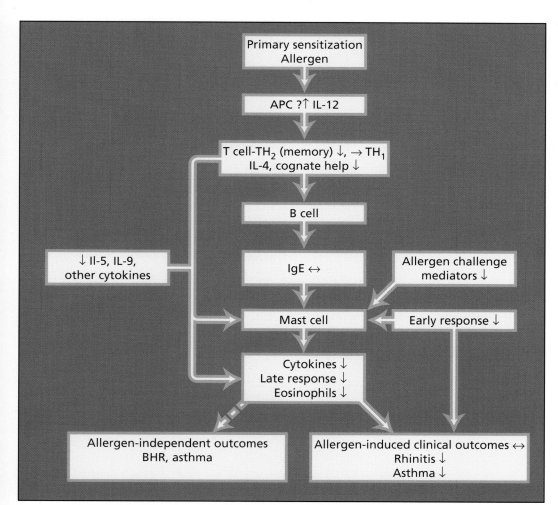

Figure 18-13.

Pathways of allergic sensitization and responses to allergen challenge. Allergen immunotherapy results in upregulated Th (T helper)-1 and downregulated Th-2 responses. Skin and nose responses of allergic individuals treated with allergen immunotherapy and submitted to allergen provocation showed increased interferon-gamma (a typical cytokine of the Th-1 response) levels. Furthermore, the same study showed an overall decrease in all CD4+ cells. Other results of allergen immunotherapy include increased production of CD8+ (suppressor) cells and increased production of interferon-gamma responding cells.

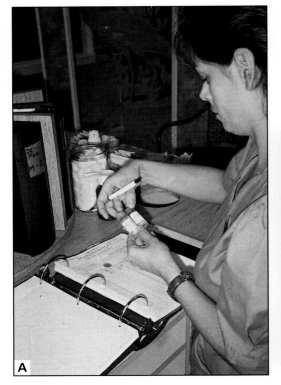

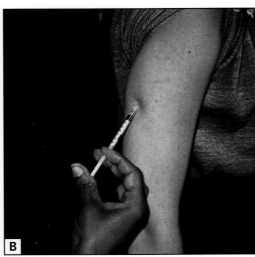

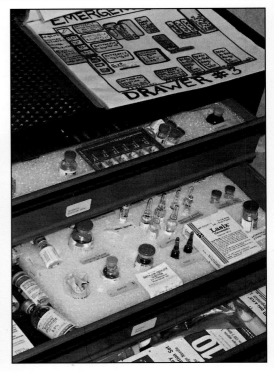

■ Figure 18-14.

Administration of allergens. **A,** Immunotherapy vaccines are individually prepared for the patient by the allergist-immunologist. The maintenance of full-strength vaccine is diluted by serial 10-fold dilutions for the build-up phase. Prior to receiving the first injection, patients should sign a consent form, which outlines the risks and benefits of allergen immunotherapy.

Physicians administering allergen immunotherapy are responsible for assuring that the injection is given correctly. First, the vials of vaccine should be checked to assure that the patient is receiving the correct vaccine. Second, the patient should be asked whether or not there have been any problems associated with the prior dose of vaccine and the healthcare professional should make sure that the appropriate dose is administered.

B, The first injection of allergen immunotherapy, usually 0.05 or 0.1 mL, is withdrawn into a 1-cc syringe with a 27- or 28-gauge needle from the most dilute vaccine vial of the build-up series. Some allergists/immunologists perform an intradermal skin test from the dilute vaccine using a 10 mm or smaller diameter wheal as the cut-off for administering the appropriate dilutions for the initial injection. Initial doses of vaccine are administered one to two times a week, spaced at least 2 days apart during the build-up schedule. The patient's maintenance dose is thereafter administered every 1 to 2 weeks until clinical improvement is noted, and thereafter, the interval between injection visits can be increased to every 3 to 4 weeks. An every 4-week schedule is recommended for inhalant allergen immunotherapy contingent on the maintenance of clinical improvement. The appropriate amount of vaccine should be carefully withdrawn from the vial and given subcutaneously in the middle half of the posterior lateral part of the arm.

■ Figure 18-15.

Emergency treatment cart. An emergency treatment cart should be available containing the following equipment and reagents: stethoscope and sphygmomanometer; tourniquets, syringes, hypodermic needles, and large-bore (14-gauge) needles; aqueous epinephrine HCl 1:1000; equipment for administering oxygen; equipment for administering intravenous fluids; oral airway; antihistamine for injection; corticosteroids for intravenous injection; vasopressor. All the emergency equipment required for clinics where allergen immunotherapy is administered is included in this cart. In addition, other medications that could be used to treat anaphylaxis or other emergencies are also included. The medications included in the cart should be catalogued and checked at least once every 3 months.

Risk Factors for Life-threatening Systemic Reactions or Fatalities

Errors in dosing

Presence of symptomatic asthma

A seasonal exacerbation of allergic rhinoconjunctivitis, particularly asthma

A high degree of skin or in vitro test sensitivity

During the initial build-up period, particularly with accelerated or "rush" schedules of immunotherapy

High-dose maintenance regimens in highly sensitive allergic subjects

Concomitant use of β-blocker drugs for the treatment of hypertension, cardiac disorders, or migraine prophylaxis

Injection from new vials

Figure 18-16.

Risk factors for life-threatening systemic reactions or fatalities.

Relative Contraindications for Immunotherapy

Serious immunopathologic and immunodeficiency diseases

Malignancy

Severe psychologic disorders

Treatment with β-blockers, even when administered topically

Poor compliance

Severe asthma uncontrolled by pharmacotherapy and/or irreversible airways obstruction (FEV$_1$ consistently under 70% of predicted after adequate pharmacologic treatment) except for Hymenoptera venom hypersensitivity

Significant cardiovascular diseases that increase the risk of side effects from epinephrine, except for Hymenoptera venom hypersensitivity

Children under 5 y of age, except for Hymenoptera venom hypersensitivity

Figure 18-17.

Relative contraindications for immunotherapy.

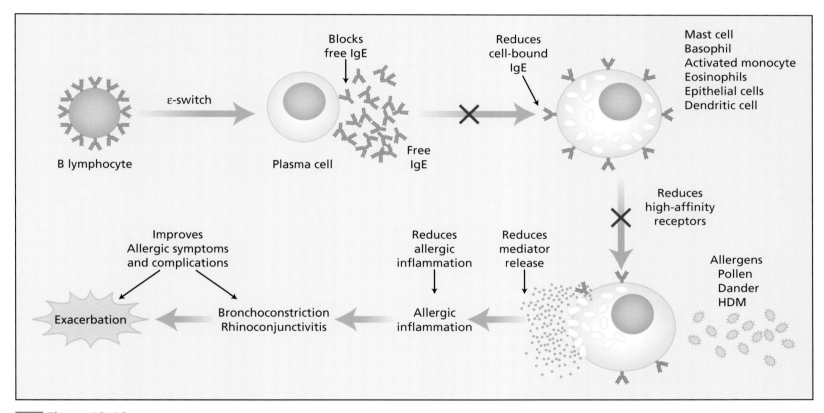

Figure 18-18.

Anti-IgE therapy. Before the therapy, IgE has circulating and anchored moieties in constant interchange, through which the immune system equips mast cells with the means of degranulating in response to cross-bridging by allergens. Anti-IgE binds to IgE at the site the immunoglobulin could otherwise use to anchor itself.

After about 4 months of monthly injections, circulating IgE has been depleted, and any IgE leaving a mast cell surface is likely to be cleared before it can re anchor itself anywhere. Mast cell expression of IgE receptors appears to decline proportionately.

References

1. Platts-Mills T, Vervloet D, Thomas W, *et al.*: Indoor allergens and asthma: report of the third international workshop. *J Allergy Clin Immunol* 1997, 100:S1–S24.

2. Sporik R, Ingram J, Price W, *et al.*: Association of asthma with serum IgE and skin test reactivity to allergens among children living at high altitude: tickling the dragon's breath. *Am J Respir Crit Care Med* 1995, 151:1388–1392.

3. Munir A, Bjorksten B, Einarsson R, *et al.*: Cat (Fel d1), dog (Can f1) and cockroach allergens in homes of asthmatic children from three climatic zones in Sweden. *Allergy* 1994, 49:508–516.

4. Peat L, Tovey C, Mellis C, *et al.*: Importance of house dust mite and *Alternaria* allergens in childhood asthma: an epidemiological study in two climatic regions of Australia. *Clin Exp Allergy* 1993, 23:812–820.

5. Halonen M, Stern D, Wright A, *et al.*: Alternaria as a major allergen for asthma in a desert environment. *Am J Respir Crit Care Med* 1997, 155:1356–1361.

6. Nelson R, DiNicolo R, Fernandez-Caldas E, *et al.*: Allergen-specific IgE levels and mite allergen exposure in children with acute asthma first seen in an emergency department and in nonasthmatic control subjects. *J Allergy Clin Immunol* 1996, 98:258–263.

7. Gelber L, Seltzer L, Bouzoukis J, *et al.*: Sensitization and exposure to indoor allergens as risk factors for asthma among patients presenting to hospital. *Am Rev Respir Dis* 1993, 147:573–578.

8. Holgate S: Asthma and allergy, disorders of civilization? *Q J Med* 1998, 91:171–184.

9. Bousquet J, Lockey RF, Malling HJ, eds.: World Health Organization position paper. Allergen immunotherapy: therapeutic vaccines for allergic diseases. *Allergy* 1998, 44:1–42.

10. Larsen JN, Wikborg T, Lombardero M, Lowenstein H: Manufacturing and standardizing allergen vaccines. In *Allergens and Allergen Immunotherapy*, edn 2. Edited by Lockey RF, Bukantz SC. New York: Marcel Dekker; 1999.

11. Trudeau WL, Fernandez-Caldas E, Fox RW, *et al.*: Allergenicity of the cat flea (*Ctenocephalides felis felis*). *Clin Exp Allergy* 1992, 23:377–383.

12. Ipsen H, Larsen JN, Niemeijer NR, *et al.*: Allergenic extracts. In *Allergy: Principles and Practice*, edn 5. Edited by Middleton E, Reed CE, Ellis EF, *et al.* St. Louis: Mosby.

13. Jiménez I, Antón E, Picans I, *et al.*: Occupational asthma caused by mink urine. *Allergy* 1996, 51:364–365.

14. Savolainen J, Vitti J, Halmepuro L, Nordman H: IgE response to fur animal allergens and domestic animal allergens in fur farmers and fur garment workers. *Clin Exp Allergy* 1997, 27:501–509.

15. Codina R, Reichmuth D, Lockey RF, Jaen C: Ferret allergy. *J Allergy Clin Immunol*, 2001, 107:927.

16. Lockey RF: Allergic reactions to insect stings. In *Conn's Current Therapy*. Edited by Rakel RE. Philadelphia: WB Saunders Co.; 1998:767–770.

17. Stanaland BE, Stablein JJ, Lockey RF: Ants and human anaphylaxis. In *Monograph on Insect Allergy*, edn 3. Edited by Levine MI, Lockey RF. Pittsburgh; Dave Lambert Associates; 43–54.

18. Noon L: Prophylactic inoculation against hayfever. *Lancet* 1911, 1:1572.

19

Latex Allergy

Dennis R. Ownby

Natural rubber latex has been used in many different ways throughout history; therefore it has been regarded as a generally safe and nearly inert material. This perception changed radically in the late 1980s with the increasing awareness that latex—or, more accurately, naturally occurring proteins within latex—could cause IgE-mediated allergic reactions. Such reactions range from mild itching of the skin to fatal anaphylaxis [1,2].

In the majority of cases, the signs and symptoms provoked by latex exposure in susceptible individuals are identical to those observed in individuals who are allergic to other substances. Such symptoms include urticaria, rhinitis, conjunctivitis, and asthma, and they manifest the same whether induced by latex or other allergens [1].

This chapter illustrates some of the unique aspects of latex allergy. These include hand dermatitis (one of the most frequent presenting symptoms of persons with occupational exposure to latex gloves) and two different types of latex reactions. Also presented are some of the many medical and household products that are made from natural rubber latex.

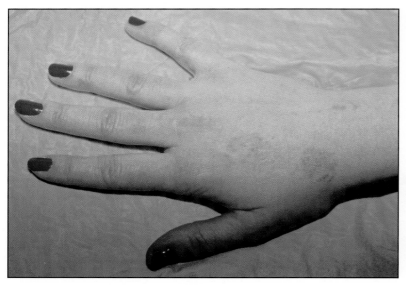

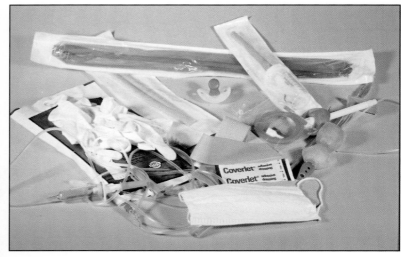

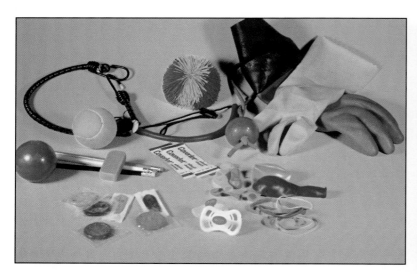

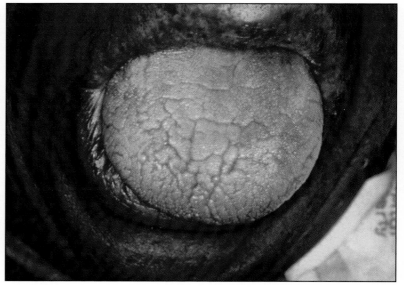

Figure 19-1.

Hand dermatitis. Many healthcare workers and others who wear latex gloves as part of their occupation may first notice itching or irritation of the hands after wearing such gloves. It is impossible by just looking at the rash illustrated here to tell the cause. The three most common diagnostic possibilities are 1) irritant dermatitis, 2) contact or type IV skin allergy, or 3) immediate or type I skin allergy (also called "contact urticaria"). In the case illustrated, in vitro and skin tests for IgE antibodies to latex were negative, as were patch tests for contact sensitivity to latex and chemicals found in rubber; thus a diagnosis of irritant dermatitis is most likely [1,3–6].

Figure 19-2.

Some of the many medical products that can contain latex or natural rubber. All products that contain or are made of highly elastic material, white to light tan in color, should be suspected of being made of natural rubber. Even when the rubber is partially covered, as in the case of the elastic bands on the facemask in the foreground, contact may lead to allergic reactions in highly sensitive individuals. This is especially true if the covering gets wet, such as with perspiration [6].

Figure 19-3.

Products commonly found in homes that contain significant amounts of latex. Although latex or natural rubber is commonly thought of in relationship to medical products, many products commonly found in homes contain significant quantities of latex. Examples include rubber bands, balloons, condoms, rubber gloves, and Koosh™ balls.

Figure 19-4.

Systemic type I allergic reactions to natural rubber can take many forms. The reaction in this patient was caused by contact with the latex balloon on a catheter used to administer a barium enema for diagnostic purposes. The reaction was limited to massive swelling of the tongue. This picture was taken several hours after the height of the reaction and after multiple doses of epinephrine and antihistamines. Note that the patient is not trying to protrude the tongue; in fact, this is a far as the patient could retract the tongue into the mouth, nearly 4 hours after the start of the reaction. The patient had no known occupational exposure to latex and did not have a history of other forms of allergic disease [7].

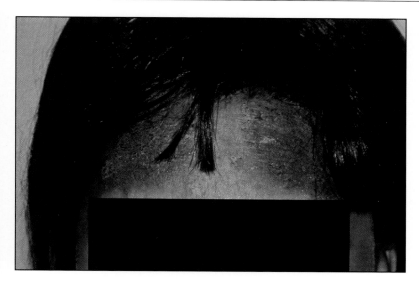

■ Figure 19-5.

Atopic dermatitis. Atopic dermatitis appears to be a risk factor for severe reactions to natural rubber. In rare patients, such as the person shown here, repeated contact with latex appeared to be a major exacerbating factor for the atopic dermatitis. This young adult had had mild atopic dermatitis from childhood that suddenly became much more symptomatic (24 months before this picture was taken). At about the same time that the atopic dermatitis flared, the patient had begun to use a latex-based glue to hold a hairpiece in place. She had a positive in vitro test for antilatex IgE antibodies, and her atopic dermatitis improved rapidly after she stopped using the hair glue. Of interest in addition to this case, a newspaper report from Great Britain described a young woman who died due to latex-related anaphylaxis brought on by the use of a latex-based hair glue [1,7].

References

1. Ownby DR: Manifestations of latex allergy. *Immunol Allergy Clin North Am* 1995, 15:31–43.

2. American College of Allergy Asthma and Immunology: Latex allergy: an emerging healthcare problem. *Ann Allergy Asthma Immunol* 1995, 75:19–21.

3. Bubak ME, Reed CE, Fransway AF, *et al.*: Allergic reactions to latex among health-care workers. *Mayo Clin Proc* 1992, 67:1075–1079.

4. Charous BL, Hamilton RG, Yunginger JW: Occupational latex exposure: characteristics of contact and systemic reactions in 47 workers. *J Allergy Clin Immunol* 1994, 94:12–18.

5. Yunginger JW: Diagnostic skin testing for natural rubber latex allergy. *J Allergy Clin Immunol* 1998, 102:351–352.

6. Cohen DE, Scheman A, Stewart L, *et al.*: American Academy of Dermatology's position paper on latex allergy. *J Am Acad Dermatol* 1998, 38:98–106.

7. Ownby DR, Tomlanovich M, Sammons N, McCullough J: Anaphylaxis associated with latex allergy during barium enema examinations. *AJR Am J Roentgenol* 1991, 156:903–908.

20

Asthma in Adults

Gnanasegaram Gnanakumaran and Stephen T. Holgate

Asthma is a major chronic disorder in adults, with an economic burden estimated to exceed that of HIV/AIDS and tuberculosis combined. The term asthma is derived from a Greek word meaning "panting." It is defined as a chronic inflammatory disease of the airways clinically characterized by recurrent episodes of wheeze, breathlessness, cough, and chest tightness. It is associated with widespread but variable airflow limitation that is at least partly reversible, either spontaneously or with treatment.

Asthma is a worldwide problem. Its prevalence varies among countries, from less than 1% to as high as 30%. In recent years the prevalence and severity of asthma is noted to be increasing. The prevalence of asthma in adults is between 5% and 10% in the industrialized countries, and about 10% of these patients have a severe disease that is not optimally treated with currently available therapies [1]. Asthma in adults can be categorized into the following three groups: 1) persistence of childhood asthma; 2) relapse of asthma during adulthood; and 3) late- or adult-onset asthma. In contrast to childhood-onset asthma, which is caused by atopy, adult-onset asthma is often associated with exposure to occupational sensitizers. Although remission is not common in adult-onset asthma, it is frequently seen in young adults, particularly those with less severe disease initially and those treated early after the onset of asthma [2]. The late-onset asthma often poses diagnostic difficulties with other chronic respiratory diseases such as chronic obstructive pulmonary disease and allergic bronchopulmonary aspergillosis.

Asthma runs in families and has a 50% to 60% heritability. The hallmark in its pathogenesis is the development of chronic airway inflammation leading to bronchial hyperresponsiveness and airway remodeling, both of which contribute toward the clinical presentation and variable phenotype. Exposure to inhalant allergen results in the activation of T lymphocytes with subsequent cascade of events leading to the release of cytokines and inflammatory mediators. The principal effector cells are eosinophils and mast cells, whereas T lymphocytes orchestrate the entire process. Other important cells involved in the inflammatory process are antigen-presenting cells, macrophages, neutrophils, and structural cells such as airway epithelial cells, endothelial cells, smooth muscle cells, and fibroblasts. Mediators such as histamine, leukotrienes, and prostaglandins produce the acute airway narrowing by bronchial smooth muscle contraction, mucosal edema, and increased mucus secretion leading to airway plugging. The inflammatory process also leads to airway remodeling, which is characterized by smooth muscle hypertrophy and hyperplasia, submucosal edema with infiltration of inflammatory cells, subepithelial fibrosis, basement membrane thickening, goblet cell hyperplasia, and disruption of the epithelial layer. It has been recognized that airway epithelial response to injury plays a major role in the pathogenesis of asthma in addition to the immunologic responses.

Asthma is often misdiagnosed because of its episodic nature and the nonspecific types of symptoms. Patients often delay seeking medical attention until their asthma restricts daily activities, *ie*, impinges on their quality of life. Diagnosis relies on a combination of a meticulous history and the objective evidence of airway lability. The latter is demonstrated by diurnal variability in peak expiratory flow (PEF) and the increase in PEF after inhalation of a bronchodilator, such as salbutamol. Presence of atopy can be shown by skin prick tests to specific allergens and serum IgE assay.

Asthma cannot be cured with currently available therapies, but it can be effectively controlled. The goal in asthma therapy is to prevent the gradual deterioration of the underlying disease, thus minimizing the chronic symptoms and preventing exacerbation. Specific pharmacotherapy and patient education to avoid the asthma triggers are key points in the management strategy. Current asthma treatment follows a graded pattern, which starts at a level appropriate to the severity of asthma and is stepped up or down by regular review. New therapeutic targets are in development with the long-term goal of achieving a cure for asthma.

Epidemiology and Etiology

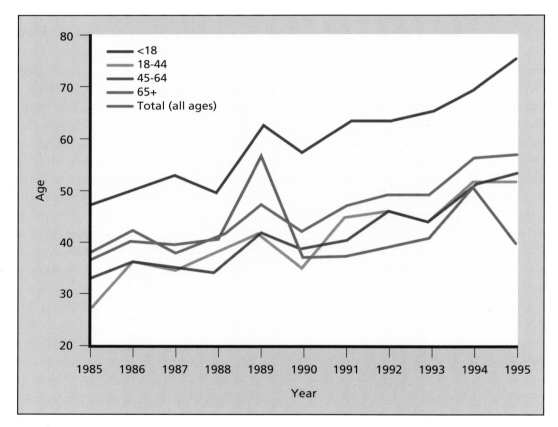

Figure 20-1.

Trends in the prevalence of asthma by age in the United States between 1985 and 1995. Worldwide, approximately 150 million people suffer from asthma. This statistic has imposed a heavy burden on health services. The prevalence of asthma is increasing in all age groups. Although some of the increase is attributable to increasing awareness of the disease by doctors and patients, it is widely accepted that the true prevalence has increased. The exact cause for this increase is not fully known, but some factors may involve early exposure to various inhalant allergens and pollutants and the fact that people now have fewer infections during childhood owing to the wide availability of antibiotics. The prevalence varies among different countries but it is difficult to compare prevalence rates because the definition of asthma varies in epidemiologic surveys. Even within a country the prevalence varies, being higher in urban than rural areas. Racial difference is noted in several countries; in the United States, a higher prevalence is noted among blacks. In adults, no difference is observed between male and female subjects. (*Data from* the Global Initiative for Asthma [http://www.ginasthma.com].)

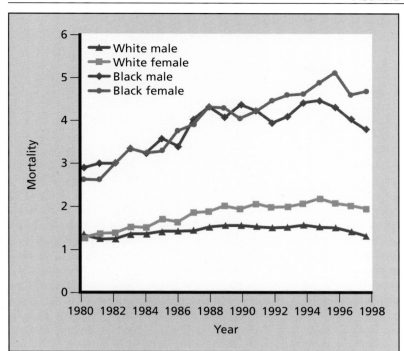

■ Figure 20-2.

Death rates for asthma by race and sex in the United States between 1980 and 1998. Since 1960, asthma mortality has been declining in most countries (except for the episodic increase noted in certain countries). However, US deaths have increased by more than 25% over the past decade; most of these deaths occurred among blacks in inner-city areas. The increase in asthma severity, reduced use of anti-inflammatory drugs, and poor compliance are some of the factors contributing to high mortality in these areas. Asthma mortality data are only available for a few countries, and such data are difficult to interpret owing to the variation in diagnostic and reporting criteria among countries. The accuracy of diagnosis on the death certificates is over 85% for patients younger than 35 years of age, but this accuracy declines with increasing age. Older patients who died from concomitant chronic obstructive pulmonary disease may have been included in asthma deaths, thus falsely increasing asthma mortality data. (*Data from* the Global Initiative for Asthma [http://www.ginasthma.com].)

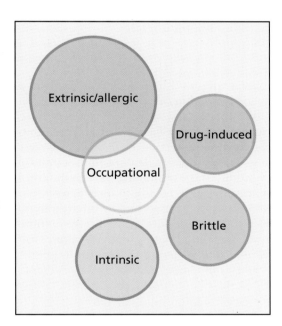

■ Figure 20-3.

Types of asthma in adults. Asthma is a clinical syndrome rather than a single disease. Therefore, grouping asthma into distinctive entities is helpful in developing appropriate management plans. Although different mechanisms are involved in the pathogenesis of the different types of asthma, all have chronic airway inflammation as the underlying abnormality. Some of these groups overlap into others. *Extrinsic or allergic asthma* forms a major portion of adult asthma, and most of the cases are of childhood onset. Late-onset asthma is often caused by sensitization to occupational agents and drugs. Aspirin and other nonsteroidal anti-inflammatory drugs are the most common causes of *drug-induced asthma*. Approximately 10% to 20% of adult asthmatic patients are sensitive to aspirin. In subjects with asthma, sinusitis, and nasal polyps, aspirin sensitivity increases to 40%. *Occupational asthma* is considered in another chapter. *Brittle asthma* is a rare type of asthma that can present in two distinctive forms. Some patients with a relatively well-controlled asthma and near-normal lung function experience sporadic severe asthma attacks. Other patients with poorly controlled asthma develop frequent severe episodes. Patients with brittle asthma are at high risk of dying from asthma. Finally, those in whom no environmental cause for asthma can be identified are considered to have *intrinsic (cryptogenic) asthma*. A higher prevalence of intrinsic asthma is noted in female patients.

Etiologic Factors in the Development of Asthma

Predisposing (host) factors
   Genetic predisposition to asthma
   Atopy
   Gender
   Race
Causative (inducing) factors
   Allergens
      House dust mites
      Pollens
      Animal dander (cat, dog)
      Mold, fungi
   Occupational sensitizers
   Aspirin and other NSAIDS
Contributing factors
   Respiratory infections
   Air pollution
   Smoking (active or passive)
   Diet
   Socioeconomic status

■ Figure 20-4.

Etiologic factors in the development of asthma. It has long been known that asthma runs in families, but the exact nature of its inheritance is not yet known. It is more likely that asthma inheritance is polygenic. Several candidate genes have been suggested for asthma and its related features (*eg*, atopy and airway hyper-responsiveness). About 50% of asthma cases are associated with atopy (the tendency to have persistent IgE-mediated responses to common allergens), which is clinically characterized by raised serum IgE levels, presence of allergen-specific IgE in serum, and positive skin-prick tests to allergens. Among the environmental factors, allergens play an important role in inducing asthma. In adult-onset asthma, occupational sensitizers play major roles in the induction of asthma. Although respiratory infections and air pollution do not directly induce asthma, they do enhance the allergens in initiating and perpetuating the disease process. There is no evidence that cigarette smoking is a risk factor for the development of asthma; however, it is associated with asthma severity and poor response to asthma treatment. NSAIDS—nonsteroidal anti-inflammatory drugs.

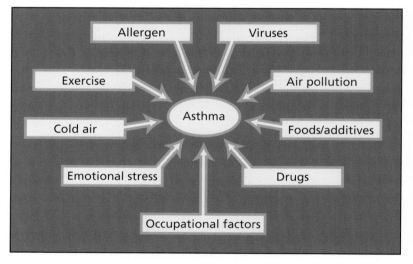

■ Figure 20-5.

Precipitating (trigger) factors in asthma. The factors shown here trigger asthma exacerbations ("attacks") by inducing inflammation or provoking acute bronchoconstriction or both. Inhaled allergens such as house dust mite, pollen, animal dander, and spores of fungi are the most common trigger factors, but ingested or injected allergens can also precipitate acute episodes. Pollens tend to cause seasonal attacks: tree pollen in spring, grass pollen in summer, and weed pollen in autumn. Cats and dogs are among the common pets known to trigger asthma attacks due to allergy to their dander, saliva, urine, and feces. Important fungi associated with asthma is *Aspergillus fumigatus*, which causes episodes mainly in late autumn and winter. Among the respiratory infections, rhinovirus is a common culprit. Exercise and associated hyperventilation can exacerbate symptoms through changes in temperature of airway mucosa and changes in osmolarity of fluid lining the airway mucosa. Drugs such as aspirin and other nonsteroidal anti-inflammatory drugs, which induce asthma development, also cause exacerbations. β-adrenergic blockers provoke bronchoconstriction in asthma patients by blocking β-receptors to endogenous catecholamines. Although asthma is not a psychosomatic disorder, emotional stress can cause exacerbation indirectly through hyperventilation.

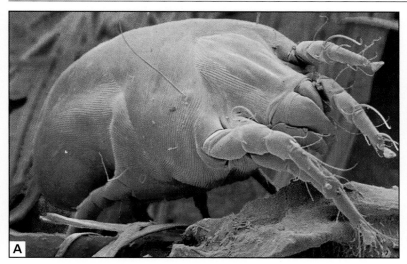

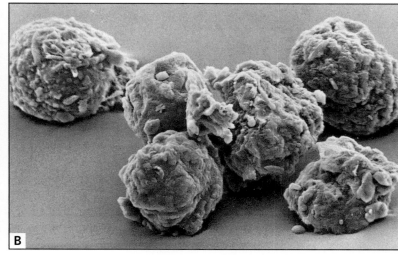

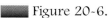 Figure 20-6.

House dust mite (HDM). In Western countries, HDMs are the most common allergen known to induce the development of asthma as well as trigger acute exacerbations. *Dermatophagoides pteronyssinus* (**A**) is the most common species; proteins in its feces (**B**), including DerP1, are the substances that induce the allergic response. These arthropods live in mattresses, soft furnishings, and carpets, and they thrive on dead human skin. They proliferate most in temperatures of 25°C and a relative humidity of 80%. Because of their ubiquitous nature and minute size, eradication is difficult but not impossible. Keeping rooms well ventilated, avoiding carpets and fabric furnishing, regular vacuuming, use of air-tight covers on mattresses and pillows, and weekly washing of bed linens in hot water are some measures to control HDMs.

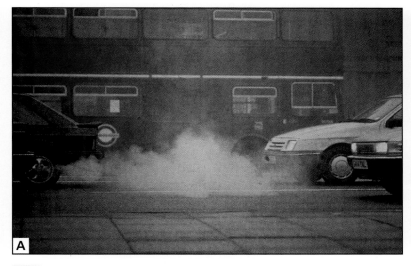

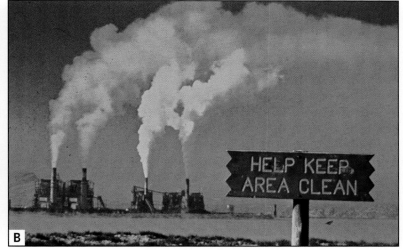

Figure 20-7.

Air pollution. Air pollution is defined as the presence of gases or particles of matter in the air that are not natural to the atmosphere at such concentrations. Although air pollution per se does not appear to increase the risk of developing asthma, it is a known trigger for asthma exacerbation, particularly in severely asthmatic patients. It is generally man-made, but could also arise from natural events such as eruption of volcanoes. Air pollution is mainly caused by combustion fuel exhaust from motor vehicles (**A**) and factory fumes (**B**). Diesel exhaust is a major source of particulate matter pollution, which also contains chemicals such as nitrogen dioxide and sulfur dioxide (SO_2), all of which trigger asthma. Diesel particles have also been shown to absorb allergens from grass pollen into their surface, thereby enhancing the antigenicity of pollen and its deposition in the lung. SO_2, nitrogen dioxide (NO_2), and ozone (O_3) are the common gaseous pollutants known to trigger asthma. (*Panel B courtesy of* Jonathan Samet, Johns Hopkins University, Baltimore.)

Pathology and Pathogenesis

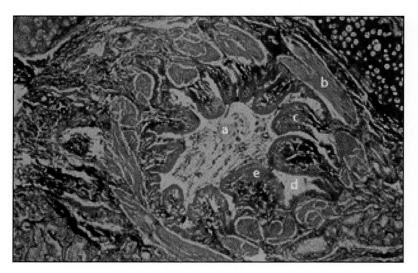

Figure 20-8.

Pathologic features of the asthmatic airway. This postmortem specimen depicts most of the characteristic features of an asthmatic airway caused by chronic inflammation. Hypertrophied and hyperplastic smooth muscle, mucosal edema, and increased mucus secretion contribute to the bronchoconstriction. Thickening of basement membrane and subepithelial fibrosis decreases the usual elasticity of the airway, leading to ineffective bronchodilation with treatment. These structural changes are collectively known as "airway remodeling." Biopsy studies have shown increased numbers of activated eosinophils, mast cells, and T lymphocytes in the airway mucosa and lumen. These changes may be present even when asthma is asymptomatic, and their extent appears to be correlated with the clinical severity of the disease [3]. a—mucus plug containing cells and debris; b—smooth muscle hypertrophy and hyperplasia; c—thickening of basement membrane and subepithelial fibrosis; d—damaged epithelium; e—hypertrophied mucous gland.

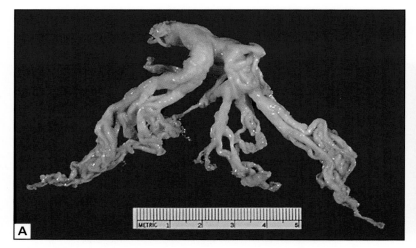

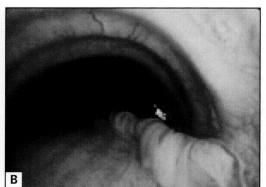

Figure 20-9.

Mucus plug. **A,** Cast of mucus plug. **B,** Bronchoscopic view showing lumen with mucus plug.

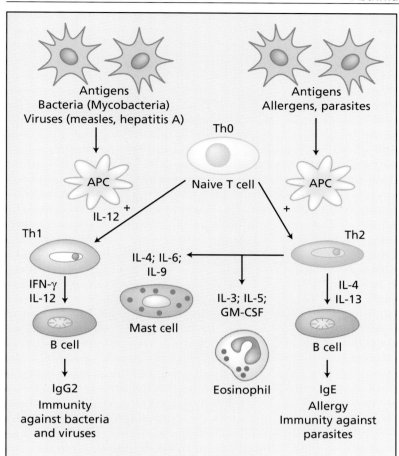

Immune response to antigens: the role of T helper (Th) imbalance. Th lymphocytes are the principal cell orchestrating the immune responses in asthma and other allergic diseases. Antigen-presenting cells (APCs), such as dendritic cells, uptake the antigens and present them to Th cells after processing them. Genetic predisposition and the nature of the antigen presented are thought to determine the direction of a naïve Th cell (Th0) toward type 1 (Th1) or type 2 (Th2) lymphocytes. Some antigens (mycobacterium, measles virus, and hepatitis A virus) induce Th0 cells toward Th1 whereas allergens and parasites induce a Th2 immune response.

Interleukin (IL)-4 and IL-13 are the principal cytokines produced by Th2 cells. They stimulate the B lymphocytes to produce IgE. Other Th2 cytokines stimulate the production and recruitment of mast cells and eosinophils. Th1 cells produce interferon gamma and IL-12, which stimulate B cells toward IgG2 production, augmenting cell-mediated immunity. Th1 cytokines also inhibit the Th2 responses. In other words, in normal healthy subjects there is a balance between Th1 and Th2 response; in asthma, including nonatopic asthma, the balance is tipped toward Th2.

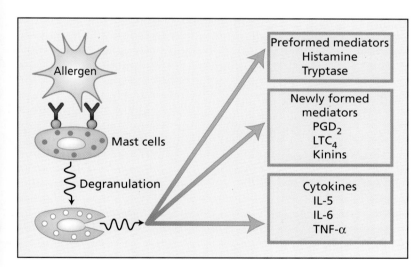

■ Figure 20-11.

Allergen-induced degranulation of mast cells and basophils. Abundant mast cells are seen in the epithelium and the submucosa of the airways. These cells contain cytoplasmic granules that act as storage for inflammatory mediators such as histamine and tryptase. Numerous IgE molecules are attached on the surface of the mast cells. Crosslinking of these IgE molecules by the specific antigen leads to degranulation of mast cells and release of preformed mediators. Crosslinking also stimulates the production of mediators such as prostaglandins, leukotrienes, and various cytokines. These mediators are responsible for the acute symptoms and the persistence of the chronic inflammatory process. IL—interleukin; LTC_4—leukotriene C_4; PGD_2—prostaglandin D_2; TNF-α—tumor necrosis factor-α.

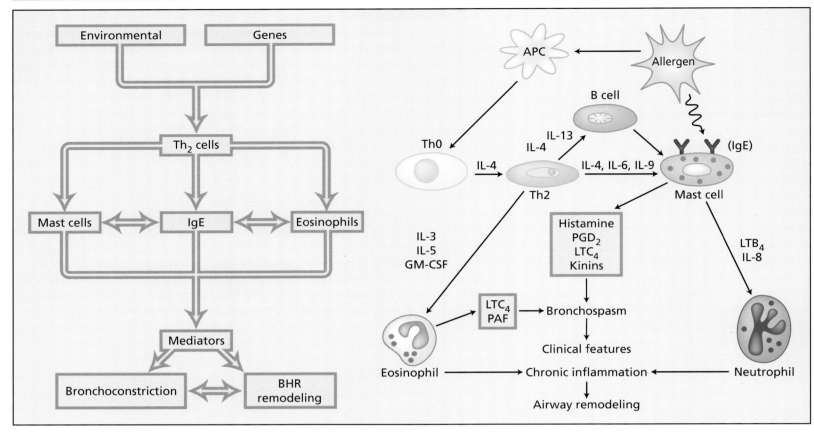

■ Figure 20-12.

The pathogenesis of asthma: the traditional paradigm of chronic inflammation. Asthma is traditionally viewed as a specific type of chronic inflammatory disease of the airways that is caused by a T helper (Th) 2-type immune response. The principal effector cells in this process are eosinophils and mast cells. These cells produce various mediators that cause bronchoconstriction and inflammation. This inflammation is central to the development of bronchial hyper-responsiveness (BHR) and is also thought to play a major part in the process of remodeling. Most asthmatics have increased numbers of activated eosinophils in their bronchi, and there is a significant association between the activation of eosinophils and the severity of asthma and BHR. Interleukin (IL)-5 is an important proinflammatory cytokine that selectively propagates eosinophil differentiation and activation and promotes eosinophil recruitment to the airway mucosa. Recent studies have shown that reducing the numbers of blood and sputum eosinophils by the use of anti–IL-5 monoclonal antibodies had no effect on BHR or clinical outcome measures such as forced expiratory volume in 1 second (FEV_1) [4]. Further study has shown that use of regular anti-inflammatory medications reduced the airway inflammation, but had no therapeutic benefit in terms of lung function [5]. These findings suggest that inflammation alone is insufficient to explain the chronic nature of the disease and its progression. APC—antigen-presenting cell; GM-CSF—granulocyte macrophage–colony-stimulating factor; LTB_4—leukotriene B_4; LTC_4—leukotriene C_4; PAF—platelet-activating factor; PGD_2—prostaglandin D_2.

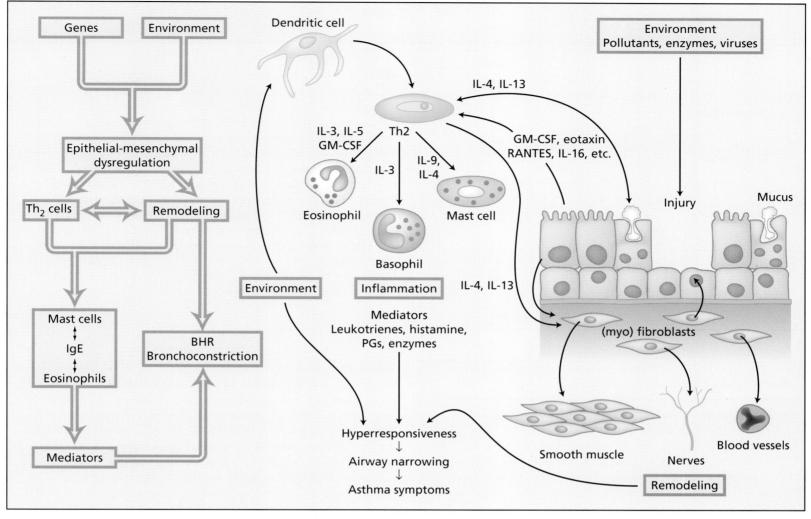

■ Figure 20-13.

The pathogenesis of asthma: an alternate paradigm involving abnormal repair response to epithelial injury. Epithelial injury is caused by exogenous factors such as allergens, viruses, and air pollutants, and endogenous factors such as proteolytic enzymes (tryptase, chymase, and MMP9 from mast cells and eosinophils). In asthmatic patients, the epithelial response to the injury appears to be impaired, leading to a prolonged and abnormal repair process that results in structural changes collectively known as airway remodeling. Epithelium and the connective tissue beneath it is known as epithelial mesenchymal trophic unit (EMTU), which responds to the injury by overproducing profibrotic growth factors such as transforming growth factor-β and stimulating the fibroblasts to differentiate into myofibroblasts. Activated myofibroblasts produce various growth factors and cytokines that promote subepithelial fibrosis, proliferation of airway smooth muscle, increase in microvascular permeability, and increased neural network. These changes have been observed in children up to 4 years before the onset of asthma. Therefore it is suggested that along with inflammation, the EMTU response to epithelial injury is fundamental, along with inflammation, in the pathogenesis of asthma. Further research is currently being done to study further the role of EMTU in the pathogenesis of asthma. BHR—bronchial hyperresponsiveness; GM-CSF—granulocyte macrophage–colony-stimulating factor; IL—interleukin; PG—prostaglandin; RANTES—regulated upon activation normal T cell expressed and secreted; Th—T helper.

Clinical Features and Diagnosis

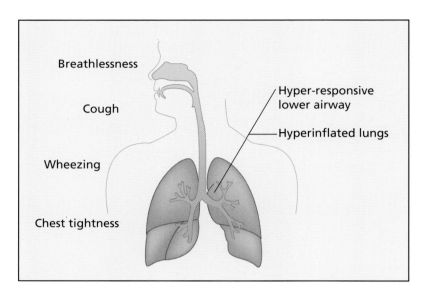

Breathlessness

Cough

Hyper-responsive lower airway

Hyperinflated lungs

Wheezing

Chest tightness

Figure 20-14.

Clinical features of asthma. Symptoms of asthma are caused by narrowing of airways, which is caused by smooth muscle contraction, edema of the airway wall, and increased mucus in the airway. Wheezing, breathlessness, chest tightness, and cough are the common symptoms of asthma. Each of these symptoms are important features of asthma, but separately they are not diagnostic. They are usually most marked at night or early hours of the morning. Patients may also experience nocturnal awakening with these symptoms. In adults, wheezing and breathlessness are more persistent features that show less spontaneous variation than childhood asthma. In long-standing asthma, hyperventilation of the chest is often noted.

Potential Therapies for Asthma

Immune modulators
    Anti-IgE (monoclonal antibody)
    Vaccines (DNA vaccine; *Mycobacterium vaccae*, CpG)
    Desensitization (allergen–specific immunotherapy including
        recombinant gene–manipulated antigens and peptides)
Cytokine modulators (targeting specific steps in the inflammatory cascade)
    Anti IL-5
    Anti IL-4, IL-13
    IL-12
    IL-10
    Transcription factor inhibitors
Others
    Selective phosphodiesterase inhibitors
    Selective tryptase inhibitors
    Potassium channel activators
    Adhesion molecule inhibitors
Gene therapy
    Targeting susceptibility genes
    Targeting polymorphism of receptors for drugs

Figure 20-15.

Potential new therapies for asthma. Target therapies for asthma are being developed owing to a better understanding of the molecular mechanisms of inflammation and of genetic techniques. Cytokine modulators selectively inhibit Th2 cytokine response by reducing their production (targeting transcription, suppressing translation of cytokine-specific mRNA, posttranslation modification) or by blocking their effect on target receptors (neutralization by cytokine-specific antibodies, blocking receptor-ligand interaction, interfering with the receptor-mediated signaling events). Genetic targeting is against the specific genes for asthma, atopy, and bronchial hyper-responsiveness, thus preventing the development of asthma. Genetic manipulation is also targeted at polymorphisms involving cellular receptors against which drugs are directed, thus enhancing drug treatment. IL—interleukin.

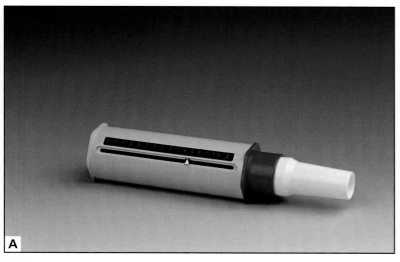

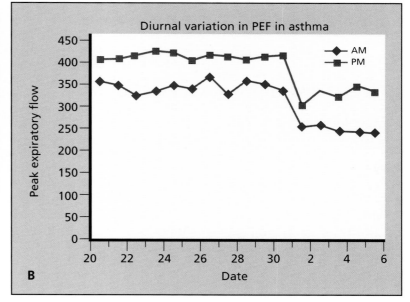

Figure 20-16.

Peak expiratory flow (PEF) meter. This is a simple, portable, and easy-to-use device (**A**). Accuracy of the results depend on the technique used. PEF is useful in the diagnosis and monitoring of asthma. It mainly assesses the larger airway function, and the results vary depending on height and age of the patient. In asthmatic patients, there is a diurnal variation in PEF that is more pronounced during an exacerbation (**B**). Regular PEF monitoring can detect any deterioration in lung function prior to a symptomatic exacerbation, thus allowing patients to take adequate control measures to prevent an attack.

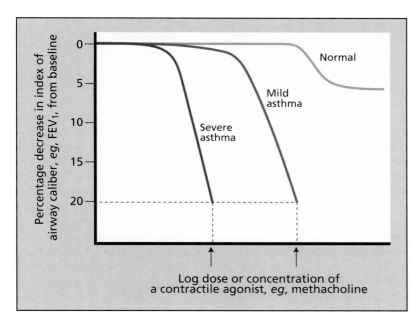

Figure 20-17.

Bronchial hyperresponsiveness (BHR). BHR is defined as the tendency of airways to constrict when exposed to various chemical (histamine, methacholine, adenosine, hypertonic saline) and physical (exercise, cold air) stimuli. This bronchoconstriction to these nonspecific stimuli is short-lived and different from a specific allergen-induced bronchoconstriction, which is prolonged and induces significant airway inflammation. BHR is a useful marker of (although not specific for) asthma. It is also noted in chronic obstructive pulmonary disease and cystic fibrosis. Also, some asthmatic patients do not have BHR. A measure of concentration (PC20) or dose (PD20) of the stimuli required to produce a 20% fall in forced expiratory volume in 1 second (FEV_1) is commonly taken as an index of BHR. This graph shows the increase of BHR with the severity of asthma. Normal subjects will react only at higher concentrations or dose of the stimuli, but they achieve a plateau state without having a 20% fall in FEV_1.

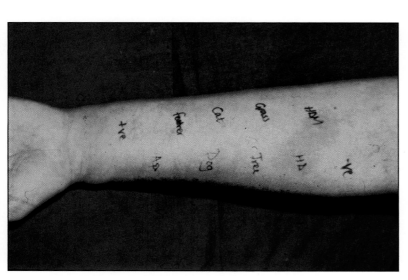

Figure 20-18.

Skin prick testing. Skin prick testing with allergens provides objective information about the atopic status, but the results should be interpreted in relation to the patient's history. In asthma, the skin prick test is done against the common aeroallergens such as house dust mite, grass pollen, cat, dog, and any putative allergens that cause asthma symptoms on their exposure. A drop of allergen solution is placed in the flexor aspect of the forearm and a prick through the solution is made using a sterile lancet. Negative saline and histamine are used as negative and positive controls, respectively. A positive test is a weal larger than 2 mm, or greater than the negative control. Skin tests should not be performed in the presence of severe eczema, and the subject should not take antihistamines during the test period.

A. Other Investigations to Measure the Severity of Asthma

Bronchoscopy (biopsy and lavage)
Examination of sputum for eosinophils and cytokines such as
        eosinophil cationic protein
NO and other "metabolic" gases

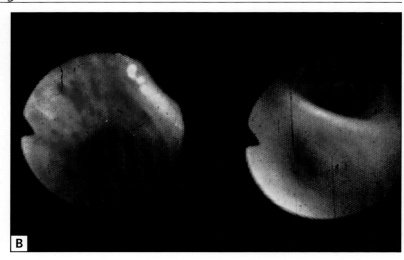

B

■ Figure 20-19.

Other investigations to measure airway inflammation. Although physiologic measures such as spirometry and peak flow are commonly used to evaluate the severity of asthma, the assessment of the airway inflammation is also a useful measure. **A,** List of techniques. **B,** Bronchoscopy. Bronchoscopy is useful to directly view the airway and obtain bronchoalveolar lavage (BAL) fluid and biopsy specimens.

Examining the sputum for various types of cells and inflammatory mediators is another useful investigation. It is particularly useful to assess the degree of inflammation in patients with severe

asthma, avoiding the need for invasive procedures such as bronchoscopy. Measuring nitric oxide (NO) in the exhaled air is an easy, noninvasive procedure to assess the airway inflammation and response to treatment; however, it requires expensive equipment.

Diagnosis of Asthma

History
    Symptoms
        Recurrent episodes of wheezing
        Cough, particularly at night
        Breathlessness
        Chest tightness
    Predisposing factors
        Personal/family history of asthma and/or atopy
        Exposure to allergens
        Medications (*eg*, aspirin and other NSAIDs, β-blockers)
        Housing condition (*eg*, carpets, dampness, pets)
Examination
    Signs (not always apparent)
        Respiratory distress
        Widespread wheeze on auscultation
        Hyperinflated chest
        Associated conditions (eczema, rhinitis)
Investigation
    PEF; spirometry (FEV$_1$)
    Histamine or methacholine bronchial provocation test
    Skin prick tests

■ Figure 20-20.

Diagnosis of asthma. Asthma can often be diagnosed on the basis of history (presence of symptoms and risk factors) and confirmed by lung function tests. In mild to moderate asthma, physical examination may be normal and physical signs apparent only during an exacerbation. In severe asthma, persistent respiratory distress can be noted even at rest. In long-standing disease, hyperinflation of the chest is noted often.

Peak expiratory flow (PEF) and forced expiratory volume in 1 second (FEV$_1$) are commonly used lung function measures in the diagnosis of asthma. A PEF variation of more than 10% (20% if patient is taking a bronchodilator) between the morning measurement and that taken 12 hours later, or an increase by more than 15% 15 to 20 minutes after inhaling a short-acting β$_2$-antagonist, is considered diagnostic of asthma. If these tests are normal, a demonstration of airway hyper-responsiveness by histamine or methacholine provocation test could help in the diagnosis. NSAIDS—nonsteroidal anti-inflammatory drugs.

Differential Diagnosis of Asthma

COPD
Congestive heart failure
Allergic bronchopulmonary aspergillosis
Gastroesophageal reflux
Neoplasm
Vocal cord dysfunction
Tracheal stenosis
Foreign bodies

Figure 20-21.

Differential diagnosis of asthma. Symptoms of asthma can be caused by any disease process leading to airway obstruction. Therefore, some other disorders with distinctive pathology can mimic asthma, particularly in older patients. One important example is chronic pulmonary obstructive disease (COPD), particularly when it has a reversible component to the airway obstruction. It is difficult to differentiate asthma from COPD when it appears for the first time in adult life. Similarly, severe asthma has been misdiagnosed as COPD when there is a fixed airflow obstruction, particularly in smokers. Measurement of diffusion capacity of carbon monoxide, exhaled nitric oxide assay, and induced sputum examination can help to distinguish between asthma and COPD.

Management

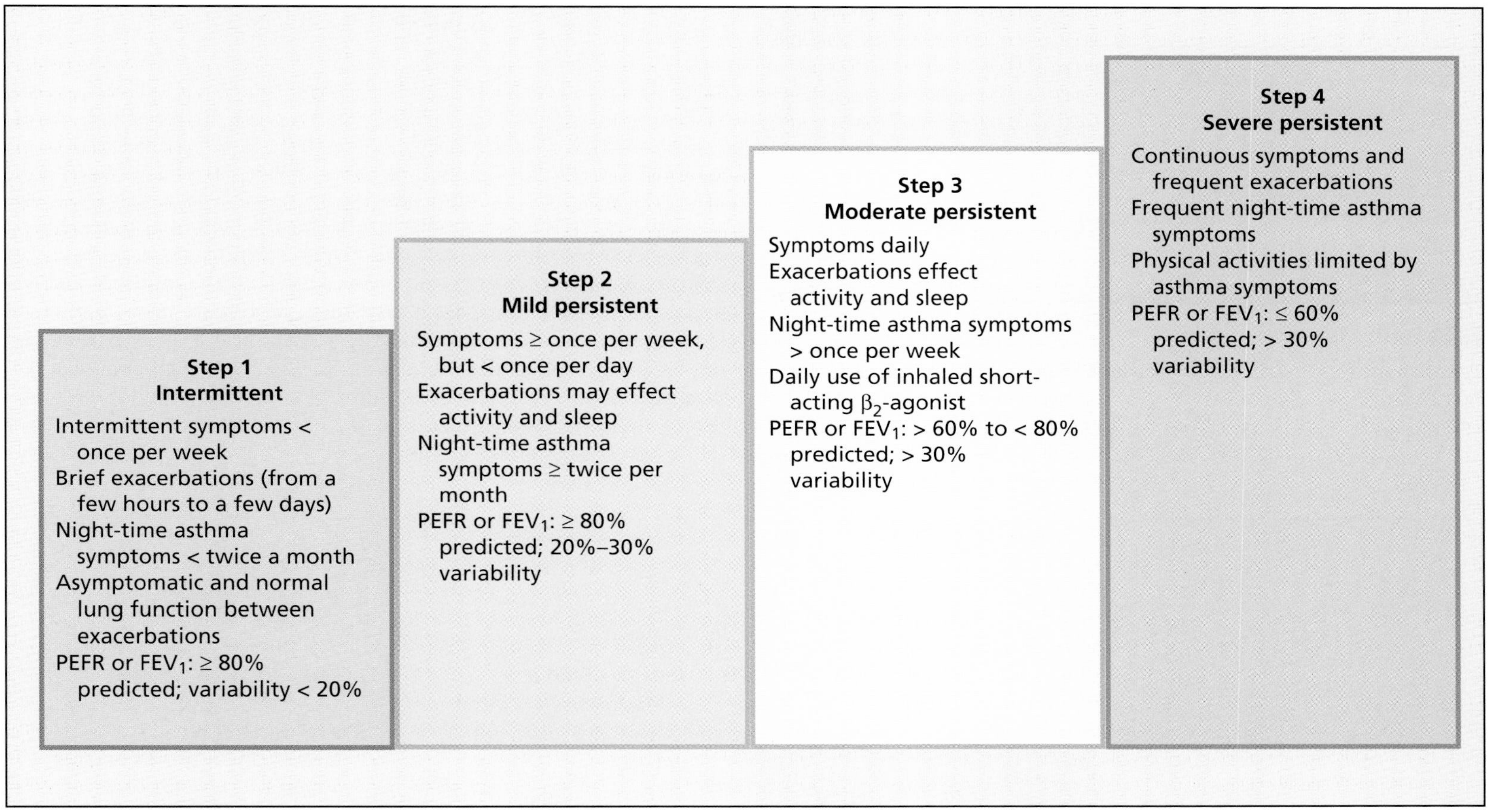

Step 1
Intermittent

Intermittent symptoms < once per week
Brief exacerbations (from a few hours to a few days)
Night-time asthma symptoms < twice a month
Asymptomatic and normal lung function between exacerbations
PEFR or FEV_1: ≥ 80% predicted; variability < 20%

Step 2
Mild persistent

Symptoms ≥ once per week, but < once per day
Exacerbations may effect activity and sleep
Night-time asthma symptoms ≥ twice per month
PEFR or FEV_1: ≥ 80% predicted; 20%–30% variability

Step 3
Moderate persistent

Symptoms daily
Exacerbations effect activity and sleep
Night-time asthma symptoms > once per week
Daily use of inhaled short-acting β_2-agonist
PEFR or FEV_1: > 60% to < 80% predicted; > 30% variability

Step 4
Severe persistent

Continuous symptoms and frequent exacerbations
Frequent night-time asthma symptoms
Physical activities limited by asthma symptoms
PEFR or FEV_1: ≤ 60% predicted; > 30% variability

Figure 20-22.

Classification of asthma severity. Severity of asthma is classified into four groups according to symptoms and lung function measurements. This method of classification is important because therapy for asthma takes a stepwise approach according to the disease severity. Generally patients have poor perception of the severity of their asthma because they tend to adapt their lifestyle to accommodate their symptoms. This in turn leads to poor control of the disease as well as poor quality of life. Classifying the disease in this stepwise fashion allows the targeting of therapy according to the severity of the disease. FEV_1—forced expiratory volume in 1 second; PEFR—peak expiratory flow rate.

Asthma Management Plan

Patient education
  Risk factor avoidance
  Adherence to regular treatment
  Regular home monitoring (PEF measurement; symptom diary)
  Recognizing worsening symptoms and the importance of seeking
    early medical attention
Optimal drug treatment
Regular medical review with lung function measurements
Public health measures
  Control of pollution
  Proper housing

Figure 20-23.

Asthma management plan. Although asthma cannot be cured with currently available therapies, it can be effectively managed with patient education and regular review by professionals. The goal of education is to keep the patient in charge of his or her disease. Regular reviews will assess inhaler techniques and adherence to therapy. The optimal drug treatment will control the daily symptoms and prevent or reduce the underlying airway inflammation. PEF—peak expiratory flow.

Medications Used for Asthma Relief and Control

Controllers	Relievers
Corticosteroids	Short-acting β_2-agonists
Cromones	Methyl xanthines
Leukotriene modifiers	Anticholinergics
Long-acting β_2-agonists	
Sustained-release methyl xanthines	
Immunosuppressants	

Figure 20-24.

Asthma medications. Drugs used in the management of asthma can be classified as *controllers* or *relievers*. The acute episodes are treated with reliever type (rescue) medications, which have immediate bronchodilator effect. The commonly used reliever medications are the short-acting β_2-agonists, such as salbutamol and terbutaline. Others include anticholinergic drugs (ipratropium and oxitropium) and the xanthines (theophylline and aminophylline). Although asthma attacks are episodic, the underlying airway inflammation is chronic; thus long-term regular treatment is achieved by controller type medications. These include inhaled corticosteroids (beclomethasone, budesonide, and fluticasone), cromogens (sodium cromoglycate and nedocromil sodium), the long-acting bronchodilators such as sustained-release theophylline and the long-acting β_2-agonists (salmeterol). Leukotriene-modifying drugs, which include the leukotriene receptor antagonists (montelukast, zafirlukast, and pranlukast) and the inhibitors of 5'-lipoxygenase (zileuton), are classified as preventers. Most asthma medications are taken as inhalers. An appropriate inhaler device is important as well as the use of a spacer device, which enhances drug delivery to the airways. Leukotriene modifiers and the xanthines are taken as oral medications.

**Step 1
Mild intermittent**

No regular medications

**Step 2
Mild persistent**

Daily inhaled corticosteroid (200–500 μg) **or** sodium cromoglycate **or** nedocromil **or** sustained-release theophylline
Antileukotrienes may be considered

**Step 3
Moderate persistent**

Daily inhaled corticosteroid (500–800 μg)
and
Daily long-acting bronchodilator (long-acting inhaled β_2 agonist **or** sustained-release theophylline)
Antileukotrienes may be considered

**Step 4
Severe persistent**

Daily inhaled corticosteroid (800–2000 μg or more)
and
Daily long-acting bronchodilator (long-acting inhaled β_2 agonist **or** sustained-release theophylline)
and
Long-term regular oral corticosteroid (on minimum effective dose)

Figure 20-25.

Stepwise treatment of asthma. The goal of drug treatment is to control chronic symptoms and prevent acute exacerbation. Patients are started on the treatment at the step appropriate to the severity of their asthma, aiming for control as quickly as possible. Once the control is achieved, the treatment is reviewed every 3 to 6 months. If control is achieved at least for 3 months, then a gradual stepwise reduction in treatment ("step-down") is considered. If control is not achieved, a "step-up" treatment is considered. Before step-up is initiated, it is important to review the medication intake technique, compliance, and measures taken to control trigger factors, such as allergen avoidance. A rescue course of prednisolone may be needed at any step of treatment.

Classification of Asthma Exacerbation

Clinical Features	Mild	Moderate	Severe	Life-threatening
Breathlessness	On walking	On talking	Even at rest	
Alertness	Normal	Usually agitated	Usually agitated	Drowsy or confused
Speaks in:	Sentences	Phrases	Words	
Wheeze	Mild; often end-expiratory	Loud throughout expiration	Loud; throughout inspiration and expiration	Silent chest
Respiratory rate	Increased	Increased	Often > 30/min	Decreased (due to fatigue)
Pulse rate/min	< 100	100–120	> 120	Bradycardia
Use of accessory muscles, suprasternal reactions	Usually not	Commonly	Usually	Paradoxical chest movement
PEF (% predicted or personal best)	> 80%	50%–80%	< 50%	
SaO_2, % (on air)	> 95%	90%–95%	< 90%	

■ Figure 20-26.

Classification of asthma exacerbation. The exacerbation of asthma can vary from a mild episode to a severe or even fatal event. It is important to recognize that even mild asthma can be associated with severe, potentially fatal exacerbation. All features may not be present in any one exacerbation. The presence of two or more characteristics places patients in the higher degree of severity. A previous history of life-threatening attacks, brittle asthma, and poor compliance with therapy are some of the factors associated with increased risk for fatal episodes. Although most asthma attacks occur suddenly, there is a gradual deterioration in lung function and symptoms prior to such an event. PEF—peak expiratory flow; SaO_2—oxygen saturation.

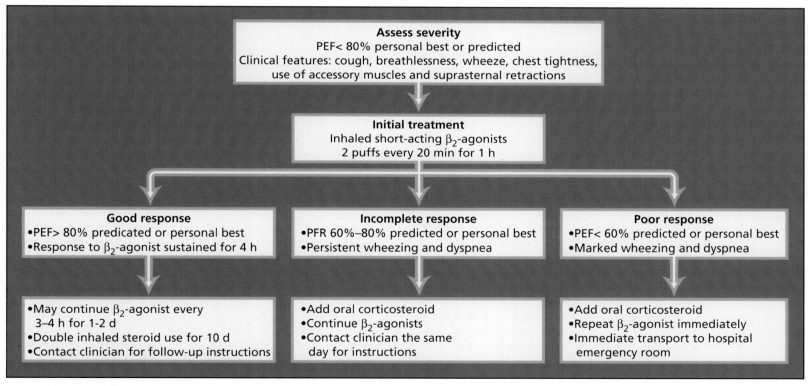

■ Figure 20-27.

Management of asthma exacerbation. The goal of initial management is to reverse the acute airflow limitation as quickly as possible with short-acting β_2-agonists as inhalers or nebulizers. If there is no immediate response to the above measures, systemic corticosteroids should be given, preferably by enteral route. Oxygen is usually given to keep the oxygen saturation (SaO_2) above 90%. A history of previous life-threatening episodes of asthma warrants low threshold for hospital admission. Once the acute attack is managed, then the long-term therapy needs to be reviewed, emphasizing self-management plans.

Asthma action plan

Name _____ Date _____

It is important in managing asthma to keep track of your symptoms, medications, and peak expiratory flow (PEF).
You can use the colors of a traffic light to help learn your asthma medications:

A. **GREEN means Go**   Use preventive (anti-inflammatory) medicine
B. **YELLOW means Caution**   Use quick-relief (short-acting bronchodilator) medicine in addition to the preventive medicine
C. **RED means STOP!**   Get help from a doctor

A. Your GREEN ZONE is _____ 80 to 100% of your personal best. GO!
   Breathing is good with no cough, wheeze, or chest tightness during work, school, exercise, or play.

   ACTION:
   ☐ Continue with medications listed in your daily treatment plan

B. Your YELLOW ZONE is _____ 50 to less than 80% of your personal best. CAUTION!
   Asthma symptoms are present (cough, wheeze, chest tightness).
   Your peak flow number drops below _____ or you notice:
   ☐ Increased need for inhaled quick-relief medicine
   ☐ Increased asthma symptoms upon awakening
   ☐ Awakening at night with asthma symptoms
   ☐ _____

   ACTIONS:
   ☐ Take _____ puffs of your quick-relief (bronchodilator) medicine _____.
      Repeat _____ times.
   ☐ Take _____ puffs of _____ (anti-inflammatory) _____ times/day.
   ☐ Begin/increase treatment with oral steroids:
      Take _____ mg of _____ every a.m. _____ p.m. _____ .
   ☐ Call your doctor (phone) _____ or emergency room

C. Your RED ZONE is _____ 50% or less of your best. DANGER!!
   Your peak flow number drops below _____ or you continue to get worse after increasing treatment according to the directions above.

   ACTIONS:
   ☐ Take _____ puffs of your quick-relief (bronchodilator) medicine _____. Repeat _____ times.
   ☐ Begin/increase treatment with oral steroids. Take _____ mg now.
   ☐ Call your doctor now (phone _____). If you cannot contact your doctor, go directly to the emergency room (phone
      _____).
   Other important phone numbers for transportation _____.

AT ANY TIME, CALL YOUR DOCTOR IF:
   ☐ Asthma symptoms worsen while you are taking oral steroids, or
   ☐ Inhaled bronchodilator treatments are not lasting 4 hours, or
   ☐ Your peak flow number remains or falls below _____ in spite of following the plan.

Figure 20-28.
Sample asthma action plan for patient self-management.

References

1. Barnes PJ, Woolcock AJ: Difficult asthma. *Eur Respir J* 1998, 12:1209–1218.

2. Panhuysen CIM, Vonk JM, Koeter GH, *et al*.: Adult patients may outgrow their asthma: a 25-year follow-up study. *Am J Respir Crit Care Med* 1997, 155:1267–1272.

3. Vignola AM, Chanez P, Campbell AM, *et al*.: Airway inflammation in mild intermittent and in persistent asthma. *Am J Respir Crit Care Med* 1998, 157:403–409.

4. Leckie MJ, ten Brinke A, Khan J, *et al*.: Effects of an interleukin-5 blocking monoclonal antibody on eosinophils, airway hyper-responsiveness, and the last asthmatic response. *Lancet* 2000, 356:2144–2148.

5. Asthma Management Program Research Group: Long-term effects of budesonide or nedocromil in children with asthma. *N Engl J Med* 2000, 343:1054–1063.

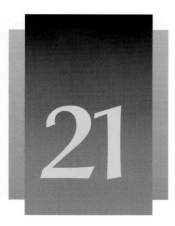

Occupational Asthma

Emil J. Bardana, Jr.

The incidence of work-related asthma far exceeds that of other causes of occupational pulmonary disease in the industrialized world. An estimated 2% to 15% of all adult asthma cases are work related, and some 250 causal agents have been identified. Compared with other industrial disorders, work-related asthma frequently results in more persistent and sometimes permanent effects.

Occupational asthma is defined as a condition characterized by reversible obstruction of the airways that originates in the inhalation of ambient dusts, vapors, gases, or fumes manufactured or used by workers (or coincidentally present in the workplace). Many cases of occupational asthma occur in association with chronic bronchitis and varying degrees of irreversible obstructive airway disease (*eg*, emphysema).

There are some basic diagnostic challenges that confront clinicians with respect to occupational asthma. The first and most important decision is to distinguish new-onset occupational asthma from a transient, irritational expression of preexisting asthma and from a never-before-encountered job-related allergen or the lasting corrosive effects of an industrial agent. The second diagnostic challenge is to distinguish the two principal pathogenetic forms of new-onset asthma (*ie*, immunologic occupational asthma and nonimmunologic occupational asthma).

Characteristics of Industrial Allergens and Inhalants

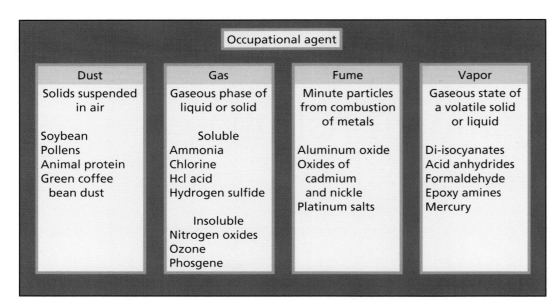

Figure 21-1.

Characteristics of inhaled work-related agents. The biologic effects of an acute exposure depend on the physiochemical properties of the specific gas, fume, vapor, or dust involved. The airborne concentration of the agent and length of exposure are also important criteria that determine the potential health effects. Irritant gases are classified according to their water solubility. The highly soluble gases are likely to cause skin burns, ocular irritation, and pharyngeal and laryngeal damage. Nasal congestion and erythema are also evident. Most of these gases are absorbed in the mucous membranes of the upper airway. Low-solubility gases such as phosgene and hydrogen sulfide generate little upper airway irritation but can produce pulmonary edema and intense inflammatory damage in the lower airways. (*Adapted from* Bardana and Montanaro [1].)

Classification of Toxic Inhalants

Irritants	**Asphyxiants**	**Neurotoxins**	**Febrile-Syndrome Inducers**
Acrolein, aldehydes	Simple (interfere with oxygen	Insecticides	Oxides of zinc fumes
Burning plastics	delivery)	Organophosphate (malathion)	Welding galvanized steel (metal
Ammonia	Carbon monoxide	Herbicides	fume fever)
Transportation accidents	Smoke in fires	Paraquat (also, lung fibrosis)	Pyrolysis of products with
Leaks in fertilizer tanks,	Methane	Fumigants	fluorocarbons (polymer
refrigeration	CO_2 in manure pits	Methylbromide	fume fever)
Chlorine	Chemical (interfere with cell	Warfare gases	Teflon
Transportation accidents	respiration)	Anticholinesterase	
Water sewage treatment	Hydrogen cyanide from burning		
Hydrogen sulfide	plastics		
Septic tanks	Hydrogen sulfide		
Methylisocyanate	Methane in manure pit		
Pesticide production (Bhopal,			
India)			
Plastic industries			
Nitrogen oxides			
Farm silos			
Explosives			
Ice-rink resurfacing			
Phosgene			
Fires			
Paint stripping			
Sulfur dioxide			
Paper mills			
Refrigeration			

Figure 21-2.

Classification of toxic inhalants. Toxic inhalants include gases, mists, fumes, and smoke. They may act as irritants, asphyxiants, or neurotoxins. Massive inhalations may occur during fires or other industrial accidents or during the transport of stored chemicals. Firefighters and industrial workers are the subsegments of the population most at risk. (*Courtesy of* Guillermo A. do Pico and Keith C. Meyer.)

Examples of Irritant Gases

Gas	Water Solubility	Predominant Site of Injury	Usual Onset of Symptoms	Comments
Acrylic aldehyde	Soluble	Airway—alveoli	Minutes	Very irritating
Ammonia	Soluble	Upper airway*	Immediate	Alkali burns, corneal burns
Chlorine	Slightly soluble	Airway—alveoli	Minutes to hours	Acid burns, strong oxidant
Hydrogen sulfide	Soluble	Airway—alveoli	Minutes to hours	Alkali irritation, central nervous system asphyxiant
Methylisocyanate		Airway—alveoli	Minutes to hours	Highly reactive, methemoglobin, carboxyhemoglobin
Nickle carbonyl	Insoluble	Alveoli	Hours	Volatile liquid, cerebral edema
Nitrogen dioxide	Insoluble	Alveoli—bronchioles	Hours	Acid burns, delayed symptoms, mild irritation, strong oxidant
Ozone	Insoluble	Airway—Alveoli	Minutes to hours	Strong oxidant
Phosgene	Insoluble	Alveoli—bronchioles	Hours	Acid burns, delayed symptoms, mild irritation
Sulfur dioxide	Very soluble	Upper airway*	Immediate	Acid burns, corneal burns

*Alveolar injury as pulmonary edema or hemorrhagic alveolitis has been reported at very high concentrations, usually hours or days after exposure.

Figure 21-3.

Examples of irritant gases. These gases, primarily found in industrial settings, may cause airway burns, central nervous system damage, and alterations of the hemoglobin molecule. Effects may be seen immediately or within 24 to 72 hours of exposure. (*Courtesy of* Guillermo A. do Pico and Keith C. Meyer.)

Classification of Selected Asthmogenic Agents by Molecular Weight

Low Molecular Weight	High Molecular Weight
Organic chemicals	Animal proteins
Acid anhydrides	Danders
Di-isocyanates	Urine
Epoxy resins	Feathers
Colophony	Saliva
Western red cedar	Insect proteins
Metal salts and inorganic compounds	Bee moth
Platinum salts	Cockroaches
Aluminum	Mites
Hard metal and cobalt	Lake flies
Nickel	Plant proteins
Vanadium	Coffee bean dust
Ammonium persulfate	Castor bean dust
Pharmaceutical agents	Gum acacia
Penicillin	Latex
Cephalosporins	Pollens
Sulfonamides	Foods and enzymes
Isoniazid	Pepsin
Tetracycline	Papain
Macrolide antibiotics	Egg powder
	Pharmaceutical agents
	Psyllium

Figure 21-4.

Classification of selected asthmogenic agents by molecular weight. Immunologic work-related asthma is usually related to sensitization to high molecular weight allergens, which primarily represent proteins derived from animals, plants, foods, and enzymes. Selected low molecular weight agents (*eg,* complex salts of platinum, nickel, penicillin, and many of the epoxy compounds) can also induce immunologic occupational asthma. The epoxy compounds have the capacity to react as haptens capable of binding to human proteins and inducing an IgE mechanism.

Predisposing Factors

Predisposing Factors that Influence the Development of Occupational Asthma

Workplace factors
  Sources of chemicals and their concentration
  Industrial hygiene practices
  Job description
Climatic factors
  Presence of oxidizing pollutants
  Incidence of temperature inversions
  Wind conditions
  Proximity of other allergens or irritants
Atopic background
Tobacco abuse
Recreational drug use
Viral upper respiratory infections
Bronchial hyperreactivity
Miscellaneous medical factors
  Aspirin idiosyncrasy syndrome
  Pharmacologic influences (*eg*, β-blocking drugs)
  Gastrointestinal reflux
  Stress or hyperventilation

Figure 21-5.

Predisposing factors influencing the development of occupational asthma. The development of occupational asthma may be influenced by a variety of genetic, industrial, meteorologic, and medical factors. Industrial factors include the extent and nature of chemical exposures as well as both the workers' and the employers' attitudes toward safety. Weather has played a role in a number of asthma epidemics in New Orleans and Barcelona. Genetic predisposition to atopic disease determines proclivity to react to sensitizing agents. The use of tobacco and other recreational drugs adversely affects the respiratory tract and may play a role in the induction to sensitization. The presence or absence of bronchial hyperreactivity and its severity determines the threshold of reactivity to industrial irritants. This may also be affected by viral infections. A variety of other factors such as medicinal agents, exercise, cold air, stress, and gastroesophageal reflux disease may provoke airway obstruction. (*Adapted from* Bardana [2].)

Rationale for Infectious Events Predisposing to the Development of Occupational Asthma

Viral infections frequently precipitate initial asthmatic episode
Viral infections are commonly associated with exacerbations of
    asthma
Viral infections damage irritant receptors in the lung
Viral-specific IgE could result in release of vasoactive amines from
    mast cells
Viral infections may depress cellular immunity
Chlamydia pneumoniae infection is associated with development of
    asthma
Chronic pyogenic sinusitis may be associated with intensification of
    bronchial asthma

Figure 21-6.

Rationale for infectious events predisposing to the development of occupational asthma. In susceptible patients, respiratory tract infections induce new-onset bronchial hyperresponsiveness, which may terminate in the development of overt bronchial asthma. In this respect, many patients evaluated for suspected work-related asthma frequently recall symptoms of a viral infection shortly before the start of their asthmatic symptoms. (*Adapted from* Bardana [2].)

Significance of Nonspecific Bronchial Hyperreactivity in the Diagnosis of Occupational Asthma

NSBHR is a cardinal feature of symptomatic bronchial asthma; it is defined as an exaggerated airway narrowing in response to a wide variety of stimuli

Sensitivity to histamine and methacholine correlate well with the severity of bronchial asthma and the presence of inflammatory cell infiltrates

NSBHR probably waxes and wanes secondary to a variety of environmental and host factors

Whereas the positive predictive value of NSBHR for the presence of asthma is only about 10%, the negative predictive value is about 90%

Figure 21-7.

Significance of nonspecific bronchial hyperreactivity (NSBHR) in the diagnosis of occupational asthma. NSBHR is frequently misinterpreted as representing a gold standard for the diagnosis of asthma and, at times, for the diagnosis of occupational asthma. However, NSBHR is found in 10% to 15% of normal asymptomatic individuals. It may also be found transiently after viral respiratory infections. It is associated with tobacco abuse or exposure to certain pollutants (ozone is well known). It is also present in patients with a variety of nonasthmatic pulmonary disorders (*eg*, hypersensitivity pneumonitis, cystic fibrosis).

Clinical and Pathogenic Features

Pathogenetic Mechanisms in the Induction of New-onset Occupational Asthma

There are two basic mechanisms implicated in the causation of OA. Most common is an immunologically induced inflammation. Less common are several nonimmunologic forms of OA (*eg*, irritant induced or pharmacologic).

Most cases of OA result from exposure and sensitization to work-related allergens (*see* Fig. 22-4)

A latent period of months or years is generally required before sensitization to a workplace allergen takes place

Rhinoconjunctivitis frequently precedes the development of immunologic OA

Rhinoconjunctivitis frequently precedes the development of immunologic OA

Nonimmunologic OA usually results from a high-level workplace exposure to a corrosive irritant

Onset is abrupt and not preceded by typical allergic upper airway or ocular complaints. This variant is known as RADS.

Any given industrial reactant can probably induce OA by more than a single mechanism, and more than a single mechanism may be operative in any given patient

Figure 21-8.

Pathogenetic mechanisms in the induction of new-onset occupational asthma (OA). From a pathogenetic standpoint, OA may be divided into two broad categories, depending on whether immunologic sensitization is believed to play a principal role. Nonimmunologic occupational asthma usually involves an acute inflammatory insult or an acute neurogenically mediated process independent of a specific immune process. In the latter instance, the clinical presentation is easier to link to an acute inhalational exposure. RADS—reactive airways dysfunction syndrome.

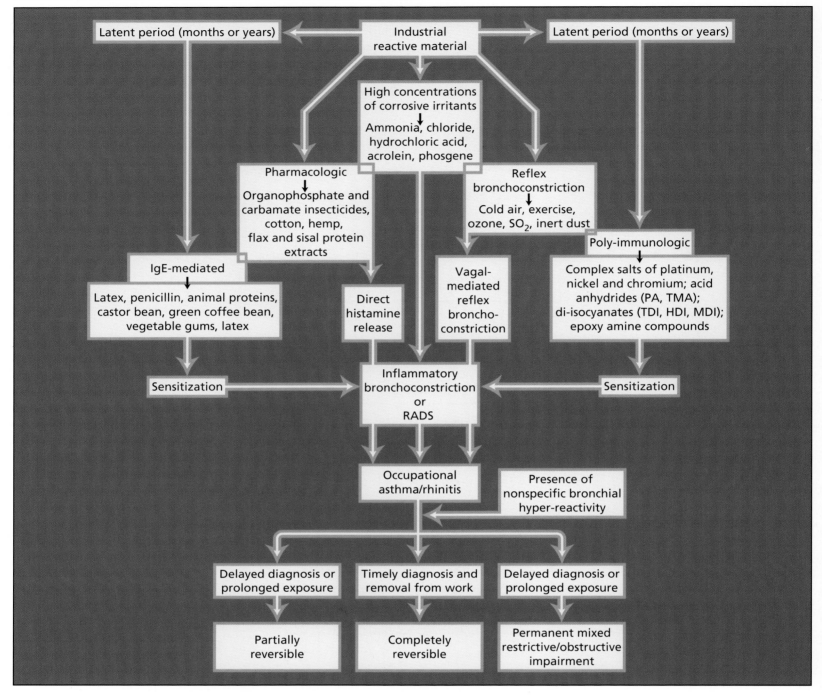

Figure 21-9.

Schematic conceptualization of overlapping pathogenetic mechanisms operative in occupational asthma (OA). This schematic portrays the classic nonimmunologic mechanism down the center of the diagram. A corrosive industrial agent induces inflammatory bronchoconstriction or reactive airways dysfunction syndrome (RADS). There are two minor subcategories of nonimmune asthma: one secondary to pharmacologic bronchospasm (*eg*, organophosphate insecticides) and one secondary to reflex bronchospasm (*eg*, SO₂, cold air, exercise). The left side of the diagram depicts classic IgE-mediated sensitivity (*eg*, animal proteins, latex), and the right side shows polyimmunologic reactions (*eg*, acid anhydrides, di-isocyanates). HDI—hexamethylene di-idocyanate; MDI—methylene diphenyldi-isocyanate; PA—phthalic anhydride; TDI—toluene di-isocyanate; TMA—trimellitic anhydride. (*Adapted from* Bardana [2].)

Diagnostic Criteria for New-onset Immunologic Occupational Asthma

Symptoms related temporally to the workplace
Established industrial asthmogenic agent
Persistent variable airway obstruction
Demonstration of variable airway obstruction to the putative work-related agent
Bronchial provocation with a controlled, subirritant dose of suspected agent
Improvement in symptoms with timely diagnosis and removal of putative agent

Figure 21-10.

Diagnostic criteria for new-onset immunologic occupational asthma. In the evaluation of patients with suspected occupational asthma, it is critical to define the parameters of diagnosis that distinguish it from a variety of closely allied conditions. Too often, these initial steps are overlooked or only partly satisfied with resultant misdiagnosis. (*Adapted from* Bardana [2].)

Criteria for the Diagnosis of Reactive Airway Dysfunction Syndrome

ACCP Consensus (major) criteria
　Documented absence of preceding respiratory complaints
　Onset of symptoms after a single exposure incident or accident
　Exposure to very high concentrations of a gas, smoke, fume, or vapor with irritant properties
　Onset of symptoms within 24 hours after exposure with persistence of symptoms for at least
　　　3 months
　Symptoms simulating asthma with cough, wheeze, and dyspnea
　Presence of airflow obstruction on PFT or presence of nonspecific bronchial hyperresponsiveness
　All other pulmonary diseases excluded
Minor criteria
　Absence of an atopic state
　Absence of peripheral or pulmonary eosinophilia
　Absence of cigarette smoking for 10 years
　Bronchial hyperactivity of moderate to severe degree (*ie,* positive at methacholine
　　　concentration ≤ 8 mg/mL)
　Histopathology and/or bronchoalveolar lavage showing minimal lymphocytic inflammation

Figure 21-11.

Criteria for the diagnosis of reactive airways dysfunction syndrome (RADS). RADS results from a high-level workplace exposure to a corrosive irritant. Criteria have been proposed for its diagnosis as adopted by the American College of Chest Physicians (ACCP). These are referred to as the major criteria. Five minor criteria have been proposed that, if met, would strengthen the diagnosis considerably. It has been suggested that satisfaction of at least four of the five minor criteria (including the first three) would exclude the significant confounding factors that surround the confident diagnosis of RADS. PFT—pulmonary function test. (*Adapted from* Bardana and Montanaro [1].)

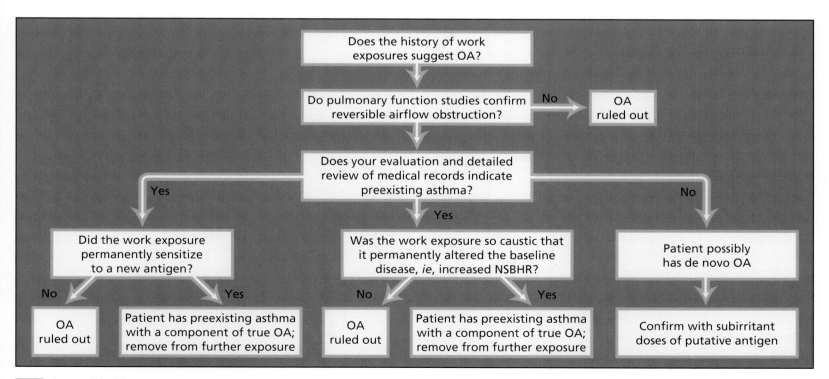

Figure 21-12.

Algorithm for the diagnosis of occupational asthma (OA). In diagnosing OA, the medical history is a critical part of the evaluation and should include a comprehensive medical record review. There should be an inquiry related to protective gear used at the worksite, chemical exposures (via material safety data sheets), whether masks have been fit tested, the number and nature of chemical spills, the available ventilation, and so on. Pulmonary function testing should reveal reversible airflow obstruction and nonspecific bronchial hyperreactivity (NSBHR). Challenge testing with subirritant doses of the putative antigen may be essential in confirming the diagnosis. (*Adapted from* Bardana and Montanaro [1].)

MATERIAL SAFETY DATA SHEET

I PRODUCT IDENTIFICATION

MANUFACTURER'S NAME	REGULAR TELEPHONE NO EMERGENCY TELEPHONE NO
ADDRESS	
TRADE NAME	
SYNONYMS	

II HAZARDOUS INGREDIENTS

MATERIAL OR COMPONENT		HAZARD DATA

III PHYSICAL DATA

BOILING POINT 760 MM HG		MELTING POINT	
SPECIFIC GRAVITY (H$_2$0•1)		VAPOR PRESSURE	
VAPOR DENSITY (AIR•1)		SOLUBILITY IN H$_2$0 % BY WT	
% VOLATILES BY VOL		EVAPORATION RATE IBUTYL ACETATE II	
APPEARANCE AND ODOR			

Figure 21-13.

Material safety data sheet (MSDS). The MSDS represents the best source of information related to a worker's exposure. The Occupational and Safety and Health Administration requires that all manufacturers and importers of chemicals prepare such forms on their products. The MSDS must include the identification of the compound and its physical hazards as well as health hazards associated with exposure to the compound. The employer must not only maintain MSDSs on file but must make them readily available to employees and health care providers. (*Adapted from* O'Hollaren [3].)

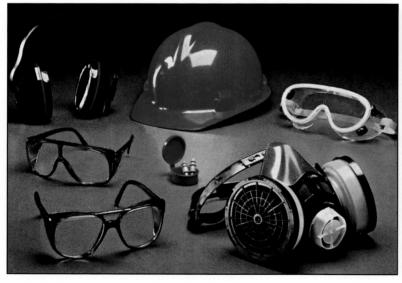

Figure 21-14.

Types of protective equipment used by workers. It is important to acquire a detailed understanding of the protective equipment used by the worker. These include a face mask, earplugs, goggles, gloves, uniform, steel-tipped shoes, and so on.

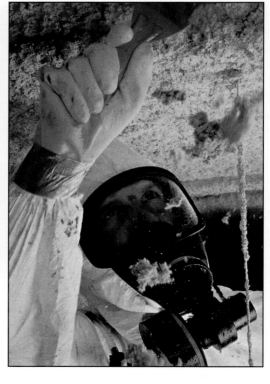

Figure 21-15.
Protective full face, enclosed respirator or air supply mask. Certain highly toxic exposures such as asbestos or isocyanate vapors require a full-face, enclosed respirator or air-supply respirator.

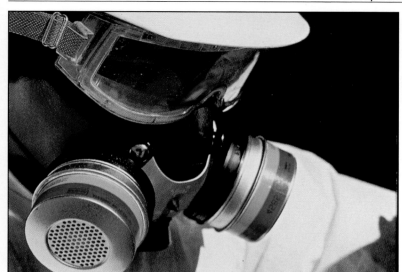

■ Figure 21-16.

Partial face respirator. It is important to acquire a detailed understanding of the protective equipment used by the patient. The examiner should inquire about the details of the mask worn, how was it fitted, the frequency of cartridge change, the presence of prefilters, and so on.

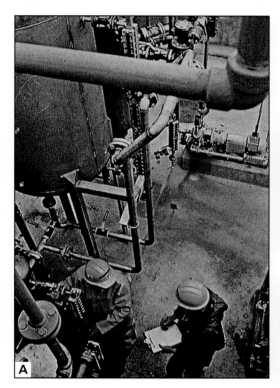

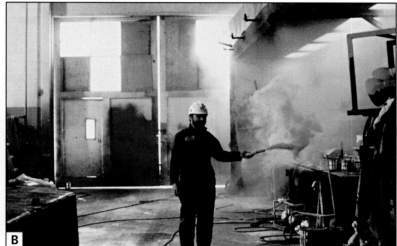

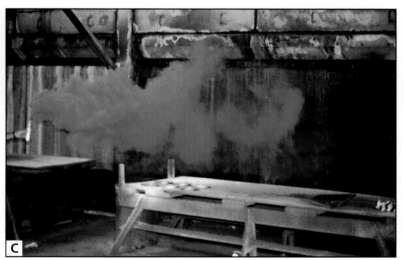

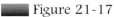 Figure 21-17

Visitation to the worksite. **A,** Isocyanate plant with evidence of an old spill. A visit to the worksite may uncover evidence of previous spills or accidents. **B** and **C,** A shipyard paint bench; testing the suction exhaust with a smoke bomb. Inspection of a waterfall exhaust system proximal to a shipyard spray paint area. A smoke bomb provides visual assurance of adequate performance. (*From* Bardana [2]; with permission.)

Diagnosis and Management

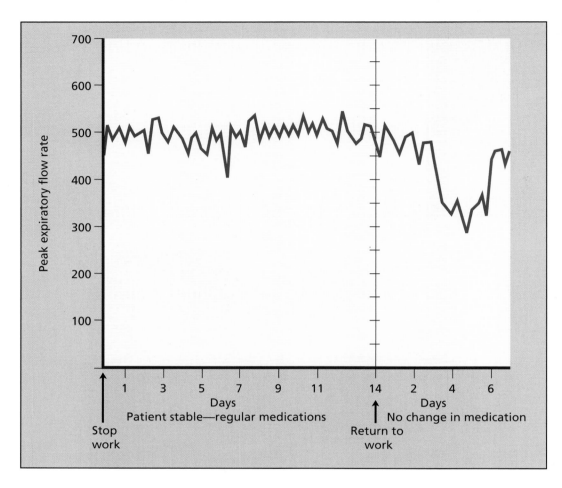

Figure 21-18.
Serial peak expiratory flow rates. Shown is a representation of serial peak expiratory flow rates charted during a period of work abstinence and after return to work. This is an excellent method of screening for potentially involved occupational allergens. Confirmation should be sought with carefully executed spirometry. (*Adapted from* Bardana [2].)

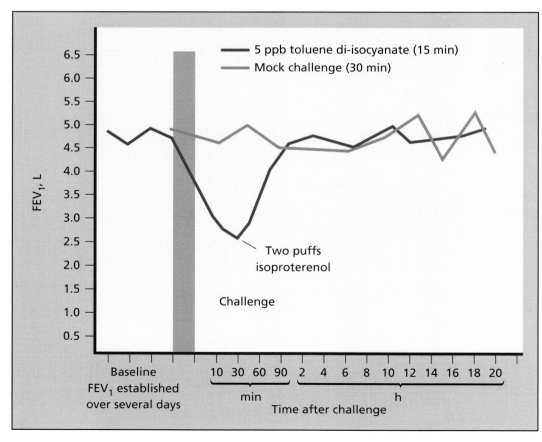

Figure 21-19.
Controlled provocation study. Spirometric results of a controlled bronchial provocation study to toluene di-isocyanate, indicating a positive immediate response. (*Adapted from* Bardana [2].) FEV_1—forced expiratory volume in 1 second.

Therapeutic Principles for Occupational Asthma
Insulate at-risk workers from potentially hazardous agents
Institute regular surveillance
After the diagnosis has been established, remove the patient from all further exposure
Treat symptoms in accordance with established guidelines for asthma

Figure 21-20.

Therapeutic principles for occupational asthma (OA). The best approach to managing a patient with OA is prevention (*ie*, maintain the highest safety standards at the worksite with the finest industrial hygiene practices). After the diagnosis of OA has been established with certainty, the patient should be removed from all further exposure. Any residual asthmatic symptoms should be treated aggressively, as one would treat any patient with asthma.

References

1. Bardana EJ, Montanaro A: Occupational asthma and related disorders. In *Clinical Immunology: Principles and Practice*, edn 2. Edited by Rich RR. St. Louis: Mosby; 2001: in press.

2. Bardana, EJ: Occupational respiratory allergy. In *Current Practice of Medicine: Allergy & Immunology*, vol 2. Edited by Lieberman PL. Philadelphia: Current Medicine; 1999:1731–1738.

3. O'Hollaren MT, Montanaro A, Bardana EJ: Evaluation of the patient with occupational asthma. In *Occupational Asthma*. Edited by Bardana EJ, Montanaro A, O'Hallaren MT. Philadelphia: Hanley & Belfus; 1992: 283–301.

Recommended Reading

Aul DJ, Bhaumir A, Kennedy AL, *et al*.: Specific IgG response to monomeric and polymeric dephenylmethane diisocyanate conjugates in subjects with respiratory reactions to isocyanates. *J Allergy Clin Immunol* 1999, 103:749.

Alberts MW, doPico GA: Reactive airways dysfunction syndrome. *Chest* 1996, 109:1618.

Bardana EJ: Occupational asthma and related respiratory disorders. *Dis Mon* 1995, 61:141.

Bardana EJ: Reactive airways dysfunction syndrome (RADS): guidelines for diagnosis and treatment and insight into likely prognosis. *Ann Allergy Asthma Immunol* 1999, 83:583.

Baur X, Chen Z, Liebers V: Exposure-response relationships of occupational inhalation allergens. *Clin Exp Allergy* 1998, 28:537.

Cartier A: Occupational asthma: what have we learned? *J Allergy Clin Immunol* 1998, 102(suppl):90.

Chan-Yeung M, Brooks SM, Alberts WM, *et al*.: Assessment of asthma in the workplace. *Chest* 1995, 108:1084.

Grammer L, Shaughnessy M, Kenamore B: Utility of antibody in identifying individuals who have or will develop anhydride-induced respiratory disease. *Chest* 1998, 114:1199.

Holgate ST: Genetic and environmental interaction in allergy and asthma. *J Allergy Clin Immunol* 1999:104:1139.

Johnson AR, Dimich-Ward HD, Manfreda J, *et al*.: Occupational asthma in adults in six Canadian communities. *Am J Resp Crit Care Med* 2000, 162:2058–2062.

Kogevinas M, Anto JM, Sunyer J, *et al*.: Occupational asthma in Europe and other industrialized areas: a population-based study. *Lancet* 1999, 353:1750.

Lemiere C, Chaboilliez S, Trudeau C, *et al*.: Characterization of airway inflammation after repeated exposures to occupational agents. *J Allergy Clin Immunol* 2000, 106:1163–1170.

Malo J-L, Trudea C, Ghezzo H, *et al*.: Do subjects investigated for occupational asthma through serial PEF measurements falsify their results? *J Allergy Clin Immunol* 1995, 96:601.

Mapp C, Boschetto P, Miotto D, *et al*.: Mechanisms of occupational asthma. *Ann Allergy Asthma Immunol* 1999, 83:645.

Montanaro A: Chemically-induced nonspecific bronchial hyperresponsiveness. *Clin Rev Allergy Immunol* 1997, 15:187.

Pattemore PK, Johnston SL, Bardin PG: Viruses as precipitants of asthma symptoms. I. Epidemiology. *Clin Exp Allergy* 1992, 22:325.

Planter RC, Smith TF: Respiratory infections, wheezing and asthma. *Immunol Allergy Clin North Am* 1993, 13:141.

Rischitelli DG: A workers' compensation primer. *Ann Allergy Asthma Immunol* 1999, 83:614.

Seaton A, Godden DJ, Brown K: Increase in asthma: a more toxic environment or a more susceptible population? *Thorax* 1994, 49:171.

Selner JC, Staudenmayer H: Psychological factors complicating the diagnosis of work-related illness. *Immunol Allergy Clin North Am* 1992, 12:909.

Siracusa A, Desrosiers M, Marabini A: Epidemiology of occupational rhinitis: Prevalence, etiology and determinants. *Clin Exp Allergy* 2000, 30:1519–1534.

Smith DD: Acute inhalation injury: how to assess, how to treat. *J Resp Dis* 1999, 20:405.

Venables KM, Chan-Yeung M: Occupational asthma. *Lancet* 1997, 349:1465.

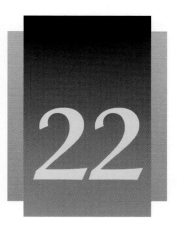

22

Food Allergy

Wesley Burks, Scott H. Sicherer, and Glenn Furuta

A basic understanding of the classification of adverse reactions to foods is critical to any discussion of food allergy and food intolerance. The use of these terms has allowed better communication regarding various reactions to food components. An *adverse food reaction* is a general term that can be applied to a clinically abnormal response to an ingested food or food additive. Adverse food reactions may be secondary to food hypersensitivity (allergy) or food intolerance.

Food hypersensitivity (allergy) is an immunologic reaction that results from the ingestion of a food or food additive. These reactions occur only in some patients, may occur after only a small amount of the substance is ingested, and are unrelated to any physiologic effect of the food or food additive. To most physicians, the term is synonymous with reactions that involve the IgE mechanism, of which anaphylaxis is the classic example.

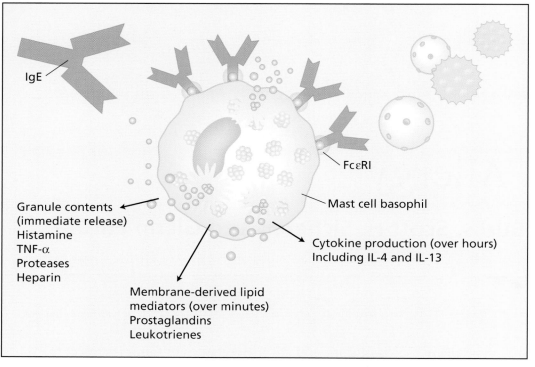

Figure 22-1.

IgE-dependent activation of mast cells and basophils. *Food intolerance* is a general term that describes an abnormal physiologic response to an ingested food or food additive. This reaction has not been proven to be immunologic in nature and may be caused by many factors, including toxic contaminants (*eg*, histamine in scombroid fish poisoning; toxins secreted by *Salmonella*, *Shigella*, and *Campylobacter* spp), pharmacologic properties of the food (*eg*, caffeine in coffee, tyramine in aged cheeses), characteristics of the host such as metabolic disorders (*eg*, lactase deficiency), and idiosyncratic responses.

The term *food intolerance* has often been overused and, similar to the term *food allergy*, has been applied incorrectly to all adverse reactions to foods. IgE-mediated (type I) hypersensitivity accounts for the majority of well-characterized food allergic reactions, but non–IgE-mediated immune mechanisms are believed to be responsible for a variety of hypersensitivity disorders. For this discussion, we examine adverse food reactions that are IgE mediated and non–IgE mediated, and entities that have characteristics of both. IL—interleukin; TNF—tumor necrosis factor.

Clinical Manifestations of Food Hypersensitivity

IgE-mediated Hypersensitivity

Oral Allergy Syndrome	
Oral manifestations	Burning
	Swelling
	Itching
	Erythema
	Immediate onset of symptoms
Age at onset	Beyond infancy
	Typically < 5 years
Proteins implicated	Heat-labile fresh fruit and vegetable allergens
	Pollen and latex cross-reactivity
Pathology	IgE antibodies
Treatment	Avoidance
	Cooking
Natural history	Unknown

Figure 22-2.

Oral allergy syndrome. The oral allergy syndrome is considered a form of contact urticaria that is confined almost exclusively to the oropharynx and rarely involves other target organs. The symptoms include rapid onset of pruritus and angioedema of the lips, tongue, palate, and throat. The symptoms generally resolve quite rapidly. This syndrome is most commonly associated with the ingestion of fresh fruits and vegetables. Interestingly, patients with allergic rhinitis secondary to certain airborne pollens (especially ragweed and birch pollens) are frequently afflicted with this syndrome. Patients with ragweed allergy may experience these symptoms after contact with certain melons (watermelons, cantaloupe, honeydew) and bananas. Patients with birch sensitivity often have symptoms after the ingestion of raw potatoes, carrots, celery, apples, and hazelnuts. The diagnosis of this syndrome is made after a suggestive history and positive prick skin test results with the implicated fresh fruits or vegetables. The convert in this syndrome is that the commercially available allergen extracts for fresh fruits and vegetables often do not have the reliability of the other food extracts. It may be necessary to use the prick-by-prick method, in which the device used for introducing the allergen into the skin may have to initially be pricked into the food. (*Adapted from* Metcalfe *et al.* [1].)

Immediate Gastrointestinal Hypersensitivity

Manifestations	Nausea, abdominal pain and vomiting within 1 to 2 hours
	Diarrhea within 2 to 6 hours
	Frequently associated with atopic disease
	Food-specific IgE antibodies
	Radiographic: gastric hypotonia and pylorospasm
Age at onset	Infancy, childhood
Proteins implicated	Milk, eggs, peanuts, soy, cereal, fish
Pathology	IgE mediated
Treatment	Protein elimination
Natural history	80% of cases resolve after protein elimination diet (except in the case of peanut and fish allergy)

Figure 22-3.

Immediate gastrointestinal (GI) hypersensitivity. Immediate GI hypersensitivity is a form of IgE-mediated GI hypersensitivity that may accompany allergic manifestations in other target organs. The symptoms vary but may include nausea, abdominal pain, abdominal cramping, vomiting, and diarrhea. In studies of children with atopic dermatitis and food allergy, the frequent ingestion of a food allergen appears to induce partial desensitization of GI mast cells, resulting in less pronounced symptoms (as suggested in the rodent model).

The diagnosis of these symptoms is made by a suggestive clinical history, positive prick skin test results, complete elimination of the suspected food allergen for up to 2 weeks with resolution of symptoms, and oral food challenge tests. After avoidance of a particular food for 10 to 14 days, it is not unusual for symptoms of vomiting to occur during a challenge test even though the patient was previously ingesting the food without vomiting every time he or she ate it. (*Adapted from* Sampson [2].)

Mixed IgE-mediated and Non–IgE-mediated Reactions

A. Allergic Eosinophilic Gastritis

Manifestations	Vomiting
	Abdominal pain
	Anorexia
	Early satiety
	Hematemesis
	Failure to thrive
	Gastric outlet obstruction
	Gastric bleeding
	50% of cases atopic
	Elevated IgE
	50% of cases with peripheral eosinophilia
	Radiographic: antral obstruction, thickened folds
	GERD
	Failure to respond to H-2 blockers
	Responds to protein elimination
Age at onset	Neonate to adolescent
Proteins implicated	Cow's milk, eggs, corn, cod, soy
	Often single antigen
	< 50% skin test specificity
Pathology	Marked eosinophilic infiltration of gastric mucosa and submucosa, especially in the gastric antrum
Treatment	Protein elimination
	Excellent response to hydrolyzed protein formula in patients younger than age 2 years
	Excellent response to L-amino acid formula
	Excellent response to low-dose, often long-term steroids
Natural history	Guarded outcome in older patients

Figure 22-4.

Characteristics of allergic eosinophilic gastroenteropathy. **A,** Allergic eosinophilic gastritis. (*continued on next page*)

B. Allergic Eosinophilic Gastroenterocolitis

Manifestations	Abdominal pain
	Anorexia
	Early satiety
	Failure to thrive
	Gastric outlet obstruction
	Gastric or colonic bleeding
	± 70% of cases atopic
	Elevated IgE
	± Food-specific IgE
	50% of cases with peripheral eosinophilia
	Radiographic: antral obstruction, Menetrier's disease, GERD, bowel wall edema, vomiting, diarrhea, protein-losing enteropathy, decreased albumin
Age at onset	Neonate to adolescent
Proteins implicated	Cow's milk, eggs, fish, soy, cereals
	< 50% skin test specificity
Pathology	Marked eosinophilic infiltration of mucosa and submucosa; gastric antrum, esophagus, and duodenum; and colon
Treatment	50% of patients respond to dietary elimination of documented allergen
	Excellent response to hydrolyzed protein formula in patients younger than age 2 years
	Excellent response to L-amino acid formula
	Responsive to steroids
Natural history	Disorder is typically prolonged

Figure 22-4. (*continued*)

B, Allergic eosinophilic gastroenterocolitis. Allergic eosinophilic gastroenteropathy is characterized by infiltration of the gastric or intestinal walls (or both) with eosinophils, absence of vasculitis, and frequently peripheral eosinophils. Patients who present with this syndrome frequently have postprandial nausea and vomiting, abdominal pain, diarrhea, occasionally steatorrhea, and failure to thrive in young infants or weight loss in adults. There appears to be a subset of patients with allergic eosinophilic gastroenteritis who have symptoms secondary to ingestion of food. These patients generally have the mucosal form of this disease with IgE staining cells in jejunal tissue, elevated IgE in duodenal fluids, atopic disease, elevated serum IgE concentrations, positive prick skin test results to a variety of foods and inhalants, peripheral blood eosinophils, iron deficiency anemia, and hypoalbuminemia.

The diagnosis of this entity is based on an appropriate history and a gastrointestinal biopsy that demonstrates a characteristic eosinophilic infiltration. Multiple sites (≤ eight) may need to be biopsied to effectively exclude eosinophilic gastroenteritis because the eosinophilic infiltrates may be quite patchy. Patients with the mucosal form of the disease may have atopic symptoms, including food allergy, elevated serum IgE concentrations, positive skin test results (or radioallergosorbent test [RAST]) and peripheral eosinophilia. Other laboratory studies consistent with this disease include Charcot-Leyden crystals in the stool, anemia, hypoalbuminemia, and abnormal D-xylose tests. An elimination diet of up to 12 weeks may be necessary before complete resolution of symptoms and normalization of intestinal histology. GERD—gastroesophageal reflux disease. (*Adapted from* Sampson and Anderson [3].)

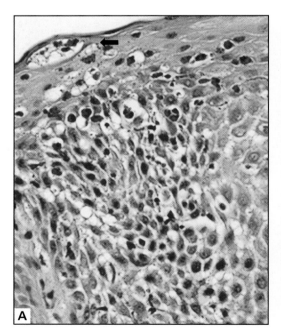 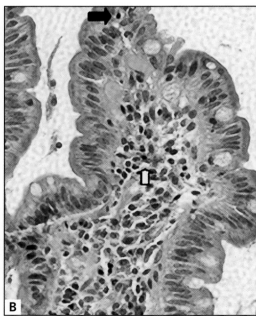 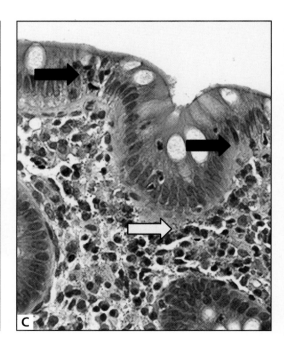

Figure 22-5.

Endoscopic pinch biopsy specimens from a patient with eosinophilic gastroenteritis. This 14-year-old female patient with the mucosal form of eosinophilic gastroenteritis reported abdominal pain and diarrhea. The physical examination was unremarkable. The peripheral blood smear showed eosinophilia. An upper gastrointestinal series with small bowel follow-through were normal. The patient's symptoms responded to dietary restriction of egg and cow's milk.

A, The esophageal squamous epithelium shows increased eosinophils, some of which are on the superficial surface (*black arrow*). (Magnification, × 40.) **B,** Duodenal biopsy specimen shows eosinophilic infiltration of the lamina propria. Eosinophils are adjacent to the basal pole of the epithelial cells (*open arrow*) and transmigrating eosinophils are seen at the villous top (*black arrow*). (Magnification, × 40.)

C, Sigmoid biopsy specimen demonstrates eosinophilic infiltration of the lamina propria. As in the duodenal biopsy specimen, eosinophils are adjacent to the basolateral surface of the epithelial cell (*open arrow*) and can be seen transmigrating through the epithelium (*black arrows*). (Magnification, × 40.)

Non–IgE-mediated Food Hypersensitivity

Dietary Protein Enterocolitis

Manifestations	Diarrhea with bleeding
	Anemia
	Emesis
	Abdominal distension
	Failure to thrive
	Hypotension
	Fecal leukocytes
	Normal IgE
	Food challenge: vomiting in 3 to 4 hours; diarrhea in 5 to 8 hours
Age at onset	1 day to 1 year
Proteins implicated	Cow's milk, soy, rice, poultry, fish
Pathology	Patchy villous injury and colitis
Treatment	≥ 80% of patients respond to hydrolyzed casein formula; symptoms clear in 3 to 10 days
	≤ 20% of patients require L-amino acid formula or temporary IV therapy
Natural history	In general, 50% of patients resolve by 18 months of treatment; 90% of patients resolve by 36 months
	Cow's milk: 50% of patients resolve by 18 months of treatment; 90% of patients resolve by 36 months
	Soy illness is often more persistent

Figure 22-6.

Dietary protein enterocolitis. Dietary protein enterocolitis, also known as protein intolerance, presents most commonly in infants between age 1 week and 3 months. The typical symptoms are isolated to the gastrointestinal tract and consist of typically recurrent vomiting or diarrhea. The symptoms can be severe enough to cause dehydration. Cow's milk and soy protein (particularly in infant formulas) are most often responsible for this syndrome, but egg sensitivity has been reported in older patients. The children often have stools that contain occult blood, polymorphonuclear neutrophils, and eosinophils and are frequently positive for reducing substances (indicating malabsorbed sugars). Prick skin test results for the putative food protein are characteristically negative. Jejunal biopsies classically reveal flattened villi; edema; and increased numbers of lymphocytes, eosinophils, and mast cells. A food challenge test with the responsible protein generally results in vomiting or diarrhea within minutes to several hours and occasionally leads to shock. It is common to find children who are sensitive to both cow's milk and soy protein. This disorder also tends to disappear by 18 to 24 months of age.

Elimination of the offending allergen generally results in improvement or resolution of the symptoms within 72 hours, but secondary disacchoridase deficiency may persist longer. Oral food challenge tests, which should be done in a medical setting because they can induce severe vomiting, diarrhea, dehydration, or hypotension, consist of administering 0.6 g/kg body weight of the suspected food allergen. IV—intravenous. (*Adapted from* Sampson and Anderson [3].)

Dietary Protein Proctitis

Manifestations	Blood-streaked, soft to loose stools
	Fecal leukocytes
	Mild peripheral eosinophilia
	Mild hypoalbuminemia
	Low risk of anemia
	Food challenge test: symptoms in 6 to 72 hours
Age at onset	1 day to 6 months
	Most cases manifest at 2 to 8 weeks
Proteins implicated	60% of reported infants exclusively breastfed
	Cow's milk, eggs, soy
Pathology	Endoscopic: focal to diffuse colitis, linear erosions
	Microscopic: eosinophilic colitis > 20 eosinophils/40 per high-power field; 20% of cases with nodular lymphoid hyperplasias
Treatment	Protein elimination
	Symptoms generally clear in 72 hours in patients given extensively hydrolyzed formula
	Resume or continue breastfeeding on maternal antigen-restricted diet
Natural history	Symptoms usually clear by 1 year

Figure 22-7.

Dietary protein proctitis. This disorder generally presents in the first few months of life and is often secondary to cow's milk or soy protein hypersensitivity. Infants with the disorder often do not appear ill and have normally formed stools. This disorder is generally discovered because of the presence of blood (gross or occult) in the patient's stools. Gastrointestinal lesions are confined to the small bowel and consist of mucosal edema with eosinophils in the epithelium and lumina propria. If lesions are severe with crypt destruction, polymorphonuclear cells are also prominent. It is believed, without a lot of well-controlled studies, that cow's milk– and soy protein–induced colitis resolves by 6 months to 2 years of allergen avoidance.

Elimination of the offending food allergen leads to resolution of hematochezia within 72 hours, but the mucosa lesions may take up to 1 month to disappear and range from patchy mucosal injection to severe friability with small aphthoid ulcerations and bleeding. (*Adapted from* Sampson and Anderson [3].)

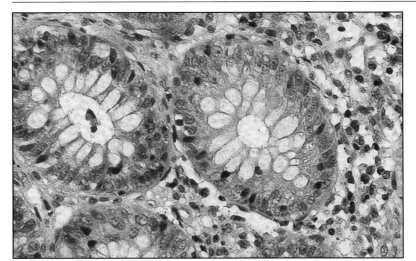

Figure 22-8.

Rectosigmoid biopsy specimen from a patient with allergic colitis. The patient, a well-appearing infant, had bloody stools despite restriction of cow's milk, soy milk, and protein hydrolysate formula. The physical examination was normal except for hemoccult-positive stools. Endoscopic biopsies revealed lymphonodular hyperplasia. The patient's symptoms responded to an amino acid–based formula. This specimen demonstrates increased numbers of eosinophils in the lamina propria, eosinophils at the basal pole of epithelial cells, and an eosinophilic crypt abscess.

Diagnosing Adverse Food Reactions

Methods Used in the Evaluation of Food Allergic Reactions
Medical history
Diet diary
Elimination diet
Prick skin testing
Radioallergosorbent test
Basophil histamine release assay
Intestinal mast cell histamine release
Double-blind, placebo-controlled food challenge

Figure 22-9.

Methods used in the evaluation of food allergic reactions. As with all medical disorders, the diagnostic approach to a patient with a suspected adverse food reaction begins with the medical history and physical examination. Based on the information derived from these initial steps, various laboratory studies may be helpful.

The true value of the medical history largely depends on the patient's recollection of symptoms and the examiner's ability to differentiate between disorders provoked by food hypersensitivity and other causes. The history may be directly useful in diagnosing food allergy in acute events (eg, systemic anaphylaxis

after the ingestion of fish). However, in many series, fewer than 50% of reported food allergic reactions could be substantiated by a double-blind, placebo-controlled food challenge (DBPCFC). Several pieces of information are important to establish that a food allergic reaction occurred: 1) the food suspected to have provoked the reaction, 2) the quantity of the food ingested, 3) the length of time between ingestion and development of symptoms, 4) a description of the symptoms provoked, 5) if similar symptoms developed on other occasions when the food was eaten, 6) if other factors (eg, exercise) are necessary, and 7) the length of time since the last reaction. Any food may cause an allergic reaction, but only a few foods account for 90% of the reactions. In children, these foods are eggs, milk, peanuts, soy, and wheat (and fish in Scandinavian countries). In chronic disorders such as atopic dermatitis, the history is often an unreliable indicator of the offending allergen.

A diet diary has been frequently used as an adjunct to the medical history. Patients are asked to keep a chronological record of all foods ingested over a specified period of time and to record any symptoms they experience during this time. The diary can then be reviewed at a patient visit to determine if there is any relationship between the foods ingested and the symptoms experienced. This method rarely detects an unrecognized association between a food and a patient's symptoms. But as opposed to the medical history, this method allows one to collect information on a prospective basis, which is not so dependent on a patient's or parent's memory.

An elimination diet is frequently used both in diagnosis and management of patients with adverse food reactions. If a certain food (or foods) is suspected of provoking the reaction, it is completely eliminated from the diet. The success of an elimination diet depends on several factors, including the correct identification of the allergen (or allergens) involved, the ability of the patient to maintain a diet completely free of all forms of the possible offending allergen, and the assumption that other factors will not provoke similar symptoms during the study period. The likelihood of all of these conditions being met is often slim. For example, in a young infant reacting to cow's milk formula, resolution of symptoms after substitution of cow's milk formula with a soy formula or casein hydrolysate is highly suggestive of cow's milk allergy but also could be caused by lactose intolerance. Avoidance of suspected food allergens before blinded challenge is recommended so the reactions may be heightened. However, elimination diets are rarely diagnostic of food allergy, particularly in patients with chronic disorders such as atopic dermatitis and asthma. IMCHR—intestinal mast cell histamine release. (*Adapted from* Metcalfe *et al.* [1].)

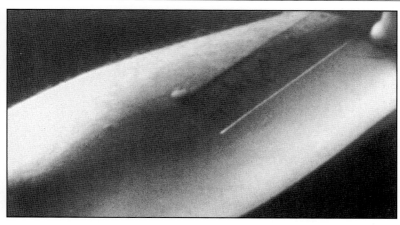

Figure 22-10.

Allergy prick skin test. Allergy prick skin tests are highly reproducible and are often used to screen patients with suspected IgE-mediated food allergies. The glycerinated food extracts (1:10 or 1:20) and appropriate positive (histamine) and negative (saline) controls are applied by either the prick or puncture technique. A food allergen that elicits a wheal (not including erythema) at least 3 mm greater than the negative control is considered a positive result; anything smaller is considered a negative one. There are two important pieces of information from the allergy prick skin test. First, a positive skin test to a food indicates the possibility that the patient has symptomatic reactivity to that specific food (the overall positive predictive accuracy is less than 50%). Second, a negative skin test confirms the absence of an IgE-mediated reaction (the overall negative predictive accuracy is greater than 95%). Both of these statements are justified if appropriate and good quality food extracts are used.

The prick skin test should be considered an excellent means of excluding IgE-mediated food allergies but are only suggestive of the presence of clinical food allergies. There are some minor exceptions to the general statement: 1) IgE-mediated sensitivity to several fruits and vegetables (*eg*, apples, oranges, bananas, pears, melons, potatoes, carrots, celery) are frequently not detected with commercial reagents, presumably secondary to the liability of the responsible allergen in the food; 2) children younger than age 1 year may have IgE-mediated food allergy without a positive skin test result, and children younger than age 2 years may have smaller wheals, possibly caused by the lack of skin reactivity and conversely; 3) a positive skin test result to a food ingested in isolation that provokes a serious systemic anaphylactic reaction may be considered diagnostic.

An intradermal skin test is a more sensitive tool than the prick skin test but is much less specific compared with a double-blind, placebo-controlled food challenge (DBPCFC). In Bock's study [3], no patient who had a negative prick skin test but a positive intradermal skin to a specific food had a positive DBPCFC result to that food. In addition, intradermal skin testing increases the risk of inducing a systemic reaction compared with prick skin testing.

Radioallergosorbent tests (RASTs) and similar *in vitro* assays (*eg*, enzyme-linked immunosorbent assays) are used for the identification of food-specific IgE antibodies. These tests are often used to screen for IgE-mediated food allergies. Although generally considered slightly less sensitive than skin tests, one study [4] comparing Phadebos (Pharmacia, Uppsala, Sweden) RAST with DBPCFCs found prick skin tests and RASTs to have similar sensitivity and specificity when a Phadebos score of three or greater was considered positive. In this study, if a two was considered a positive result, there was a slight improvement in sensitivity, but the specificity decreased significantly. In general, *in vitro* measurements of serum food-specific IgE performed in high-quality laboratories provide information similar to that provided in prick skin tests. The newest generation of *in vitro* studies for specific IgE include the CAP-FEIA. For patients with suspected food allergy, there are now accepted levels of specific IgE that are greater than 95% predictive of a patient's being allergic to that food. This test is best used for patients with possible allergic reactions to milk, eggs, and peanuts.

Food Challenge Setting from Highest to Lowest Risk for Reactions
Intensive care unit
Hospital room
Office (within hospital)
Office (isolated)

Figure 22-11.

Food challenge settings. The double-blind, placebo-controlled food challenge (DBPCFC) has been labeled the "gold standard" for the diagnosis of food allergies. This test has been used successfully by many investigators in both children and adults for the past several years to examine a wide variety of food-related complaints. The foods to be tested in the oral challenge are based on patient history or positive prick skin test (radioallergosorbent test [RAST]) results or both.

A DBPCFC is the best means of controlling for the variability of chronic disorders (*eg*, chronic urticaria, atopic dermatitis), potential temporal effects, and acute exacerbations secondary to reducing or discontinuing medications. Particularly, psychogenic factors and observer bias are eliminated. There are the rare false-negative challenges in a DBPCFC. This may occur when a patient receives insufficient challenge material during the challenge to provoke the reaction or the lyophilization of the food antigen has altered the relevant allergenic epitopes (*eg*, fish). Overall, the DBPCFC has proven to be the most accurate means of diagnosing food allergy at the present time.

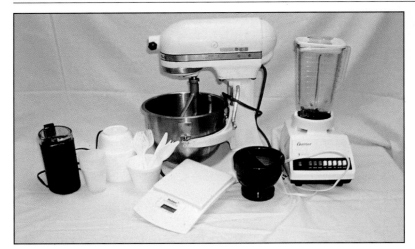

Figure 22-12.

Food preparation. A number of different food processing techniques will be helpful in preparing allergenic foods for use in blinded food challenges.

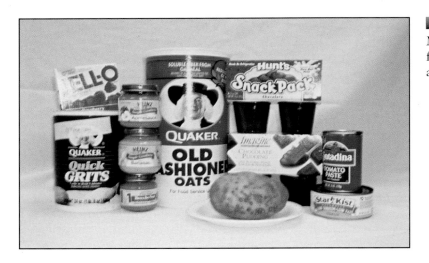

Figure 22-13.

Masking agents. Because of the taste and odor of certain allergenic foods, it may be necessary to utilize other foods to mix with the allergenic food to mask its presence.

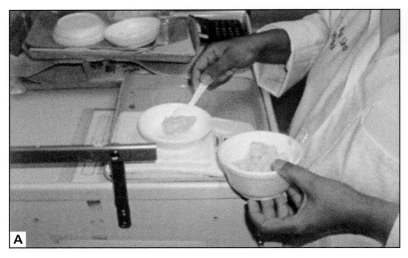

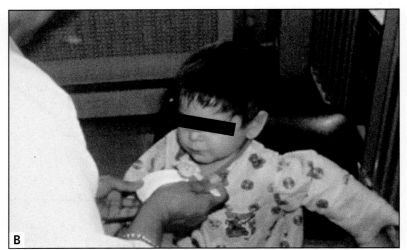

Figure 22-14.

Administration of a food challenge test (**A and B**). The patient will receive the suspected food in increasingly larger amounts over approximately 1 to 2 hours. Generally, the challenge will start with 100 mg of the suspected food. The entire challenge consists of ingestion of 10 g of the suspected food.

Management

Acute Management

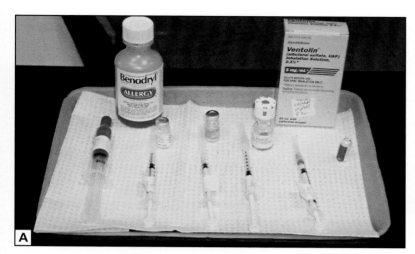

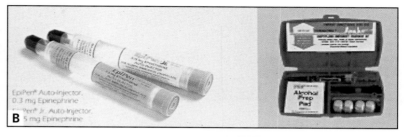

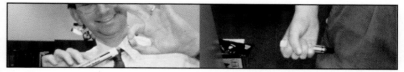

D. Directions for Using the Epinephrine Auto-Injector

1. Pull off gray safety cap
2. Place black tip on thigh at right angle to leg; always apply to thigh
3. Using a quick motion, press hard into thigh until auto-injector mechanism functions and hold in place for several seconds. The injector should then be removed and discarded. Massage the injection area for 10 seconds.

See Figure 22-13C for photographic representation.

Figure 22-15.

Emergency medications for the treatment of patients with food allergy. **A,** Benadryl (Warner-Lambert Consumer Group, Morris Plains, NJ) and albuterol sulfate (Ventolin; GlaxoSmithKline, Research Triangle Park, NC). Fatalities may occur if treatment of a food-induced anaphylactic reaction is not immediate. Initial treatment must be preceded by a rapid assessment to determine the extent and severity of the reaction, the adequacy of oxygenation, cardiac output, and tissue perfusion, any potential confounding medications (*eg*, β-blockers), and the suspected cause of the reaction. Initial therapy should be directed at the maintenance of an effective airway and circulatory system. Epinephrine (adrenaline) is the drug of choice in the treatment of patients with anaphylaxis. The first step in the management of anaphylaxis is the subcutaneous or intramuscular (IM) injection of 0.01 mL/kg of aqueous epinephrine 1:1000 (maximal dose, 0.3 to 0.5 mL or 0.3 to 0.5 mg). Recent reports indicate that IM administration may achieve a faster and higher rate of absorption.

The importance of epinephrine in the treatment of patients with anaphylaxis is best seen in the cases of fatal and near-fatal food-induced anaphylaxis. In general, patients who die from anaphylatic reactions have received no epinephrine or have received an inadequate dose during their acute reaction. In contrast, patients who have survived a near-fatal anaphylactic reaction generally received epinephrine early in the course of their reaction, and many have received repeated doses of epinephrine.

In order to ensure that patients receive epinephrine as early as possible, it is important that they, their family members, and other care providers are instructed in the self-administration of epinephrine (**B** through **D**). Preloaded syringes with epinephrine are available and should be given to any patients at risk for food-induced anaphylaxis (*ie*, patients with a history of a previous anaphylactic reaction and those with asthma and food allergy, especially if they are allergic to peanuts, nuts, fish, or shellfish). In the United States, premeasured doses of epinephrine can be obtained by either Epi-Pen or Epi-Pen Jr. (**C**; distributed by Center Laboratories, Port Washington, NY).

Long-term Management

Factors Indicating Increased Risk for Severe
Anaphylactic Reactions

History of previous anaphylactic reaction
History of asthma, especially if poorly controlled
Allergy to peanuts, nuts, fish, and shellfish
Beta-blockers or angiotensin-converting enzyme inhibitors
Female gender (?)

Figure 22-16.

Factors indicating increased risk for severe anaphylactic reactions. The life-threatening nature of anaphylaxis makes prevention the cornerstone of therapy. If the causative food allergen is not clearly delineated, an evaluation to determine the etiology should be promptly initiated so a lethal recurrence can be prevented, as discussed previously. The central focus of prevention of food-induced anaphylaxis requires the appropriate identification and complete dietary avoidance of the specific food allergen.

An educational process is imperative to ensure that the patient and family understands how to avoid all forms of the food allergen and the potential severity of a reaction if the food is inadvertently ingested. The Food Allergy & Anaphylaxis Network is a nonprofit organization located in Fairfax, Virginia (phone: 800-929-4040; www.foodallergy.org) that can assist in providing patients with information about food allergen avoidance. This organization has several programs for schools and parents of children with food allergies and at high risk for anaphylaxis.

Prognosis

Strategies to "Desensitize" Allergic Patients to Foods

Recombinant "mutated" allergen immunotherapy
Peptide immunotherapy
Bacterial-encapsulated allergen immunotherapy
ISS-conjugated allergen immunotherapy
Cytokine-modulated immunotherapy
Anti-IgE therapy (general, not specific allergen treatment)

Figure 22-17.

"Desensitization" strategies. For many young children diagnosed with anaphylaxis to foods such as milk, egg, wheat, and soybeans, there is a good possibility that the clinical sensitivity may be outgrown after several years. Children who develop their food sensitivity after 3 years of age are less likely to lose their food reactions over a period of several years. Allergies to foods such as peanuts, tree nuts, fish, and seafood are less likely to be outgrown, no matter at what age they develop. These individuals appear likely to retain their allergic sensitivity for a lifetime. Consequently, several groups are evaluating new strategies to "desensitize" patients to these foods.

References

1. Metcalfe DD, Sampson HA, Simon RA: *Food Allergy: Adverse Reactions to Foods and Food Additives*. Cambridge: Blackwell; 1997.
2. Sampson HA: Food allergy. *J Allergy Clin Immunol* 1989, 84:1062–1067.
3. Sampson HA, Anderson JA: Summary and recommendations: classification of gastrointestinal manifestations due to immunologic reactions to foods in infants and young children. *J Pediatr Gastroenterol Nutr* 2000, 30 (suppl 1):587–594.
4. Sampson HA, Albergo R: Comparison of results of skin tests, RAST, and double-blinded placebo-controlled food challenges in children with atopic dermatitis. *J Allergy Clin Immunol* 1984, 74:26–33.

Recommended Reading

Anderson JA, Sogn DD (eds): *Adverse Reactions to Foods*. American Academy of Allergy and Immunology Committee on Adverse Reactions to Foods and the National Institute of Allergy and Infectious Disease. Washington, DC: US Department of Health and Human Services (NIH Publication No. 84-2442); 1984.

Bock SA: Natural history of severe reactions to foods in young children. *J Pediatr* 1985, 107:676.

Bock SA: Patterns of food hypersensitivity during sixteen years of double-blind, placebo-controlled food challenges. *J Pediatr* 1990, 117:561.

Bock SA: Prospective appraisal of complaints of adverse reactions to foods in children during the first 3 years of life. *Pediatrics* 1987, 79:683.

Burks AW, Sampson HA: Diagnostic approaches to the patient with suspected food allergies. *J Pediatr* 1992, 121(suppl):64.

Bush RK, Taylor SL: Adverse reactions to food and drug additives. In *Allergy: Principles and Practice*, edn 4. Edited by Middleton Jr E, Reed CE, Ellis EF, *et al*. St. Louis: Mosby-Year Book; 1998:1183–1198.

Crowe SE, Perdue MH: Gastrointestinal food hypersensitivity basic mechanisms of pathophysiology. *Gastroenterology* 1992, 103:1075.

Jenkins HR, *et al*.: Food allergy: the major cause of infantile colitis. *Arch Dis Child* 1984, 59:326.

Sampson HA, Mendelson L, Rosen, JP: Fatal and near-fatal anaphylactic reactions to food in children and adolescents. *N Engl J Med* 1992, 327:380.

Sampson HA: Adverse reactions to foods. In *Allergy: Principles and Practice*, 4th edn. Edited by Middleton Jr E, Reed CE, Ellis EF, *et al*. St. Louis: Mosby-Year Book; 1998:1162–1182.

Terr AI: Unconventional theories and unproven methods in allergy. In *Allergy: Principles and Practice*, 4th edn. Edited by Middleton Jr E, Reed CE, Ellis EF, *et al*. St. Louis: Mosby-Year Book; 1998:1235–1249.

Yunginger JW: Lethal food allergy in children. *N Engl J Med* 1992, 327:421–422.

Zeiger RS: Secondary prevention of allergic disease: an adjunct to primary prevention. *Pediatr Allergy Immunol* 1995, 6(suppl 3):127–138.

23

Insect Allergy

Robert P. Nelson, Jr. and Richard F. Lockey

Arthropod bites and stings inflicted by different species of insects, arachnids (spiders), and acarids (mites) cause two kinds of reaction in humans: 1) trauma inflicted by the puncture of the skin and feeding, and 2) reaction to the irritating toxic substances, antigenic substances, or both introduced into the host. The most serious of these reactions, anaphylaxis, is caused by sensitization of the host to antigenic substances found in either the saliva or the venom.

Sensitization of the host can also lead to large local reactions that are thought to be caused by one or more allergic mechanisms. The first is IgE-mediated hypersensitivity, as in the cutaneous late-phase reaction; the second, cell-mediated hypersensitivy. Rarely, neurologic sequelae occur, and they also seem to be mediated by IgE or by an immune complex reaction.

Bites

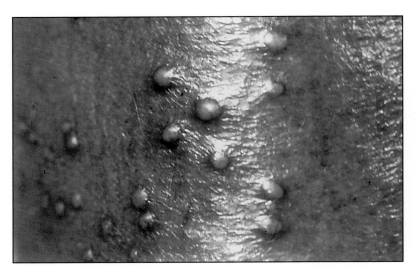

■ Figure 23-1.

The sting of the imported fire ant results in an immediate wheal-and-flare response; within 24 hours, a characteristic sterile pustule appears at the sting site. If left undisturbed, the pustule usually resolves over 10 days. (*From* Wright and Lockey [1]; with permission.)

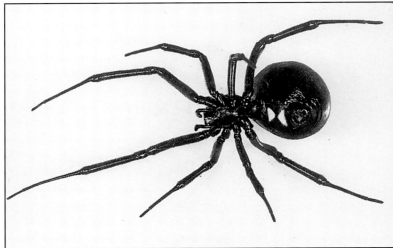

■ Figure 23-2.

Black widow spider (*Latrodectus mactans*). Black widow spiders are usually found near buildings. Note the characteristic hour-glass configuration on the abdomen, which is red. These spiders like abandoned houses, water meter boxes, and areas under park benches or tables. The poison, primarily a neurotoxin, affects the nervous system. Antivenom for black widow spiders is available, although it is rarely necessary because most bites are self-limited. (*From* Wright and Lockey [1]; with permission.)

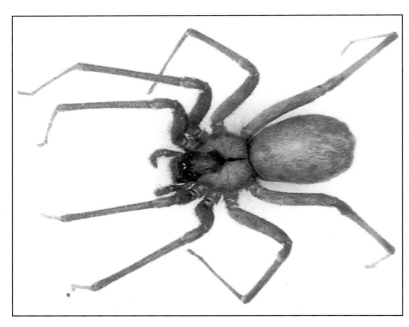

■ Figure 23-3.

Brown recluse spider (*Loxosceles reclusa*). The venom of the brown recluse spider (also known as the fiddleback spider) is primarily cytotoxic, causing local tissue destruction and delayed wound healing. Treatment is symptomatic. (*From* Lockey *et al.* [2]; with permission.)

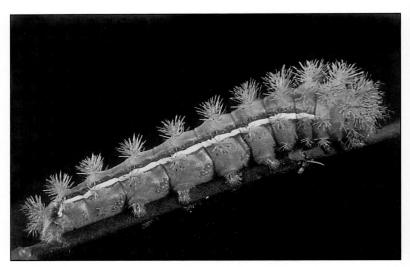

■ Figure 23-4.

Io caterpillar (*Automeris io*). The io caterpillar is a beautiful caterpillar that is about 2 inches long. It is pale green with yellow spines, and along each side are a red stripe and a yellow stripe. The stiff spines contain a poison that can cause a severe stinging injury. Supportive care is indicated. (*From* Lockey *et al.* [2]; with permission.)

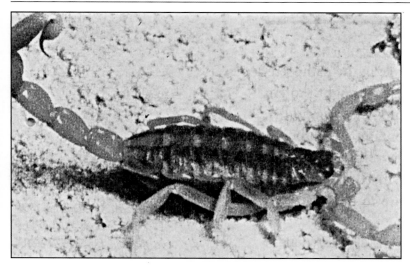

Figure 23-5.

Scorpion (*Centruroides gracilis*). Scorpions are predaceous, feeding on small insects. They are not aggressive but, if touched, with strike with their tail and inject venom into the skin. The pain from a large scorpion's sting is similar to that of a wasp, is usually benign, and should be treated in a similar fashion to a wasp sting. This is only true of scorpions native to Florida. Stings from scorpions in the southwestern United States are more serious and may require antivenom therapy. Ice packs to the area will help to eliminate pain and swelling. (*From* Lockey *et al.* [2]; with permission.)

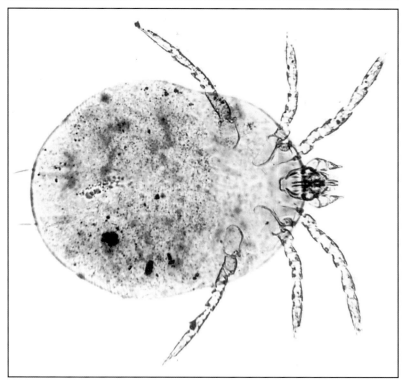

Figure 23-6.

Chigger or red bug (*Trombicula* sp.). Chiggers or red bugs prefer damp areas where the vegetation is thick. In these locations, they climb on plants and wait for a host to pass. Red bugs usually congregate on one's body where clothing is close to the body, such as under a belt or garter or shoe tops. They attach themselves to the skin with their mouth parts and inject salivary juices into the tissue. The mites feed on the damaged tissue, causing erythematous pruritic papules. Avoidance and supportive therapy are indicated. (*From* Lockey *et al.* [2]; with permission.)

Systemic Allergic Reactions

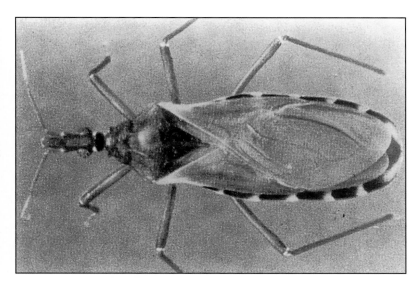

Figure 23-7.

Kissing bugs, cone-nose bugs, or assassin bugs of the order Hemiptera, genus *Triatoma*, are commonly found from Texas to California in the United States. They typically bite at night, when the victim is asleep. IgE sensitization to the insect's saliva can occur, with subsequent anaphylaxis.

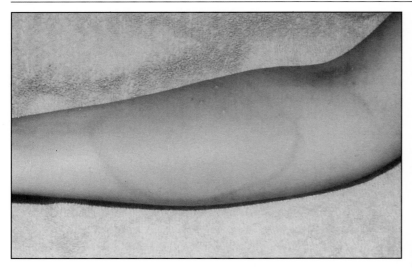

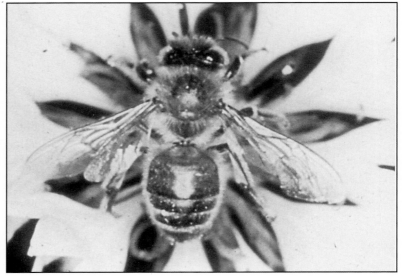

Figure 23-8.

Large local reactions often result from the sting of the imported fire ant. In this patient, shown 6 hours after three stings from a single fire ant, much of the forearm is covered with an erythematous and edematous lesion that is pruritic and painful. The reaction peaked in size at 48 hours. (*From* Lockey [1]; with permission. *Courtesy of* R. deShazo, Mobile, AL.)

Figure 23-9.

Honeybee (*Apis mellifera*). This Hymenoptera insect has a barb on its stinger and may leave its stinger in its victim's skin. The barbed stinger and the poison sac are torn from the bee after most stings. Care must be used in removing the stinger and the venom sac—grasping the venom sac can squeeze remaining venom into the victim. The sting apparatus should be carefully scraped away with a fingernail or a knife blade. (*Courtesy of* Bayer Corporation, Spokane, WA).

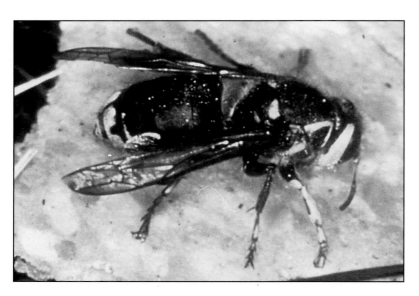

Figure 23-10.

Hornet (*Vespa, Vespula*). Hornets and yellow jackets are closely related insects. (*Courtesy of* Bayer Corporation, Spokane, WA).

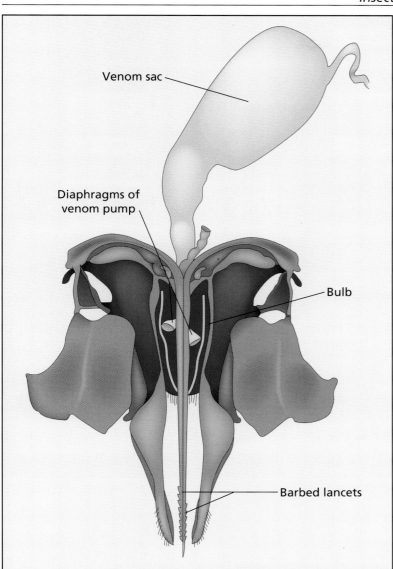

Figure 23-11.
The sting apparatus of a honeybee.

Venom sac

Diaphragms of venom pump

Bulb

Barbed lancets

Figure 23-12.
Identified Hymenoptera venom contents. Hymenoptera venoms are complex mixtures of pharmacologically and biochemically active substances. These substances comprise enzymes, peptides, and biogenic amines. (*Adapted from* Stafford [4].)

Identified Venom Contents

Honeybee	Yellow Jacket	Hornet	Wasp*
Phospholipase A	Phospholipase A	Phospholipase A	Phospolipase A
Hyaluronidase	Phospholipase B	Phospholipase A	Phospholipase B
Acid phosphatase	Hyaluronidase	Hyaluronidase	Serotonin
Melittin	Acid phosphatase	Acid phosphatase	Histamine
Apamin	Kinin	"Hornet kinin"	Hyaluronidase
Mast cell–degranulating peptide	Histamine	Histamine	Kinin
Minimine (?)†	Serotonin	Serotonin	
Norepinephrine	Dopamine	Acetylcholine	
Dopamine	Norepinephrine	Dopamine	
Histamine	Epinephrine	Norepinephrine	
	Cholinesterase	Epinephrine	
	Histidine decarboxylase	Protease	
	Protease		

*Small number of identified components probably reflects limited studies.
†Minimine has been described as a minor polypeptide that retards the development of *Drosophila*. Its existence has not been confirmed.

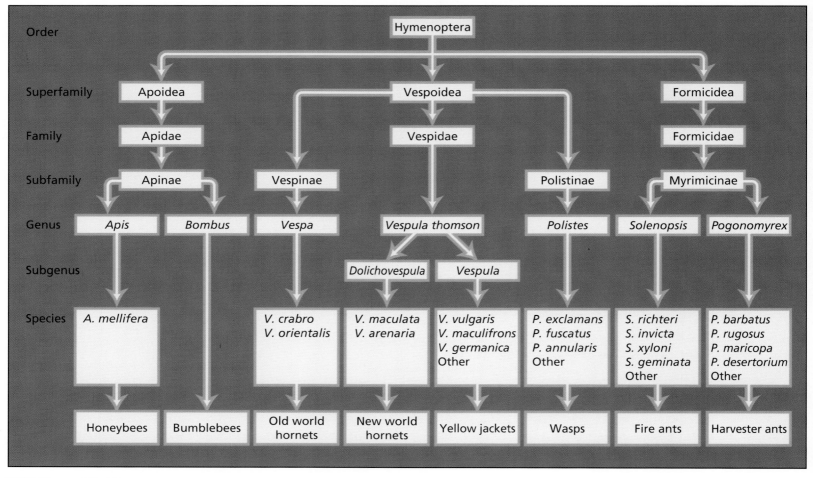

Figure 23-13.

Taxonomy of medically important Hymenoptera. The entomologic differences have significance with regard to allergenic specificity.

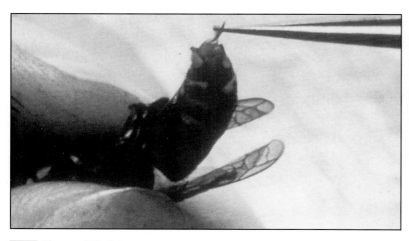

Figure 23-14.

Venom sac dissection. The venom sac is a thick-walled muscular reservoir that stores the venom produced in the acid glands. It is egg-shaped and approximately 1 to 2 mm in diameter. For vespid (yellow jacket, paper wasp, and hornet) venom production, thousands of nests must first be collected. Venom sac dissection is tedious and labor intensive. (*Courtesy of* Bayer Corporation, Spokane, WA).

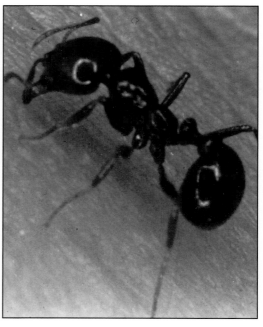

Figure 23-15.

Imported fire ant (*Solenopsis invicta*). The fire ant worker is from 0.125 to 0.25 inches long and varies in color from reddish-brown to dark brown. A sterile pustule forms at the site of each sting. Allergic reactions and secondary infections can be serious and cause death. Neurologic problems are rare and transient.

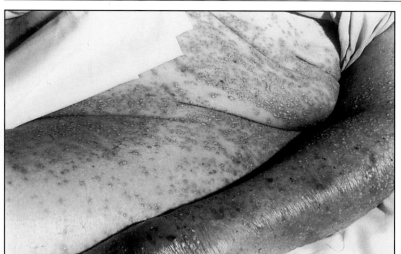

Figure 23-16.

Fire ant stings. Fire ants invaded the home of this 84-year-old woman with senile dementia who was confined to bed because of her history of multiple hip fractures. She was stung at least 10,000 times, as shown by the typical pustular eruptions. She developed neither toxic nor immunologic sequelae from the stings. Lesions such as these can become secondarily infected. Patients can also become sensitized and develop subsequent anaphylaxis on re-sting. Transient neurologic sequelae from imported fire ant stings have also been reported. (*From* Diaz *et al.* [3]; with permission.)

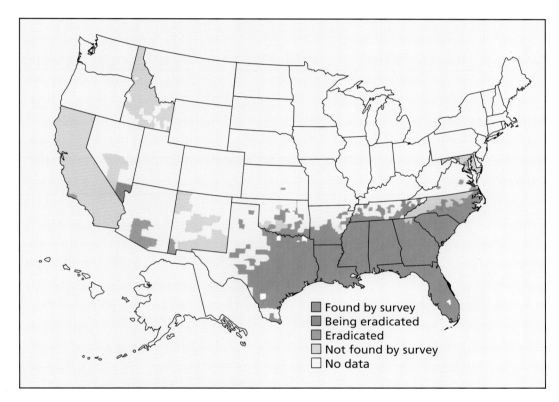

Found by survey
Being eradicated
Eradicated
Not found by survey
No data

Figure 23-17.

Reported distribution of *Solenopsis invicta* and *Solenopsis richteri* as of March 1996. Note that the areas distinguished as "being eradicated" include the tip of Nevada, almost all of North Carolina, and parts of Tennessee. These areas also include places where the fire ant has been eradicated. (*Adapted from* Stafford [4].)

Treatment of Local Reactions to Hymenoptera Stings

Reaction	Treatment
Nonallergic local	Remove stinger, if present
	Apply ice to slow rate of venom absorption and reduce edema and pruritus
	Cleanse with soap and water
	Lidocaine (topically or intradermally) for pain
	Oral or topical H1-antagonist for edema and pruritus
Large local (allergic)	Ice, elevation of affected extremity, analgesics, and oral H1-antagonist (possibly an H2-antagonist)
	Prednisone (1 mg/kg/day) for 3–5 days, starting as soon as possible after sting

Figure 23-18.

Treatment of local reactions to Hymenoptera stings. (*Adapted from* Wright and Lockey [1].)

Selection of Patients for Venom Immunotherapy

Sting reaction	ST/RAST	Venom immunotherapy
Systemic, non-life-threatening (child), immediate, generalized, confined to skin (urticaria, angioedema, erythema, pruritus)	+ or –	No
Systemic, life-threatening (child), immediate, generalized, may involve cutaneous symptoms, but also has respiratory (laryngeal edema or bronchospasm) or cardiovascular symptoms (hypotension/shock)	+	Yes
Systemic (adult)	+	Yes
Systemic*	–	No
Large local	+ or –	No
≤2 inches in diameter		
≤24 h in duration		
Normal local	+ or –	No
≥ in in diameter		
≥24 h in duration		

*The patient should be skin retested, with reconstituted extract, in 4 to 6 weeks. If still negative. RAST should be repeated to confirm the negative skin test. The opposite is true for a RAST-negative individual, in whom the skin test should confirm negative RAST results.

Figure 23-19.

Selection of patients for venom immunotherapy. There is evidence that adults with cutaneous reactions may be at minimal risk for a life-threatening reaction on a subsequent sting even without treatment [5]. RAST—radioallergosorbent test; ST—skin test.

Avoidance of and Protective Measures Against Insect Stings

Wasps usually nest under the eaves of homes or on overhangs, bushes, or trees.

Hornets nest in trees, and yellow jackets nest underground or in cavities of buildings.

The honeybee stinger is barbed. The honeybee venom sac remains in the skin of the stung victim. It should be removed carefully with a flick of the finger.

Insects seem to be less attracted to white or light khaki-colored clothing than to dark brown or black clothing.

Bright floral colors on clothing appear to attract insects and should be avoided.

Wearing long-sleeve shirts, socks, and shoes decreases the chances of being stung, whereas going barefoot increases the chances of being stung.

Scented sprays, soaps, suntan lotion, perfumes, and other cosmetics may increase the likelihood of attracting Hymenoptera insects.

Sweat bees are attracted to perspiration.

Food and beverages served outdoors attracts insects.

Lawn mowing, trimming hedges, sanding and painting homes, emptying garbage cans, and walking in wooded areas increases a person's chances of being stung.

Flower beds, fields covered with clover or other flowering plants, blooming fruit trees or trees that are bearing fruit, and areas in which fruits and vegetation are rotting should be avoided.

Windows should be closed and air conditioning used, whenever possible, while driving in a car.

Homes and cottages should be carefully screened and windows and doors checked for areas through which insects can enter the home.

Insects should be sprayed, whenever possible, around the home, particularly under the eaves.

Garbage cans should be kept clean, sprayed with insecticide where appropriate, and kept covered at all times.

When an insect is in the area, an individual should avoid sudden, rapid movements, which appear to antagonize Hymenoptera insects. The potential victim should slowly move away from an insect in an attempt to avoid an attack.

Subjects with a history of insect hypersensitivity who are not receiving treatment or who have not yet reached maintenance immunotherapy should carry an emergency sting kit containing aqueous epinephrine in a prefilled syringe. Instructions on how to use it should be provided by health care professionals.

Figure 23-20.

Avoidance of and protective measures against insect stings.

References

1. Wright DN, Lockey RF: Local reactions to stinging insects (Hymenoptera). *Allergy Proc* 1990, 11:23–28.

2. Lockey RF, Stewart GE II, Maxwell LS: *Florida's Poisonous Plants, Snakes, Insects*, edn 3. Tampa, FL: Lewis S. Maxwell; 1992.

3. Diaz JD, Lockey RF, Stablein JJ, Mines HK: Multiple stings by imported fire ants (*Solenopsis invicta*, Buren), without systemic effects. *South Med J* 1989, 82:775–777.

4. Stafford CT: Hypersensitivity to fire ant venom. *Ann Allerg Asthma Immunol* 1996, 77:87–95.

5. Reisman RE: Natural history of insect sting allergy: relationship of severity of symptoms of initial sting anaphylaxis to re-sting reactions. *J Allergy Clin Immunol* 1992, 90:335–339.

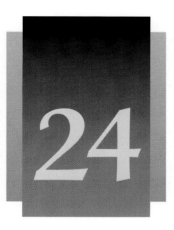

Otitis Media

Deborah A. Gentile and David P. Skoner

Otitis media is the most common disease for which children receive medical care in the United States [1]. Although the life-threatening complications of the disease were significantly decreased after the introduction of antibiotics, other complications continue to contribute to pediatric morbidity. These include the persistence of hearing loss for months to years, which can cause impaired speech and language acquisition, educational deficits, and poor social adjustment [2]. Sequelae of otitis media include cholesteatoma, ossicular erosion, and facial nerve paralysis [3,4]. More than 25% of prescriptions for oral antibiotics are for otitis media, and the most common surgical procedure requiring general anesthesia (*ie*, tympanostomy tube insertion) and the most common major surgical procedure (*ie*, adenoidectomy) are performed to treat or prevent otitis media [5]. The costs of treating patients with otitis media, including physician visits and medical and surgical treatments, are estimated at between $2 billion to $3 billion a year. Moreover, the parent or caregiver of a child with otitis media is typically absent from work 2 days per each illness episode, at an estimated additional cost of $500 million. Therefore, the total annual costs associated with otitis media ranges between $2.5 and $4.5 billion [6].

Otitis media is characterized by active inflammation of the middle ear mucosa and related structures. New episodes can be either symptomatic or asymptomatic in presentation. Both can progress to an asymptomatic persistent stage, chronic otitis media with effusion, in which the mucosal inflammation and middle ear effusion persist long after eradication or neutralization of the inciting stimulus. The cause of otitis media has been shown to be multifactorial, with eustachian tube dysfunction, bacterial or viral infection of the middle ear, and nasal inflammation resulting from allergy or viral upper respiratory infections acknowledged as being contributing factors [7–9]. Virus–allergen interactions may also play a role in predisposing patients with allergic rhinitis to otitis media. Because viruses and allergens may have an individual impact on eustachian tube obstruction, it is conceivable that the two have additive or synergistic effects that produce otitis media in allergic individuals.

The history and physical examination using the pneumatic otoscope are, in most instances, sufficient to establish the diagnosis of otitis media [10]. However, tympanometry has become established as an important tool in assessing the status of the middle ear. Audiometry is essential to determine the effect of middle ear effusion on hearing. If allergic rhinitis is suspected by history and physical examination as a risk factor for the development of otitis media, an allergy evaluation should be performed [11]. Prick skin testing is preferred to serologic tests for the detection of IgE antibodies to specific allergens because of increased sensitivity and lower costs of these tests. If an immune deficiency is suspected based on a history of recurrent, chronic, severe, or unusual infections, an immunologic assessment is indicated [12]. The initial laboratory tests performed should include quantitation of serum IgG, IgA, and IgM, as well as a complete blood cell count, including a leukocyte and differential to ascertain the absolute lymphocyte count.

Medical management of patients with otitis media includes choosing appropriate antibiotics [13,14]. Amoxicillin is the treatment of choice for initial therapy. For recurrence or suspected resistance, either high-dose amoxicillin, amoxicillin with clavulanate, erythromycin with sulfa, or a cephalosporin is suggested. Antiviral agents may have a beneficial effect in

the treatment of patients with viral-induced otitis media; however, they are not currently indicated because their role has not been fully established [15,16]. If allergic rhinitis is documented in association with otitis media, then allergy management should be instituted [11]. Surgical management of patients with otitis media includes insertion of tympanostomy tubes to promote drainage of persistent unresolved effusions and improve hearing [5,17]. Adenoidectomy has also been recommended to relieve extrinsic eustachian tube obstruction caused by peritubular lymphoid tissue [18,19]. Preventive strategies include immunizations, avoidance of exposure to tobacco smoke and allergens, avoidance of daycare facilities (if possible), and handwashing [11,20–23].

Anatomy

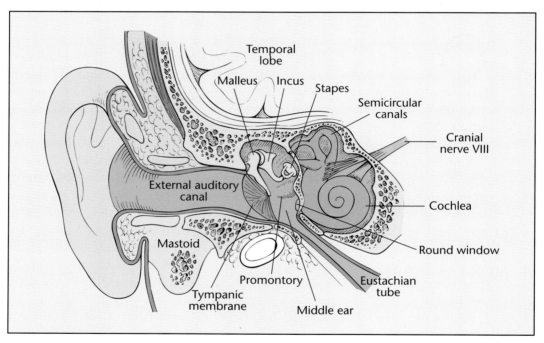

■ Figure 24-1.

Normal cross-sectional anatomy of the ear. The external, middle, and inner ear comprise a compact group of components situated in the temporal bone. Sound is funneled by the pinna into the external auditory canal, where it causes vibration of the tympanic membrane. Attached to the tympanic membrane is the malleus, which, with the incus, increases sound pressure by 30%. The stapes articulates with the long process of the incus, and the stapes footplate acts as a piston to transfer the sound vibrations to the cochlea, where the vibratory stimuli are transformed to nerve impulses. The inner ear also houses the semicircular canals, which, via a portion of the eighth cranial nerve, give dynamic and static information on the motion and position of the head.

Classification

Classification of Otitis Media

Subtype	Diagnostic Criteria
Acute otitis media	Rapid onset of symptoms or signs of inflammation (fever, otalgia, irritability)
	Opacification, fullness or bulging, or poor or no mobility of tympanic membrane because of effusion
Recurrent acute otitis media	Three or more episodes of acute otitis media within 6 months or four or more episodes of acute otitis media within 1 year
Otitis media with effusion	Effusion in middle ear without symptoms or signs of acute inflammation
	Often accompanied by hearing loss
Chronic otitis media with effusion	Otitis media with effusion persisting for 3 months or more
Chronic suppurative otitis media with effusion	Prolonged or intermittent drainage through a tube or perforation in the tympanic membrane

Figure 24-2.

Classification of otitis media. Otitis media is characterized by inflammation of the middle ear and is usually associated with middle ear effusion, which can be serous, mucoid, or purulent. Middle ear mucosa is thickened and edematous. Microscopically, there is glandular hypertropy, engorgement of capillaries and small venules, and a cellular infiltrate of lymphocytes and neutrophils. Otitis media is usually classified into several subtypes. Based on epidemiologic studies, the pathogenesis of otitis media may best be viewed as a disease continuum. This suggests that each of the subtypes of otitis media may represent a stage in the continuum of a single middle ear disease process [12].

Pathogenesis

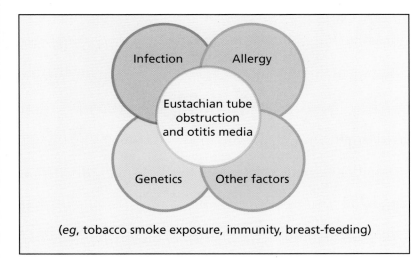

(*eg*, tobacco smoke exposure, immunity, breast-feeding)

Figure 24-3.

Interaction between predisposing factors and the development of otitis media. Eustachian tube obstruction plays a prominent role in the pathogenesis of otitis media [12]. The most common causes of eustachian tube obstruction are viral upper respiratory infections and allergic rhinitis. Other less common causes of eustachian tube obstruction are tumors, enlarged adenoid glands, or abnormalities in the structure or function of the eustachian tube. Rarely, otitis media may be caused by host defense defects, including primary immune deficiencies, infection with HIV, or ciliary defects. Risk factors for the development of otitis media include age younger than 2 years, male gender, exposure to tobacco smoke, allergic rhinitis, daycare facility attendance or older siblings, bottle feeding rather than breast-feeding, congenital craniofacial defects such as cleft palate or Down syndrome, family history of otitis media, and Native American, Eskimo, or Australian Aborigine ethnicity.

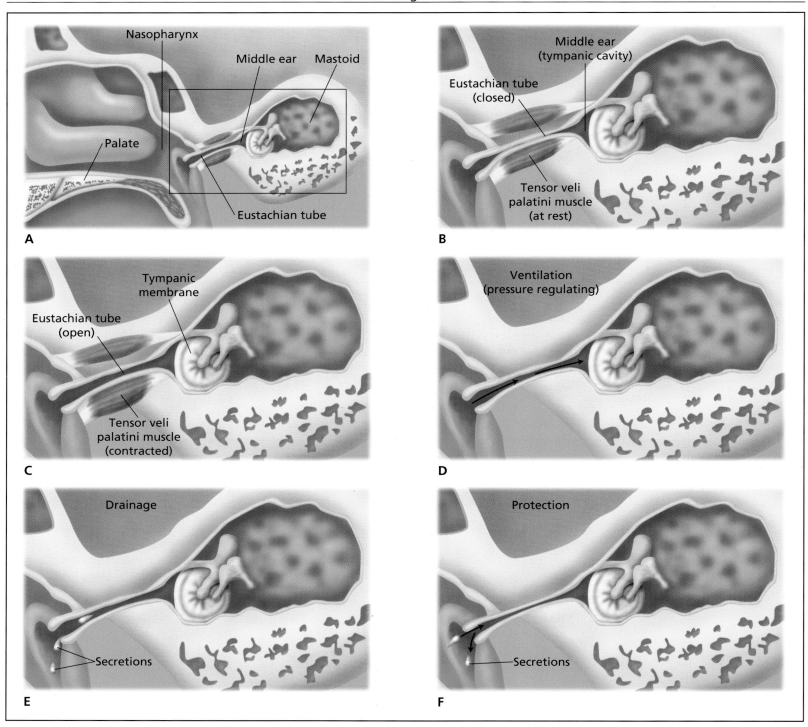

Figure 24-4.

Role of eustachian tube dysfunction in the development of otitis media. The eustachian tube (**A**) connects the middle ear and the nasopharynx; its function is partially controlled by the tensor veli palatini muscle. When the muscle is at rest, the tube is almost always closed (**B**). When the muscle contracts during swallowing, yawning, or crying, the tube opens (**C**). Functions of the eustachian tube include ventilation of the middle ear to regulate pressure (**D**), drainage (**E**), and clearance of middle ear secretions and protection (**F**) of the middle ear from nasopharyngeal secretions. The use of animal models has documented that experimental obstruction of the eustachian tube results in middle ear underpressures and middle ear effusion by transudation, which are hallmark features of otitis media [12].

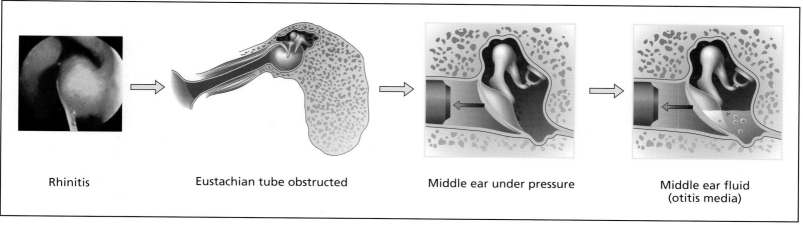

Rhinitis   Eustachian tube obstructed   Middle ear under pressure   Middle ear fluid (otitis media)

Figure 24-5.

Role of allergic rhinitis in the development of otitis media. Several lines of evidence support the hypothesis that allergic rhinitis contributes to the development of otitis media. Allergic rhinitis has been shown to be present in approximately 50% of patients in whom otitis media with effusion was diagnosed, and otitis media with effusion has been shown to be present in approximately 20% of patients in whom allergic rhinitis was diagnosed [12]. Elevations of IgE and inflammatory mediators released during IgE-mediated degranulation reactions, including prostaglandin D$_2$, tryptase, histamine, eosinophil products, and cytokines, have been detected in middle ear effusions of children with otitis media.

Experimental histamine and allergen inhalation by allergic patients has been shown to result in both early (within 30 minutes) and late (2 to 12 hours after challenge test) eustachian tube dysfunction. The results of this laboratory model were confirmed in a natural history model, in which untreated patients allergic to grass followed during grass pollen season also developed eustachian tube dysfunction. A similar study [12] showed the development of middle ear underpressures during pollen season. Despite the confirmed phenomenon of allergen-induced eustachian tube dysfunction and middle ear underpressures, conclusive evidence of allergen-induced middle ear fluid has not been forthcoming in either human or animal models. However, it is conceivable that an interaction between allergy and viral upper respiratory infections may play a role in predisposing to otitis media in patients with allergic rhinitis. This possibility is strengthened by the regular, extensive overlap between respiratory viral and allergen seasons.

Figure 24-6.

Role of viruses in the development of otitis media. The most well-supported immediate cause of otitis media is a preceding or concurrent viral upper respiratory infection. Indeed, otitis media is one of the most frequent complications of viral upper respiratory infections, with epidemiologic studies [8,9,24,25] documenting that more than 50% of new episodes of otitis media are diagnosed immediately after or concurrent with a viral upper respiratory infection. A causal relationship between the two disorders was documented in experimental studies. Using an adult experimental model of infection, otitis media has been observed as a complication of rhinovirus and influenza virus in approximately 3% and 20% of subjects, respectively [16]. In these studies, there was a sequential development of nasal inflammation, impaired eustachian tube function, abnormal middle ear pressures, and the development of otitis media. In clinical studies, a significantly lower incidence of acute otitis media was reported for infants and children immunized with an influenza virus vaccine compared with nonimmunized controls during a seasonal influenza epidemic [21].

Respiratory virus

Increased eustachian tube obstruction
Abnormal immune/ inflammatory response

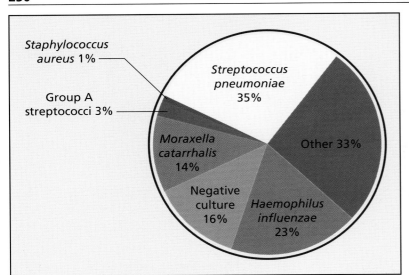

■ Figure 24-7.

Distribution of bacterial pathogens in otitis media. Bacteria are frequently isolated from middle ear fluids of children with otitis media and less frequently from children with chronic otitis media [26]. The bacteriology of acute otitis media in adults is very similar to that in children. A number of bacteria cultured from middle ear aspirates have developed mechanisms of resistance against commonly used antimicrobial agents [27]. Certain strains of *Haemophilus influenzae* and *Moraxella catarrhalis* produce the enzyme capable of degrading the β-lactam ring of penicillin-like antibiotics. Penicillin-resistant *Streptococcus pneumoniae* is also recognized as an increasingly significant and geographically variable problem. (*Adapted from* McBride *et al.* [10].)

Evaluation

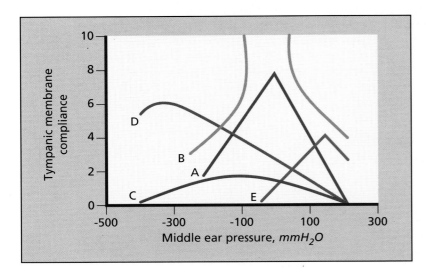

■ Figure 24-8.

Tympanometry. Tympanometry is a useful tool for evaluating the middle ear. It is useful for assessing middle ear pressure and tympanic membrane compliance [10]. This procedure is easy to perform and is highly sensitive to middle ear dysfunction but has a low specificity (*ie*, high false-positive rate). *Curve A* is typical of normal ears. *Curve B* shows high compliance but is a normal variant in young children. With these curves, there is only a 1% to 2% probability of a middle ear effusion. *Curve C* represents decreased compliance or mobility and is seen in patients with otitis media or thickened or scarred tympanic membranes. With this flattened curve, there is an 82% probability of a middle ear effusion. *Curve D* represents increased negative middle ear pressure. Otoscopy in such patients may show retraction or movement, primarily on negative pressure. This curve has a 67% probability of middle ear effusion. *Curve E* represents increased positive pressure in the middle ear. This curve has a 57% probability of middle ear effusion and is commonly seen in patients with early acute otitis media.

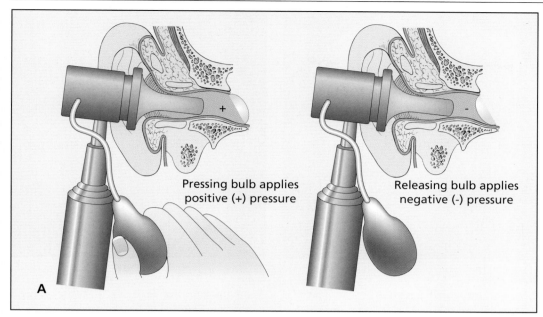

A, Pressing bulb applies positive (+) pressure

Releasing bulb applies negative (-) pressure

B. Clinical Significance of Findings in Pneumatic Otoscopy

Tympanic membrane moves to applied negative pressure		Tympanic Membrane Moves to Applied Positive Pressure	
		Yes	**No**
	Yes	Normal middle ear pressure	Negative middle ear pressure
	No	Positive middle ear pressure	Middle ear effusion or very high negative pressure

Figure 24-9.

Pneumatic otoscopy. Pneumatic otoscopy is essential for diagnosing otitis media. This procedure is used to assess the major characteristics of the tympanic membrane, including its thickness, degree of translucence, position, and mobility to applied pressure. **A,** A pneumatic otoscope head and an appropriately sized speculum are required. The speculum is inserted into the ear canal to form a tight seal. The bulb is then gently pressed (*ie*, positive pressure) and slowly released (*ie*, negative pressure) while the mobility of the tympanic membrane is assessed. A normal drum moves inward and then back. In cases of acute otitis media in which the middle ear is filled with purulent material, the tympanic membrane bulges outward and moves minimally. In cases of otitis media with an air fluid level (including chronic otitis media and some cases of acute otitis media), although the tympanic membrane may be retracted and mobility on positive pressure may be reduced, mobility on negative pressure is normal or only mildly decreased. In cases of high negative pressure and no effusion, mobility on positive pressure is absent, but the drum billows outward on negative pressure. **B,** Clinical significance of findings in pneumatic otoscopy. (*Adapted from* Skoner and Casselbrant [12].)

Diagnosis

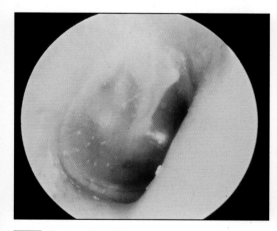

Figure 24-10.

Normal tympanic membrane. The tympanic membrane is thin, translucent, neutrally positioned, and mobile. The ossicles, particularly the malleus, are easily visualized. (*From* McBride *et al.* [10]; with permission.)

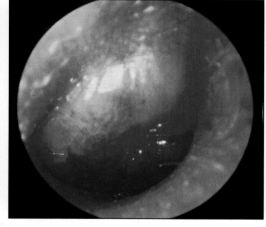

Figure 24-11.

Acute otitis media. The tympanic membrane is erythematous, opaque, and bulging. The landmarks are not visualized, and mobility is markedly decreased. In infants and young children, the most common symptoms include tugging at the ear, fever, irritability or fussiness, and crying when lying down. In older children and adults, the most common symptoms are otalgia, fever and chills, fullness in the ear, and muffled hearing. Nausea and vomiting may also occur. (*From* McBride *et al.* [10]; with permission.)

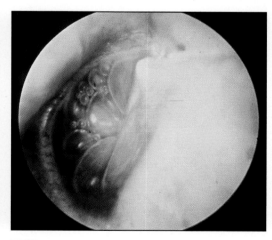

Figure 24-12.

Acute otitis media with air fluid levels. Bubbles formed by the presence of both air and fluid and separated by grayish-yellow menisci are readily visible. The combination of this finding with fever and otalgia is consistent with an acute infection. (*From* McBride *et al.* [10]; with permission.)

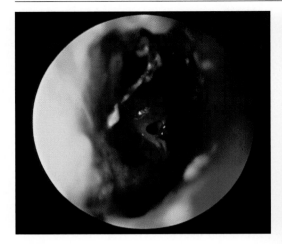

■ Figure 24-13.

Acute otitis media with perforation. Increased middle ear pressure associated with acute otitis media may result in perforation of the tympanic membrane. The tympanic membrane is erythematous and thickened. Acute otorrhea through a perforation of the tympanic membrane is common. (*From* McBride *et al*. [10]; with permission.)

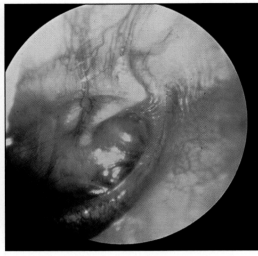

■ Figure 24-14.

Chronic otitis media with effusion. The tympanic membrane is retracted and thickened. A clear, yellow effusion is visible behind the tympanic membrane. Mobility is decreased. Patients with chronic otitis media with effusion are not acutely ill but often have decreased hearing. (*From* McBride *et al*. [10]; with permission.)

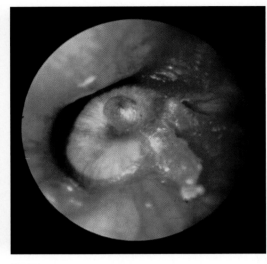

■ Figure 24-15.

Tympanosclerosis. Scarring and thickening of the tympanic membrane are common sequelae of recurrent acute or chronic otitis media. If large, tympanosclerosis may cause a mild conductive hearing loss. (*From* McBride *et al*. [10]; with permission.)

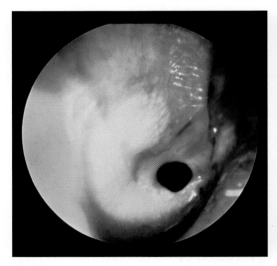

■ Figure 24-16.

Chronic perforation. Chronic perforation of the tympanic membrane is another sequela of recurrent acute or chronic otitis media or may persist after tympanostomy tubes have extruded. This tympanic membrane is also markedly thickened and scarred in a large arc. A large perforation may interfere with hearing. Also, an opening in the tympanic membrane may allow water to enter the middle ear during bathing and swimming, which may cause infection with discharge from the ear. (*From* McBride *et al*. [10]; with permission.)

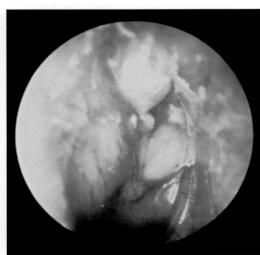

■ Figure 24-17.

Cholesteatoma. This is the most common and one of the most serious mass lesions of the tympanic membrane [3]. It is an accumulation of desquamated epithelium or keratin that often appears as a white mass behind or involving the tympanic membrane. It may be congenital or acquired. The acquired type is commonly caused by recurrent acute or chronic otitis media but can also be iatrogenic (*ie*, occurring after tympanostomy tube placement or other procedures). Cholesteatoma may enlarge and erode the bone, including the ossicles, causing hearing loss. They may also become infected, leading to a foul-smelling discharge from the ear. A cholesteatoma needs to be removed surgically. The recurrence rate is high, which necessitates long-term follow-up. (*From* McBride *et al*. [10]; with permission.)

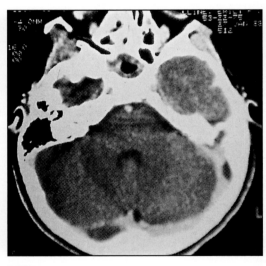

■ Figure 24-18.

Mastoiditis. This disorder may occur as a complication of otitis media [4]. This CT image shows acute left-sided mastoiditis with an associated epidural abscess. Signs of mastoiditis include displacement of the pinna away from the skull, erythema and edema of the pinna and the skin overlying the mastoid, exquisite tenderness on palpation of the mastoid process, purulent otorrhea, and fever. This condition is mainly seen in patients with long-standing, untreated, or inadequately treated otitis media. Prompt recognition, institution of intravenous antibiotics, and myringotomy are crucial to prevent extension to the central nervous system. (*From* McBride *et al*. [10]; with permission.)

Immune Evaluation

Clues That Suggest the Need for Evaluation of the Immune System in the Otitis-prone Patient

Allergy evaluation warranted if:

Family history	Positive for allergy and/or asthma
Sneeze, rhinorrhea, congestion	Prominent and present year-round or seasonally; interfere with normal activity
Symptom triggers	Pets, indoor allergens; or symptoms coincident with pollination
Nasal mucosa	Pale and boggy in appearance
Response to antiallergy medical therapy	Relief with antihistamines or intranasal cromolyn or corticosteroids

Immune deficiency evaluation warranted if:

Family history	Positive for early unexplained death or specific immune deficiency diagnosis
Frequency of infection	Elevated (> 8 respiratory infections/y)
Chronicity of infection	Present
Severity of infection	High level (meningitis, sepsis)
Complication of infection	Present (*eg*, mastoiditis complicating otitis media)
Site of infection	Multiple, not single, sites
Infecting organism	Opportunistic
Response to therapy	Poor, or recurring after discontinuation
Other signs	Failure to thrive, dermatitis, diarrhea

Figure 24-19.

Clues in an otitis-prone patient that suggest the need for evaluation of the immune system. If there is a history of frequent, chronic, or severe otitis media, a main consideration is whether an immune deficiency exists. Coincident symptoms and signs of children with otitis media that should alert the clinician to the need for such an evaluation and the type of evaluation are summarized. (*Adapted from* Skoner and Casselbrant [12].)

Management

Medical Management of Otitis Media

Condition	Treatment	Prophylaxis
Otitis media	Antibiotics 　Amoxicillin 　Amoxicillin with clavulanate 　Erythromycin with sulfa 　Cephalosporins 　Trimethoprim with sulfa 　Azithromycin or clarithromycin	Immunizations 　*Haemophilus influenzae* type B 　*Streptococcus pneumoniae* Avoid tobacco smoke
Viral upper respiratory infections	Antiviral agents 　Zanamivir 　Oseltamivir	Immunizations 　Influenza 　Respiratory syncytial virus Frequent handwashing Avoid daycare centers (if possible)
Allergic rhinitis	Antihistamines Decongestants Intranasal topical steroids Immunotherapy	Allergen avoidance

Figure 24-20.

Medical management of otitis media. Most physicians recommend antimicrobial therapy for episodes of otitis media [13,14]. Effective antimicrobial treatment should be based on the age of the patient, recent history of otitis media and antimicrobial treatment, and knowledge of the bacteriology and susceptibility patterns in the community. Amoxicillin is still the preferred drug for initial treatment of an episode of otitis media because it is active against most strains of *Streptococcus pneumoniae* and *Haemophilus influenzae*. However, because of the increasing frequency of penicillin-resistant organisms, treatment should be changed to a broad-spectrum antimicrobial agent if there is no clinical improvement within 48 to 72 hours of starting treatment [26]. Cephalosporins may be prescribed in patients allergic to penicillin but not to these agents. Macrolides, erythromycin-sulfisoxazole, or trimethoprim-sulfamethaxozole are recommended for patients allergic to penicillin and cephalosporins. Patients with documented allergic rhinitis should receive the full spectrum of available allergy therapies [11]. However, few, if any, specific allergy treatments have been evaluated in allergic patients with otitis media.

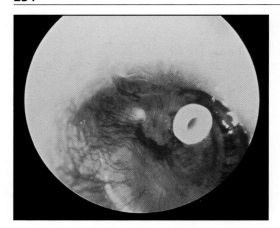

■ Figure 24-21.

Surgical management of otitis media. In patients with recurrent episodes of acute otitis media or chronic otitis media with effusion persisting for more than 3 months, tympanostomy tube insertion has been shown to be efficacious [5,17,27,28]. The tubes serve to vent the middle ear, improve hearing, and reduce the frequency of infection. Adenoidectomy has also been shown to be efficacious in treating chronic otitis media with effusion [18]. (*From* McBride *et al.* [10]; with permission.)

References

1. Daly KA, Giebink GS: Clinical epidemiology of otitis media. *Pediatr Infect Dis J* 2000, 19(suppl):31–36.

2. Roberts JE, Burchinal MR, Jackson SC, *et al.*: Otitis media in early childhood in relation to preschool language and school readiness skills among black children. *Pediatrics* 2000, 106:725–735.

3. Cohen JT, Hochman II, DeRowe A, Fliss DM: Complications of acute otitis media and sinusitis. *Curr Infect Dis Rep* 2000, 2:130–140.

4. Kaplan SL, Mason EO, PhD J, *et al.*: Pneumococcal mastoiditis in children. *Pediatrics* 2000, 106:695–699.

5. Berman S, Bondy J, Byrns PJ, Lezotte D: Surgical management of uncomplicated otitis media in a pediatric Medicaid population. *Ann Otol Rhinol Laryngol* 2000, 109:623–627.

6. Capra AM, Lieu TA, Black SB, *et al.*: Costs of otitis media in a managed care population. *Pediatr Infect Dis J* 2000, 19:354–355.

7. Skoner DP: Complications of allergic rhinitis. *J Allergy Clin Immunol* 2000, 105(suppl):605–609.

8. Heikkinen T, Thint M, Chonmaitree T: Prevalence of various respiratory viruses in the middle ear during acute otitis media. *N Engl J Med* 1999, 340:260–264.

9. Hirano T, Kurono Y, Ichimiya I, *et al.*: Effects of influenza A virus on lectin-binding patterns in murine nasopharyngeal mucosa and on bacterial colonization. *Otolaryngol Head Neck Surg* 1999, 121:616–621.

10. McBride TP, Davis HW, Reilly JS: Otolaryngology. In *Atlas of Pediatric Physical Diagnosis*, edn 3. Edited by Zitelli BJ, Davis HW. St. Louis: Mosby-Wolfe, 1997:683–728.

11. Dykewicz MS, Fineman S, Skoner DP, *et al.*: Diagnosis and management of rhinitis: complete guidelines of the Joint Task Force on Practice Parameters in Allergy, Asthma and Immunology. American Academy of Allergy, Asthma, and Immunology. *Ann Allergy Asthma Immunol* 1998, 81:478–518.

12. Skoner DP, Casselbrant M: Diseases of the ear. In *Allergy, Asthma, and Immunology from Infancy to Adulthood*, edn 3. Edited by Bierman CW, Pearlman DS, Shapiro GG, Busse WW. Philadelphia: WB Saunders; 1996:411–427.

13. Kozyrskyj AL, Hildes-Ripstein GE, *et al.*: Treatment of acute otitis media with a shortened course of antibiotics: a meta-analysis. *JAMA* 1998, 279:1736–1742.

14. Solis G, Ochoa C, Perez Mendez C: The variability and appropriateness of the antibiotic prescription of acute otitis media in childhood. *Int J Pediatr Otorhinolaryngol* 2000, 56:175–184.

15. Whitley RJ, Hayden FG, Reisinger KS, *et al.*: Oral oseltamivir treatment of influenza in children. *Pediatr Infect Dis J* 2001, 20:127–133.

16. Doyle WJ, Skoner DP, Alper CM, *et al.*: Effect of rimantadine treatment on clinical manifestations and otologic complications in adults experimentally infected with influenza A (H1N1) virus. *J Infect Dis* 1998, 177:1260–1265.

17. Rovers MM, Krabbe PF, Straatman H, *et al.*: Randomized controlled trial of the effect on ventilation tubes on quality of life at age 1-2 years. *Arch Dis Child* 2001, 84:45–49.

18. Paradise JL, Bluestone CD, Colborn DK, *et al.*: Adenoidectomy and adenotonsillectomy for recurrent acute otitis media: parallel randomized clinical trials in children not previously treated with tympanostomy tubes. *JAMA* 1999, 282:945–953.

19. Cook SP, Brodsky L, Reilly JS, *et al.*: Effectiveness of adenoidectomy and laser tympanic membrane fenestration. *Laryngoscope* 2001, 111:251–254.

20. Ilicali OC, Keles N, Deger K, Savas I: Relationship of passive cigarette smoking to otitis media. *Arch Otolaryngol Head Neck Surg* 1999, 125:758–762.

21. Belshe RB, Mendelman PM, Treanor J, *et al.*: The efficacy of live attenuated, cold-adapted, trivalent, intranasal influenza virus vaccine in children. *N Engl J Med* 1998, 338:1405–1412.

22. Eskola J, Kilpi T, Palmu A, *et al.*: Efficacy of a pneumococcal conjugate vaccine against acute otitis media. *N Engl J Med* 2001, 344:403–409.

23. The Impact-RSV Study Group: Palivizumab, a humanized respiratory syncytial virus monoclonal antibody, reduces hospitalization from respiratory syncytial virus infection in high-risk infants. *Pediatrics* 1998, 102:531–537.

24. Pitkaranta A, Jero J, Arruda E, *et al.*: Polymerase chain reaction-based detection of rhinovirus, respiratory syncytial virus, and coronavirus in otitis media with effusion. *J Pediatr* 1998, 133:390–394.

25. Chonmaitree T, Henrickson KJ: Detection of respiratory viruses in the middle ear fluids of children with acute otitis media by multiplex reverse transcription: polymerase chain reaction assay. *Pediatr Infect Dis J* 2000, 19:258–260.

26. Commisso R, Romero-Orellano F, Montanaro PB, *et al.*: Acute otitis media: bacteriology and bacterial resistance in 205 pediatric patients. *Int J Pediatr Otorhinolaryngol* 2000, 56:23–31.

27. Nagai K, Davies TA, Dewasse BE, *et al.*: In vitro development of resistance to ceftriazone, cefprozil and azithromycin in *Streptococcus pneumoniae*. *J Antimicrob Chemother* 2000, 46:909–915.

28. Franklin JH, Marck PA: Outcome analysis of children receiving tympanostomy tubes. *J Otolaryngol* 1998, 27:293–297.

29. Rovers MM, Straatman H, Ingels K, *et al.*: The effect of ventilation tubes on language development in infants with otitis media with effusion: a randomized trial. *Pediatrics* 2000, 106(suppl E):42.

25 Aerosols and Inhaler Therapy

Todd Mahr and Ketan Sheth

In addition to choosing appropriate medication for the treatment of patients with asthma, clinicians must also choose the best method for delivering the medication to the lungs. With recent advances in medications, an array of inhalation devices and methods are available to deliver these new medications. In addition, as more inhalation devices become available, clinicians must not only recognize the difference between types of delivery systems but also which delivery system will be optimal for each particular patient.

Many of the changes that have taken place are in response to the Montreal Protocol, which mandates the elimination of chlorofluorocarbon (CFC) use. The target date for the phaseout is between 2005 and 2007. At present, most metered-dose inhalers (MDIs) use CFCs as their propellants. With the impending phaseout, many current medications are being developed in either alternative propellants, such as hydrofluoroalkane (HFA) and dry powder inhalers (DPIs).

Due to this shift in delivery systems, it is important for clinicians taking care of patients with asthma to know about the various types of inhalers, both new and old. Because the shift away from CFC-containing inhalers is inevitable, learning the new delivery methods prepares clinicians and patients for appropriate treatment for the future.

Basic Aspects of Drug Delivery to the Lung

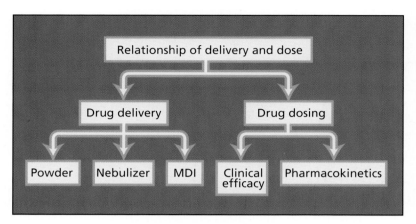

Figure 25-1.

Drug delivery to the lungs. As clinicians evaluate which medications to treat patients who have asthma, drug dosing is most often evaluated. Both clinical efficacy and pharmacokinetics are included within drug dosing. Clinical efficacy is most often studied by reviewing carefully designed studies that compare medications with placebo to examine their effect on a certain disease state. In patients with asthma, improvement in lung function is most often used as the best parameter of clinical efficacy. Pharmacokinetics is often studied to determine the dosing frequency and metabolism of medications. Equally important to dosing is drug delivery, whether by the oral, injectable, or inhaled route. Drug delivery is often overlooked; however, optimal delivery of medication is just as important as dosing to obtain the best therapeutic effect.

Drug delivery to the lung includes three major areas: powder formulations, nebulized formulations, and metered-dose inhalers (MDIs).

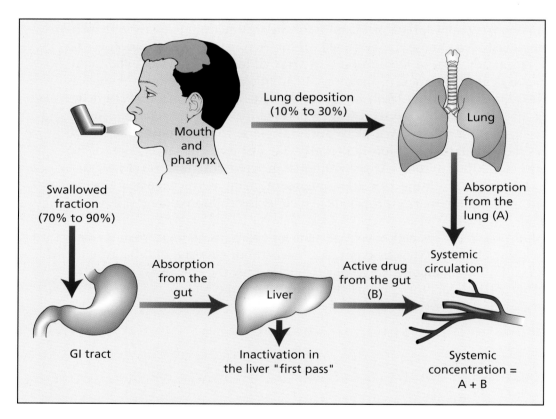

Figure 25-2.

Systemic absorption. The amount of drug actually delivered to the patient is affected by the formulation of the drug, the specific delivery device used, the technique of inhalation, and the presence or absence of a spacer. Variations in formulations in the delivery device may produce a greater than twofold difference in lung deposition of the same microgram dose. Specifically, inhaled corticosteroids (ICS) can be absorbed into the systemic circulation through the airway and gastrointestinal (GI) routes. Most of the ICS dose is swallowed, and systemic bioavailability is determined by the absorption from the GI tract and the degree of first-pass hepatic inactivation. The absorption of the fraction that is deposited in the lung can vary from drug to drug. It is known that almost all of a drug delivered to the terminal airway is absorbed into the systemic circulation. (*Adapted from* the National Asthma Education and Prevention Program [1].)

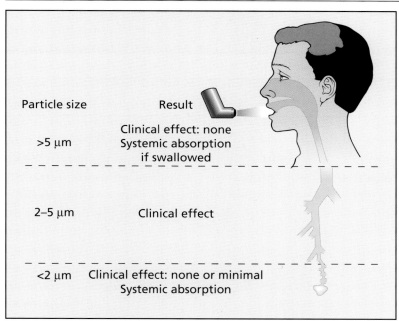

Particle size	Result
>5 µm	Clinical effect: none Systemic absorption if swallowed
2–5 µm	Clinical effect
<2 µm	Clinical effect: none or minimal Systemic absorption

Figure 25-3.

Particle size and airway deposition. The size of the particles delivered to the lungs is an important component of how effective a medication will be. The size of the particle directly relates to amount of lung deposition; however, not all lung deposition is always beneficial. Particles smaller than 2 µm generally have limited clinical benefit and can cause systemic absorption and potential side effects. Large particle size (> 5 µm) also has limited clinical benefit and may lead to systemic side effects, especially if the medication is absorbed. The most benefit comes from the ideal particle size of 2 to 5 µm [2–6].

Characteristics of an Ideal Respiratory Inhalation Drug Delivery System

Reproducible dose delivery to lungs across a wide range of inspiratory flows
Small particle size (1 to 5 µm)
Ease of use
Small size, easy to carry
Multiple-dose capability
Cost effectiveness
Dose counter

Dose-to-Lung Control

Patient Variables	Device Variables
Inspiratory flow	Concentration and particle droplet
Inspiratory volume	size distributions
Breath hold	Metered aerosols are
Disease or patient type	nonhomogeneous
Education and compliance	Unstable aerosols evaporate, impact, and sediment

Figure 25-4.

Dose-to-lung (DTL) control. DTL is simply predicted from the knowledge of the drug concentration in the air multiplied by the volume inhaled (concentration times the volume equals the drug dose inhaled), multiplied by the fractional deposition. The difficulty with this model is the number of confounding factors that are not as well controlled as desired. This table suggests some of the confounding factors. The patient variables can sometimes be improved with education, practice, and compliance. From the device standpoint, different devices provide drug aerosols in different concentrations and different size distributions. Metered aerosols (both pressurized or powder systems) are inhaled as boluses as opposed to the homogeneous aerosols, which are distributed throughout inhaled air by nebulizers [7].

Figure 25-5.

Characteristics of an ideal respiratory inhalation drug delivery system [5,8,10].

Dry Powder Inhaler Delivery

Comparison of Dry Powder Inhalers

	Date of US Introduction	Containment System	Actuations, n	Dose Counter	Reusable	Excipient for Dispersion or Taste	Molecule Available
Spinhaler (Fisons Pharmaceuticals, San Diego, CA)	1971	Discrete	1	Single dose	Yes	No	Cromolyn sodium
Rotahaler (GlaxoSmithKline, Research Triangle Park, NC)	1988	Discrete	1	Single dose	Yes	Yes; lactose	Albuterol
Turbuhaler (AstraZeneca Pharmaceuticals LP, Wilmington, DE)	1997	Reservoir	200	No	No	No	Budesonide
Diskus (GlaxoSmithKline)	1997	Discrete	60	Yes	No	Yes; lactose	Salmeterol; fluticasone; salmeterol and fluticasone combination
Diskhaler	1998	Discrete	4	Yes	Yes	Yes; lactose	Fluticasone propionate
(GlaxoSmithKline)	2001	Discrete	1	Single dose	Yes	Yes; lactose	Formoterol fumarate
Aerolizer* (Novartis)	2002?	Reservoir	60,120	Yes	No	Yes; lactose	Mometasone
Twisthaler (Schering-Plough, Kenilworth, NJ)*							

*Pending Federal Drug Administration approval.

▬ Figure 25-6.

Comparison of dry powder inhalers (DPIs). This table reviews many of the important features of various DPI inhalers available or pending approval in the United States. All of these systems rely on the patient as the power source. These devices only deliver the drug when the patient inhales. The delivery device allows the particles to be deagglomerated by the energy created by the patient's own inspiratory flow or, in some DPIs under development, by a battery-operated impeller.

The advantages of DPIs are that they are breath actuated and thus require minimal patient coordination. Similar to metered-dose inhalers (MDIs), they are relatively simple, compact, and portable. But unlike MDIs, they do not require a propellant system. An added benefit is that the empty condition of the device is usually more apparent, which alerts the patient to the need for a replacement. DPIs also can have some disadvantages. Some of the DPIs require relatively high flow rates (approximately 60 L/min) to deagglomerate the powder and, therefore, can be a problem for some children and patients (this is not true for all DPIs) [9].

The two major types of drug containment systems are the reservoir and discrete dose types. In reservoir systems, all the medication sits within a drug reservoir; when the inhaler is actuated, a mechanism allows some of the medicine to be deposited in the dosing area. The patient then inhales. Examples of reservoir devices include the Turbuhaler and Twisthaler. Reservoir devices may be susceptible to humidity or moisture, especially if the lid is left off. With some reservoir devices, there may be dose variation, and if the inhaler is dropped or gets wet, the entire inhaler may be affected.

In discrete dose containment systems, each dose is individually wrapped and either has to be loaded or is self-contained and opened by actuation of the DPI. Examples of individual doses include Rotocap and Aerolizer. Examples of discrete dose devices with multiple doses are Diskhaler and Diskus. For a discrete dose device, each individual dose is opened just before use of the medication. If there is humidity or moisture or if the device gets wet or is dropped, only that dose is affected; the patient can re-actuate the inhaler and use the next dose [2].

Another important feature of DPIs is whether they have lactose as an excipient for the medication. If lactose is present, the patient often gets a slight sweet taste sensation to confirm that he or she has received the medication. (In such devices, the amount of lactose is small enough to provide taste but not enough to cause problems for a lactose-intolerant patient.) Other DPIs do not have lactose as an excipient, so no dose sensation is experienced by the patient.

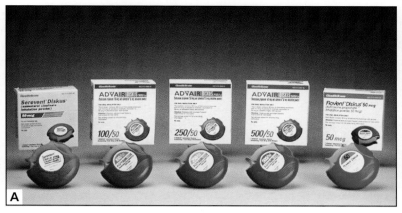

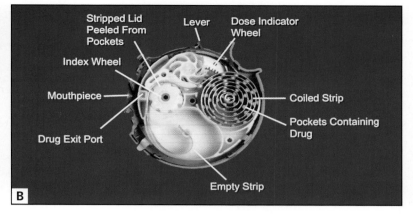

Figure 25-7.

Discrete dose systems. As previously described, a discrete dose device has each of its doses individual wrapped. **A,** The Diskus (GlaxoSmithKline, Research Triangle Park, NC) is one of the more popular examples of such a device. The device is used in three different products approved in the United States. It has 60 doses of medication in individually wrapped foil blisters on a strip. **B,** A cutaway illustration shows how the inside is engineered. The device has been shown to deliver consistent doses through the life of the device across a range of flow rates. When the lever is actuated or advanced, the blister strip rotates and is peeled, allowing the medication to sit at the drug exit port, which is adjacent to the mouthpiece. The patient then inhales. Air enters through the drug exit port and carries the drug through the mouthpiece into the patient. When the Diskus is closed, the unit is primed for actuation of the next dose. An integral cover protects the mouthpiece and inner workings from contamination or damage, and a dose counter indicates the exact number of doses remaining in the device. The last five doses are shown in red to remind the patient that it is time to get a new device.

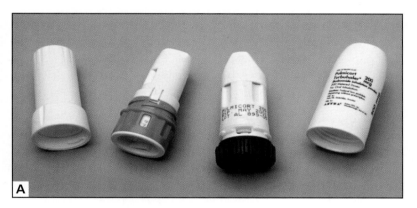

Figure 25-8.

Reservoir device. **A,** The Twisthaler (*left*) (Schering-Plough, Kenilworth, NJ) and Turbuhaler (*right*) (AstraZeneca Pharmaceuticals LP, Wilmington, DE). **B,** Corresponding cutaways. In the United States, the Turbuhaler contains 200 doses and a dose indicator wheel. This wheel does not reveal the exact number of doses remaining; rather, it turns red when 20 doses are left. Outside the United States, this device has a numerical dose counter. The Twisthaler contains 60 doses and 120 doses. It contains a dose counter integrated into the base of the device. Within the cutaway, the medication reservoir is shown.

Removal of the Twisthaler cap meters a precise dose of medication from the reservoir into the single-dose hole in the dose plate. The patient inhales rapidly and deeply to draw the metered dose up the inhalation channel. As the drug particles pass through the mouthpiece, they collide with the walls of the nozzle, causing deagglomeration into particles of respirable size. The cap is integral to the unit and is required to be replaced. The replacement process reprimes the unit for actuation of the next dose.

With actuation of the Turbuhaler, by turning the bottom, the dose drops into the drug dosing wheel and the patient then inhales to deliver the medication. Again, as the drug particles pass through the mouthpiece, they collide with the walls, causing deagglomeration. The lid must be replaced to protect the reservoir drug unit from contamination and humidity.

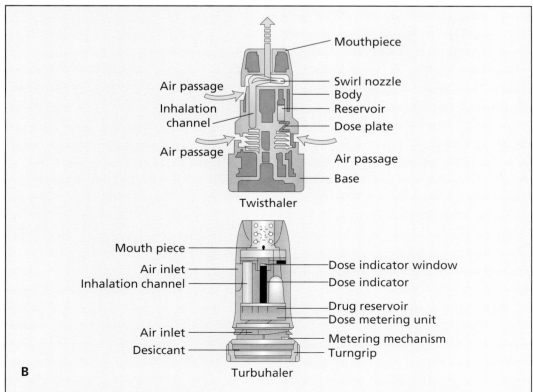

Nebulized Delivery

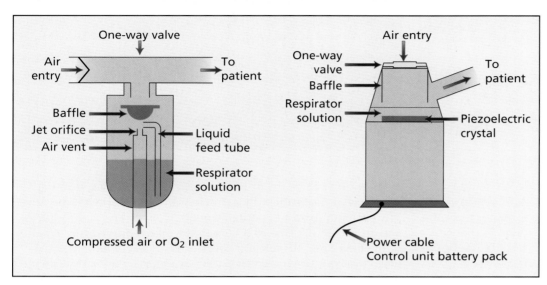

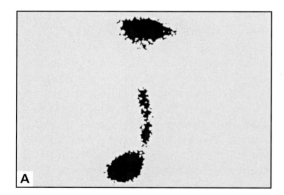

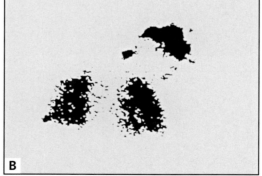

Figure 25-9.

Jet nebulizer and ultrasonic nebulizer. Shown is a typical handheld "jet" nebulizer. These devices are the most likely to be used clinically for delivery of nebulized solutions. Nebulizers are used to deliver quite large doses to the lung (*ie*, milligrams as opposed to the microgram amounts in metered dose inhalers). Jet nebulizers can work well in producing sub-5 μm, highly respirable, easily lung penetrating droplet aerosols for delivery of compounds that are placed in the nebulizer reservoirs. In most designs, air is forced from a nozzle (or jet) at high velocity past a small liquid feed capillary so the liquid nebulizer solution is atomized at the capillary exit. The majority of the aerosol mist, which may be traveling at up to sonic velocity, impacts against the baffle, drains back into the reservoir in the base, and recirculates. Only very small droplets (< 5 μm) escape the baffle and are inhaled along with "dilution air"

through the T-piece arrangement. The patient usually exhales 50% of any aerosol produced because they are breathing tidally. Some newer nebulizers are designed to minimize drug losses during patient exhalation. This is accomplished by ducting the exhaled sidestream out of the nebulizer before it can dilute the newly produced aerosol. The ultrasonic nebulizer is shown on the *right*. The piezoelectric crystal, vibrated by a high frequency oscillator, produces standing waves in the fluid above the crystal. These waves disintegrate, forming droplets, which are swept out of the nebulizer by either a fan or the patient's inspiratory breath [7,9].

Advantages of nebulizers include the lack of special timing or coordination with inspiration. Additionally, no propellant is needed, and a variety of drugs can be delivered. Large doses of medication can be delivered conveniently, but a sizable portion is wasted because of rain-out in the nebulizer and tubing. As a result, the respirable dose actually delivered to the patient is usually no greater than that delivered from a metered-dose inhaler. Disadvantages of nebulizers include their bulk, expense, and inconvenience. There is also a wide variability in the output characteristics of different nebulizers [9].

Figure 25-10.

Deposition from a nebulizer. There are many factors that affect deposition of aerosol in the lung. The ventilatory parameters for deposition efficiency include inspiratory volume, inspiratory flow rate, breath hold time, and respiratory rate. In the study by Murakami *et al.* [11] shown here, the effect that breathing pattern has on lung delivery is seen. This shows a composite of two scans obtained after inhalation of a radiolabeled drug by a crying infant and a sleeping infant. **A,** Ventilation scan in an 8-month-old girl with asthma. The scan was taken while she was crying. Lung deposition was 4% of the total body dose. Very little aerosol was deposited in the infant's lung; most of the aerosol was swallowed and was detected in the stomach. **B,** Ventilation scan taken when a 1-year-old girl with

asthma was sleeping and breathing at a lower flow rate, with possibly a greater tidal volume. Lung deposition was 21.9% of the total body dose. A greater amount of aerosol was deposited in the lung than in **A**. The aerosol was also more evenly distributed throughout the lung.

Ryan *et al.* [12] saw similar results in adults in a study in which the deposition was markedly reduced when the aerosol was inhaled rapidly compared with a slower inhalation via quiet breathing or slow vital capacity breathing. Everard *et al.* [13] compared nose and mouth breathing using a facemask for delivery of aerosol to the lung. The total dose delivered with only mouth breathing was double that in nasal breathing (75% vs 38%). The study also showed that lung deposition was more variable with nasal breathing than with mouth breathing [11–13].

Metered-Dose Inhaler Delivery

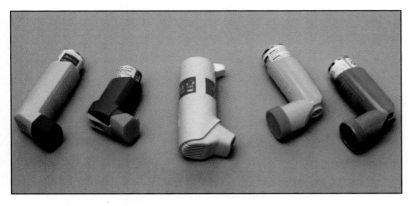

■ Figure 25-11.

Chlorofluorocarbon–metered-dose inhaler (CFC-MDI) and hydro-fluoroalkane–metered-dose inhaler (HFA-MDI) devices. Until the Montreal Protocol takes effect, CFC-MDIs remain the most commonly used inhalers in the United States. Several of the currently available CFC-MDIs are the press-and-breathe MDIs (*left*), a breath-actuated MDI (*middle*), and an HFA-MDI (*right*). Many medications are being developed with an HFA propellant. Currently two major types of HFA propellants are being used, and each has different properties with regard to particle size, taste, and flow from the mouthpiece. The HFA-MDIs currently approved in the United States contain HFA-134a.

As new HFA-MDIs become available, it is important to review the characteristics of that particular propellant to ensure understanding of the delivery mechanics of that specific inhaler. For the beclomethasone-HFA, reported lung deposition is 59%; however, this is an extra-fine aerosol with a median particle size of 1.1 μm, which leads to concern that unwanted systemic absorption may occur because the particles are smaller than 2 μm (*see* Fig. 25-3). In contrast, the fluticasone-HFA (not yet approved in the United States) uses an alternative HFA propellant and has a median particle size of 2.5 μm, which is within the desired 2 to 5 μm range [14].

Metered-dose inhalers have a number of advantages. They are compact, rugged, portable, and fairly simple to use. MDIs have a multidose capacity of 80 to 400 doses per canister. Dosing is rapid and convenient, with delivery of therapeutic doses in two inhalations or fewer, which is relatively reproducible. The major disadvantage of MDIs is that efficient dosing is highly technique dependent, which requires considerable hand–eye coordination and a slow, deep inhalation technique to prevent impaction of aerosol particles in the oropharynx or central airways. Other disadvantages include lack of a counter that would alert the user to an empty inhaler [9].

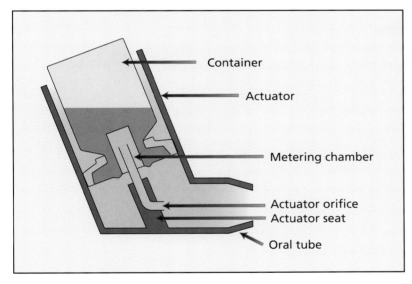

■ Figure 25-12.

Metered-dose inhaler (MDI) cutaway. Pressurized MDIs generate small boluses of drug aerosol with each actuation. The MDI consists of micronized drug in suspension or solution, together with propellant (or propellants) pressurized within an aluminum canister. Each metered dose of the drug is delivered from a metering chamber when the canister is depressed into the actuator. Droplets of propellant and drug are sprayed from the actuator orifice; the droplets are 30 to 40 μm in size and travel at velocities of up to 40 m per second. At about 10 cm from the mouthpiece, the diameter of these aerosol droplets has decreased by evaporation to about 14 μm. Because more time and distance are needed to reduce this 14-μm size to an even smaller size, spacers and chambers are used as compliance aids.

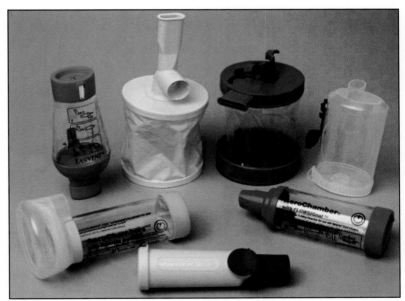

■ Figure 25-13.

Metered-dose inhaler (MDI) spacers and chambers. MDIs generate small boluses of drug aerosol. Spacers and chambers have been developed to reduce the deposition of drug in the oropharynx and allow extra time for evaporation to occur, which decreases the particle size. Waste drug that would have impacted on the posterior orophaynx can be retained in the spacer or chamber. Chambers (reservoirs), rather than spacers, often contain valves and are able to contain the aerosol for a short period of time before inhalation. These can assist patients who have difficulty coordinating the mechanics of MDI actuation and their own inhalation.

Inhalation Techniques

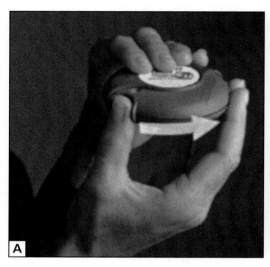 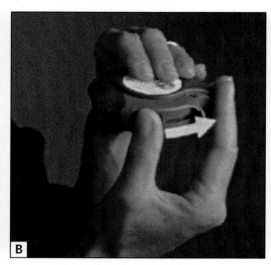 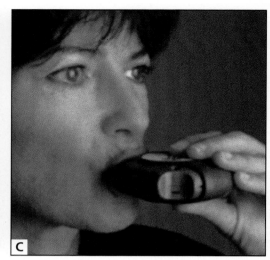

■ Figure 25-14.

Dry powder inhaler (DPI) technique. Although the use of a DPI is generally easier because DPIs are breath activated, it is still important to teach patients appropriate inhaler techniques. As an example, the use of the Diskus device is shown here. To use it, the patient opens the inhaler (**A**), clicks the lever back to activate the dose and peel it from its foil blister (**B**), and then inhales the medication (**C**). All DPIs have the same basic method: the patient starts receiving medication with breath inhalation, so coordination is not necessary. Each individual device may have specific steps, so the healthcare providers must be familiar with the DPI's recommended inhaler technique.

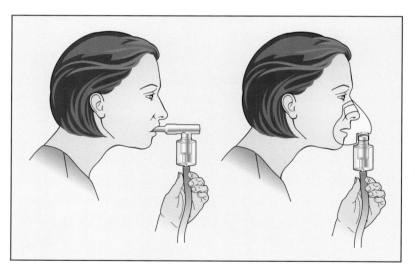

■ Figure 25-15.

Nebulizer technique. Nebulizers can take more time to set up, and patients or their parents need to be trained in the individual machine's use and care instructions. Most (except ultrasonic nebulizers) use a compressor unit that connects to the reservoir with tubing. Solution is placed in the cup per the manufacturer's recommendations, and the patient can use the mouthpiece or mask to deliver the mist (*left*). The patient should place the mouthpiece on top of the tongue and inhale through the mouth. If a mask is used, it should be tightly held or secured to the face and the patient should inhale with the mouth open (*right*). Nasal inhalation should be discouraged.

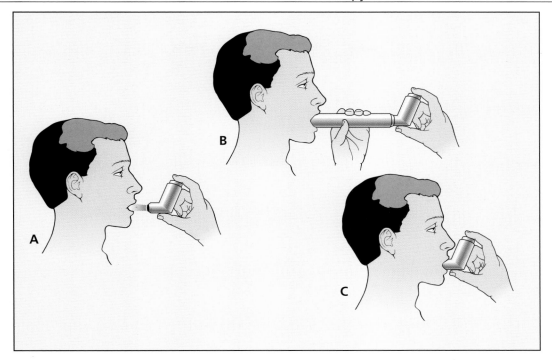

Figure 25-16.

Metered-dose inhaler (MDI) technique. The steps are as follows:

1. Remove the cap and hold the inhaler upright.
2. Shake the inhaler.
3. Tilt the head back slightly and breathe out.
4. Place the inhaler as shown in **A**, **B**, or **C** (**A** or **B** is best, but **C** is acceptable for those who have difficulty with **A** or **B**).
5. Press down on the inhaler to release the medication and at the same time, start to breathe in.
6. Breathe in slowly for 3 to 5 seconds.
7. Hold your breath for 10 seconds to allow medicine to reach deeply into lungs.
8. Repeat the puff according to the directions, waiting 1 minute between puffs.

Spacers or chambers are useful for all patients. They are particularly recommended for young children and older adults and for use with inhaled steroids [1].

References

1. National Asthma Education and Prevention Program: Expert Panel Report 2. *Guidelines for the Diagnosis and Management of Asthma.* Publication no. 97-4051. Rockville, MD: National Institutes of Health, National Heart, Lung, and Blood Institute; 1995.

2. Sheth KK, Kelly HW, Mitchell BH: *Innovations in Dry Powder Inhalers.* CME Monograph. Bala Cynwyd, PA: Meniscus Limited; 2000.

3. Tansley I. The technical transition to CFC-free inhalers. *Br J Clin Pract* 1997, 89 (suppl):22–27.

4. Ariyananda PL, Agnew JE, Clarke SW: Aerosol delivery systems for bronchial asthma. *Postgrad Med J* 1996, 72:151–156.

5. Wolff RK, Niven RW: Generation of aerosolized drugs. *Aerosol Med* 1994, 7:89–106.

6. Bisgaard H: Drug delivery from inhaler devices. *Br Med J* 1996, 313:895–896.

7. Byron PR: *Respiratory Drug Delivery.* Edited by Byron PR. Boca Raton, FL: CRC Press Inc; 1990.

8. Schlaeppi M, Edwards K, Fuller RW, Sharma R: Patient perception of the Diskus inhaler: a comparison with the Turbuhaler inhaler. *Br J Clin Pract* 1996, 50:14–19.

9. Tashkin DP: New devices for asthma. *J Allergy Clin Immunol* 1998, 101(suppl):409–441.

10. Targeting drugs to the lung. *Respir Med* 1997, 91(suppl).

11. Murakami G, Igarashi T, Adachi Y, *et al.*: Measurement of bronchial hyperactivity in infants and preschool children using a new method. *Ann Allergy* 1990, 64:383–387.

12. Ryan G, Dolovich MB, Obminski G, *et al.*: Standardization of inhalation provocation tests: influence of nebulizer output, particle size and method of inhalation. *J Allergy Clin Immunol* 1981, 67:156–162.

13. Everard ML, Clark AR, Milnar AD: Drug delivery from jet nebulizers. *Arch Dis Child* 1992, 67:586–591.

14. Vanden Burgt JA, *et al.*: Efficacy and safety overview of new inhaled corticosteroid, QVAR, in asthma. *J Allergy Clin Immunol* 2000, 1209–1226.

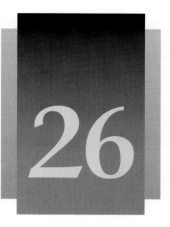

26 Immunodeficiency Disorders

Larry W. Williams and Joseph L. Roberts

Primary immunodeficiency diseases are genetically determined impairments of immune response. Our knowledge of these disorders dates only to the 1950s, when Colonel Ogden Bruton applied electrophoretic analysis to the serum of a young boy with recurrent pneumonia. No γ-globulin band was present. Antibody activity had been localized to the γ-globulin band only a decade previously. Bruton's case linked suscepti- bility to infection to absent γ-globulin and to absent antibody. Since then, a large number of syndromes of immunodeficiency have been described. As few as 15 years ago, we knew the molecular and genetic basis for no more than a handful of these diseases. Now many more than 20 disorders have established genetic causes.

Demonstration of B and T cell functional dichotomy in the 1960s led to a common clas- sification of immunodeficiency by functional defect. We have followed this scheme in the simplified classification of disorders in Figures 26-1 through 26-3. In reality, there is a good deal of overlap in functional defects between the B- and T-cell disorders because B cells require help from T cells for antibody production. However, the patterns of common infections in the B- and T-cell disorders is fairly consistent. Disorders dominated by inad- equate antibody production (ie, B-cell disorders) are marked by invasive infection with high-grade, encapsulated bacterial pathogens. These patients have less difficulty with viral infection, with the important exception of enteroviral meningoencephalitis in patients with X-linked agammaglobulinemia (see Fig. 26-4). In T-cell deficiency, there is risk of similar bacterial infection, but the clinical picture is dominated by susceptibility to virus- es and opportunistic organisms such as *Pneumocystis carinii* and fungi. In addition, a number of the T- and B-cell disorders show evidence not only of immunodeficiency but also of autoimmunity caused by the dysregulation of the components that are present.

The last group of disorders includes problems of nonspecific defenses including granu- locytes and complement. These disorders do not involve immunologic memory, but the importance of these arms of the innate immune system is proven by the severe infections that affected patients suffer.

This sample of images from immunodeficient patients is certainly not a comprehensive treatise on the disorders; rather, it is intended to illustrate some of the important features of the diseases. For a full discussion of the diseases, see Stiehm [1] or recent reviews of specific disorders.

Disorders of T- and B-cell Function

Disorders of B-cell Function

Disorder	Characteristics
X-linked agammaglobulinemia	Near absence of B cells and immunoglobulin
	Usually no palpable lymph nodes
	Risk of pneumonia, sepsis, and other invasive bacterial diseases
	Risk of chronic enteroviral meningitis
Selective IgA deficiency	IgA < 5 mg/dL (adults) with other isotypes normal
	Risk of reaction to IgA in blood products in some patients
Common variable immunodeficiency	B cells and lymph nodes usually present
	Variable decrease in serum immunoglobulin concentrations
	Poor production of specific antibody
	Autoimmune problems common
X-linked hyper-IgM syndrome	Failure to switch immunoglobulin production from IgM to other classes
	Poor specific antibody production
	Autoimmunity, neutropenia common; frequent poor outcome
Autosomal recessive hyper-IgM syndrome	Less guarded prognosis
	Similar immune picture but frequent long survival
X-linked lymphoproliferative syndrome	Inadequate response to EBV infection
	May die of EBV-driven lymphoproliferative process
	Survivors of EBV have antibody deficiency

Figure 26-1.

Disorders of B-cell function. These disorders result from deficient function of B cells. Note that in IgA deficiency, production of specific antibody of other isotypes is normal. Thus, most individuals with IgA deficiency are thought to be asymptomatic.

Disorders of T-Cell and Combined T- and B-cell Function

Disorder	Characteristics
Severe combined immunodeficiency	Several known genetic defects
	Profound T- and B-cell dysfunction
	Presents in infancy with lymphopenia, failure to thrive, opportunistic infections
	Fatal without immune reconstitution
	Risk of fatal GVHD from unirradiated blood products
Combined immunodeficiency	Presentation: failure to thrive, recurrent infections, autoimmune phenomena
	Diminished, but not absent, T-cell function and variable B-cell function
	Purine nucleoside phosphorylase deficiency responsible for many reported cases
DiGeorge syndrome	Multisystem disorder resulting from third and fourth pharyngeal pouch dysgenesis
	Most patients have chromosome 22q11 deletions
	Often present with neonatal hypocalemia, congenital heart disease, dysmorphic features
	Interrupted aortic arch type B and truncus arteriosus are common
	Variable thymic dysplasia can lead to normal, partially defective, or absent T-cell function
	Patients with significant T-cell dysfunction require irradiation of blood products
Wiskott–Aldrich syndrome	X-linked syndrome of eczema, thrombocytopenia, and recurrent infections
	Variable T- and B-cell dysfunction (often with elevated IgA and IgE, low IgM, normal IgG)
	Increased incidence of autoimmune diseases and malignancy
	Milder hereditary XLT from mutations in same *WASP* gene
Ataxia telangiectasia	Complex syndrome of progressive cerebellar ataxia and occulocutaneous telangiectasias
	Recurrent sinopulmonary infections with variable defects in T- and B-cell function
	Thymic hypoplasia and IgA deficiency are characteristic features
	Predisposition to develop lymphoid and other malignancies
	Defective protein kinase–like gene, *ATM*, cloned and mapped to chromosome 11q22.3
Chronic mucocutaneous candidiasis	Clinical syndrome of persistent or recurrent skin, nail, and mucosal candida infections
	Autosomal recessive disease in some from mutations in *AIRE* gene, described as APECED
	Pedigrees suggesting an autosomal dominant form also described
	Variable defects in B-cell function and candida-specific T-cell responses
Hyper-IgE syndrome	Syndrome of marked elevation of serum IgE and tendency to invasive staphylococcal infection
	Infections with other bacteria seen but not as often as *Staphylococcus*
	Almost always develop staphylococcal pneumonia and pneumatoceles
	Primary dentition often not normally shed
	Elevated IgE and presence of eczematoid rash believed evidence of dysregulated T-cell function

■ Figure 26-2.

Disorders of T-cell and combined T- and B-cell function. AIRE—autoimmune regulator; APECED—autoimmune polyendocrinopathy-candidiasis-ectodermal dystrophy; CID—combined immunodeficiency; SCID—severe combined immunodeficiency; WAS —Wiskott-Aldrich syndrome; XLT—X-linked thrombocytopenia.

Disorders of Granulocytes and Complement

Disorders of Granulocytes and Complement

Disorder	Characteristics
Granulocyte disorders	
Chronic granulomatous disease	Defective respiratory burst (NADPH oxidase) in granulocytes
	Poor microbial killing
	Infections with common catalase-positive bacteria
	Many infections with unusual, low grade pathogens such as *Serratia* or *Aspergillus* spp.
Leukocyte adhesion deficiency	Leukocyte surface lacks adhesion protein CD11/18
	Cells cannot firmly adhere to vascular endothelium
	Defective egress of leukocytes from vascular space to site of inflammation
Chediak-Higashi syndrome	Abnormal cytoplasmic granules and poor bacterial killing
Complement disorders	
Specific component absence (homozygous defects)	
Total absence of C1, C2, C3 or C4	Infection with encapsulated bacteria
	Clinically may mimic agammaglobulinemia
	Heterozygotes have half-normal component levels, are not immunodeficient
Absence of a terminal component (C5-C9)	Restricted tendency to *Neisseria meningitidis* and disseminated *N. gonorrhoeae* infection
Absence of alternative pathway proteins	Extremely rare disorders

Figure 26-3.

Disorders of granulocytes and complement. Phagocytes and complement are not components of acquired immunity, but they are necessary effectors of some aspects of acquired immunity. The poor microbial killing of chronic granulomatous disease results from the abnormal respiratory burst.

X-linked Agammaglobulinemia

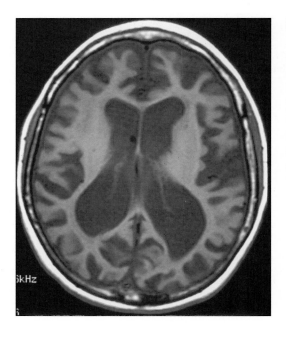

Figure 26-4.

X-linked agammaglobulinemia (XLA) and chronic encephalitis. This 15-year-old boy was found to have XLA at age 3 years. At about age 7 years, poor school performance was noted. Chronic enteroviral meningoencephalitis was suspected, but viral cultures of cerebrospinal fluid repeatedly showed negative results. Cerebral atrophy was evident by age 9 years, and enterovirus was demonstrated on brain biopsy. By age 15 years, impressive atrophy is present as seen in this magnetic resonance image, and marked cognitive and motor deterioration continued. Chronic enteroviral meningoencephalitis occurs almost solely in patients with XLA. It may present as a sudden neurologic syndrome that mimics stroke or with slow cognitive deterioration, as in this case.

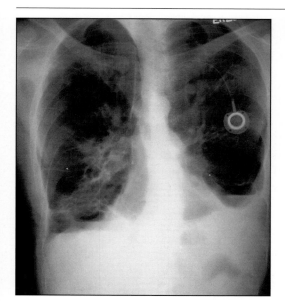

Figure 26-5.

X-linked agammaglobulinemia (XLA) and lung disease. Recurrent pneumonia with scarring and progressive loss of function may be seen in patients with absent antibody, as in this 30-year-old man with XLA. He discontinued γ-globulin replacement for about 10 years in his teens. During this lapse in therapy, he developed a chronic productive cough, dyspnea with moderate exertion, and scarring and cystic changes, as seen on this radiograph. He has bronchiectasis confirmed by chest CT scan and a mixed obstructive and restrictive pattern on pulmonary function testing. His lung disease has been slowly progressive despite resumption of regular immunoglobulin administration and physical and medical therapy for bronchiectasis.

Common Variable Immunodeficiency

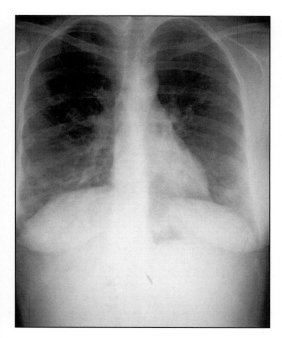

Figure 26-6.

Common variable immunodeficiency (CVID) and lung disease. This 18-year-old girl with CVID developed dyspnea and a dry cough over several months. Chest radiographs showed a pattern of increasing interstitial disease. Lung biopsy was required for diagnosis. The biopsy was negative for infectious processes; however, lymphoid interstitial pneumonitis (LIP) was seen on microscopic examination. The LIP did not improve with high-dose intravenous immune globuline but rapidly remitted on prednisone 2 mg/kg/d. Patients with CVID may exhibit a wide range of autoimmune diseases, including LIP, autoimmune hepatitis, thrombocytopenia, neutropenia, thyroiditis, and others. Because such patients lack specific antibody production, they are also at risk of invasive bacterial infection.

Combined Immunodeficiency and Severe Combined Immunodeficiency

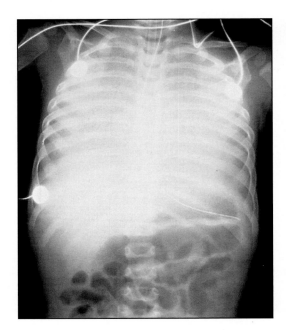

Figure 26-7.

Pneumocystis carinii pneumonia (PCP) in severe combined immunodeficiency (SCID). The complete absence of T-cell function in patients with SCID renders them highly susceptible to severe infections with opportunistic organisms such as *P. carini*. Such infections typically present in the first few months of life, often as the presenting illness in SCID. Early diagnosis, typically via bronchoscopy and lavage, antibiotic treatment and prophylaxis are vital for successful management of PCP in SCID. Isolated tachypnea often precedes development of the depicted fulminant pneumonitis and should alert the clinician to consider PCP in a patient with known primary or secondary T-cell dysfunction. Note also the characteristic absence of a detectable thymic shadow in the chest radiograph of this infant with SCID.

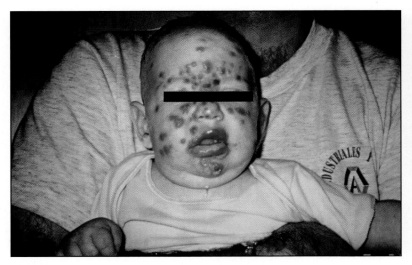

Figure 26-8.

Herpes simplex virus infection in severe combined immunodeficiency (SCID). In addition to being highly susceptible to opportunistic organisms, T-cell–deficient patients are also at risk for developing unusually severe infections with more common viral, bacterial, or fungal pathogens. This patient with SCID has disseminated cutaneous herpes simplex virus. The lesions are superinfected with *Staphylococcus aureus*. Such patients would have lethal herpes simplex disease without antiviral therapy. Varicella-zoster virus infection would have a similar appearance and, if left untreated, a lethal course in SCID.

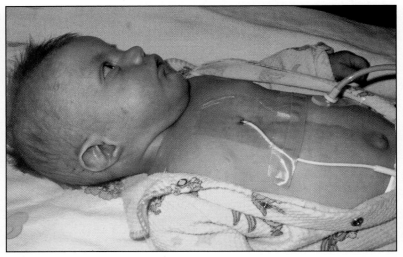

Figure 26-9.

DiGeorge syndrome. A number of abnormalities that involve structures from the face to the thorax may be seen in this syndrome. Involvement of the thymus is variable. Patients with typical heart lesions and a microdeletion of 22q11 may have perfectly normal immune function. If the thymus is absent, the patient will have essentially no T cells and no response to mitogen stimulation of peripheral blood mononuclear cells. This situation is referred to as complete DiGeorge syndrome. This infant had complete DiGeorge syndrome and also a number of nonimmunologic and noncardiac problems. He demonstrates the small mandible and low-set, simple ears sometimes seen in those with the syndrome. He also has a severe swallowing disorder and gastroesophageal reflux that required fundoplication and feeding by the gastric tube shown. Swallowing difficulties, reflux, and aspiration are common among babies with DiGeorge syndrome.

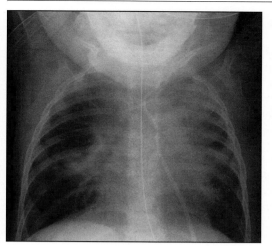

■ Figure 26-10.

Combined immunodeficiency (CID) and autoimmune lung disease. This infant girl presented in the first few months of life with failure to thrive and recurrent urinary tract infections. By age 6 months, she had persistent infiltrates on chest radiographs. No organism or etiology was apparent from bronchoscopy. Evaluation of immune status revealed low numbers of T cells, very low but not absent lymphocyte response to mitogen stimulation *in vitro*, and elevated immunoglobulins but absent isohemagglutinins and no specific antibody production after diphtheria and tetanus immunization. These findings led to a diagnosis of CID. She developed an oxygen requirement, and an open lung biopsy was performed. Microscopic examination of the tissue showed histiolymphocytic interstitial (autoimmune) pneumonitis without evidence of infection. Her lung disease improved with prednisone. Bone marrow transplantation was required for definitive therapy. Patients with CID may have a variety of autoimmune processes and infections. The diagnosis is often suspected because of autoimmune disease rather than infection. The presence of low—but not absent —T-cell function *in vitro* distinguishes such patients from those with severe combined immunodeficiency.

Chronic Mucocutaneous Candidiasis

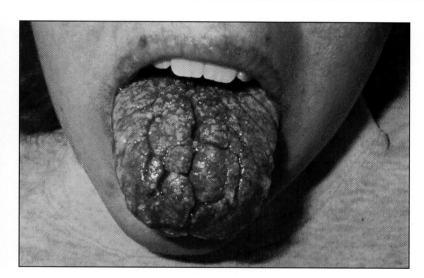

■ Figure 26-11.

Chronic mucocutaneous candidiasis. Patients with this disorder usually have a fairly restricted immune deficit. They typically handle infections normally except for surface infection with *Candida* spp. Tissue invasion is rare, in contrast to patients with more broadly based deficits in T-cell function. This 17-year-old girl has had persistent oral and perioral candidiasis from the first 2 years of life. She has not had tissue invasive candidiasis, but the oral disease was uncontrolled with nystatin and amphotericin topically and with oral imidazoles. Intense perioral inflammation from the candida infection has resolved with investigational antifungal agents, but residual mucosal disease on the tongue is obvious.

Hyper-IgE Syndrome

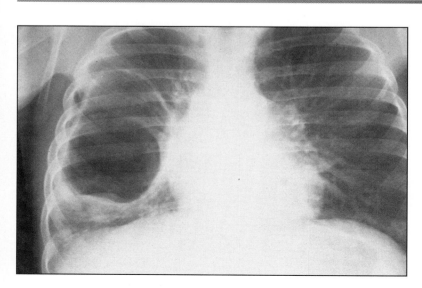

■ Figure 26-12.

Hyper-IgE syndrome. Other than often extreme elevation of serum IgE, the most typical feature of this syndrome (perhaps even a requisite for the diagnosis) is the presence of pneumatoceles after staphylococcal pneumonia, as seen in this young child. Patients with the syndrome are especially prone to furuncles and deep tissue staphylococcal abscesses. Patients with severe atopic dermatitis and very elevated IgE may be mistakenly thought to have hyper-IgE syndrome because of superficial staphylococcal infection. However, the diagnosis of hyper-IgE syndrome is excluded in patients with atopic dermatitis by the absence of invasive staphylococcal infection and pneumatoceles.

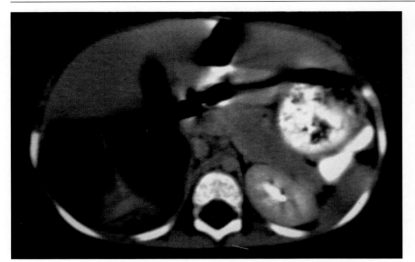

Figure 26-13.

Hyper-IgE syndrome. Large staphylococcal abscesses may occur in patients with this syndrome. This CT scan of the abdomen shows a normal left kidney, but the right kidney is pushed entirely out of the plane of the image by a multiloculated mass in the right paravertebral area. This mass was a perinephric abscess from which 750 mL of pus was obtained by CT-guided puncture. The drainage grew *Staphylococcus aureus*. The patient was a 4-year-old child who presented with increasing abdominal girth without fever or tenderness. Some, but not all, staphylococcal abscesses in patients with hyper-IgE syndrome may present without "heat" in this fashion. A typical inflammatory process with *dolor, calor, et rubor* develops with most infections in these patients.

Chronic Granulomatous Disease

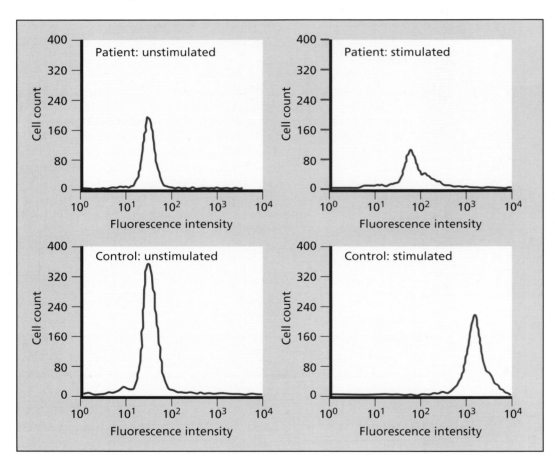

Figure 26-14.

Chronic granulomatous disease (CGD) and respiratory burst. The diagnosis of CGD was made in the past with the nitroblue tetrazolium test (NBT). This manual microscopic test has been replaced by flow cytometric measurement of the neutrophil respiratory burst. Leukocytes are first loaded with a nonfluorescent precursor compound. On stimulation of the cells with phorbol ester, the intact respiratory burst reduces the nonfluorescing compound to a polar, fluorescent form. The polar compound cannot escape the cell. After washing to remove fluorochrome from the medium, several thousand cells are analyzed on the cytometer for fluorescence and compared with similarly handled but unstimulated cells. A normal respiratory burst shifts the mean fluorescence peak after stimulation strongly to the right (brighter), as shown in the control. Little or no peak shift is seen in the patient sample here, an example of autosomal recessive CGD.

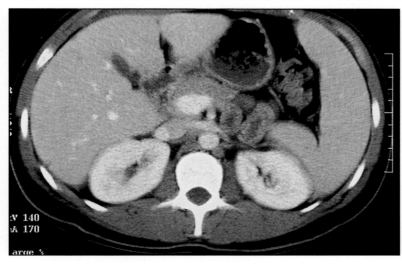

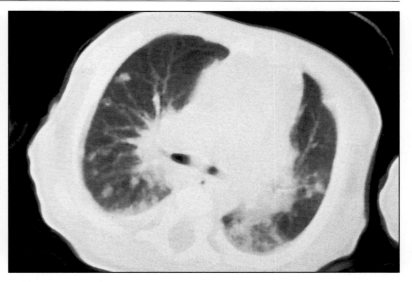

■ Figure 26-15.

Systemic aspergillus infection in patient with chronic granulomatous disease (CGD). This 22-year-old man with known autosomal
recessive CGD presented with several weeks of fever, a decrease in
hemoglobin from baseline, and an erythrocyte sedimentation rate
of 105 mm/h. He had a history of aspergillus infection in the lung
and in thoracic lymph nodes and was maintained on chronic itra-
conazole. The examination did not reveal a focus of infection. His
abdominal CT scan reveals a number of discrete lesions in the liver.
Percutaneous, ultrasonically guided aspiration of a peripheral
lesion yielded material that grew *Aspergillus* spp. This case demonstrates the difficulty of eradicating systemic aspergillus in patients
with CGD. Organisms apparently survive for long periods after
ingestion by phagocytes and may seed recurrent symptomatic infection in the original site or distantly.

■ Figure 26-16.

Chronic granulomatous disease (GCD) and effect on the lungs. A
CT scan of the chest and abdomen was obtained in this 4-month-
old infant boy because of daily fever for 2 weeks and mild
splenomegaly. A sister had died suddenly of probable sepsis at 2
months of age. The parents were consanguineous. A subsequent
test of neutrophil respiratory burst was consistent with CGD. The
chest CT scan shows lesions in the lung periphery that may be
infectious foci or granulomatous lesions. The abdominal CT scan
was thought to show massive prevertebral lymphadenopathy; however, at laparoscopy for biopsy of nodes, diffuse peritonitis was discovered. Cultures grew *Candida lusitania*. This presentation and
the presence of an uncommon organism are not unusual for CGD.
Family genetic analysis revealed autosomal recessive CGD.

Leukocyte Adhesion Deficiency

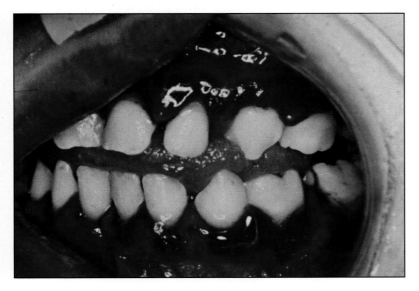

■ Figure 26-17.

Leukocyte adhesion deficiency (LAD) and gingivitis. If expression
of the leukocyte adhesion molecules CD11/18 is low but not totally
absent, patients may develop severe periodontal disease in the first
decade of life but avoid more disastrous complications. This 3-
year-old child has severe gingivitis, as seen by the intense erythema
of the gums. The molars and premolars were mobile ("floating")
because of periodontitis with bone loss that was obvious on dental
radiographs. LAD should be included in the differential diagnosis
of young children with periodontal disease. True periodontitis in
preschool children is rare in the absence of LAD, even if there is
gingivitis related to poor hygiene.

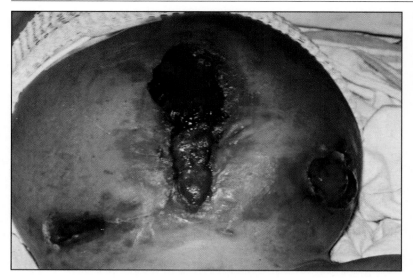

■ Figure 26-18.

Leukocyte adhesion deficiency (LAD). In LAD, there is severe impairment of the migration of leukocytes to areas of inflammation or infection. If the CD11/18 complex is totally (or nearly) absent from leukocytes, circulating leukocytes are unable to firmly adhere to the capillary endothelium and pass into tissues. With such severe deficiency of CD11/18, infection may begin in the first weeks of life. Omphalitis extending to peritonitis may occur and is likely to be severe or fatal. The umbilical cord is slow to separate, but the features most suggestive of LAD are omphalitis and extreme elevation of the absolute neutrophil count, often more than 50,000 per mm^3. This picture demonstrates necrotic, nonhealing surgical incisions and colostomy in a 2-year-old boy. Before it was known that he had LAD, he had an abdominal exploration for surgical abdomen that was actually peritonitis. Several subsequent procedures were attempted because of poor healing. The lesions shown improved with granulocyte transfusions.

Chediak-Higashi Syndrome

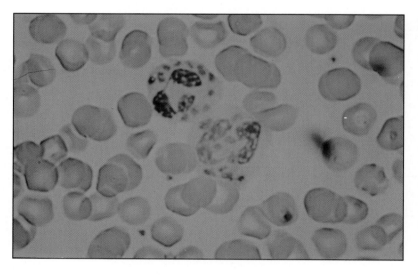

■ Figure 26-19.

Chediak-Higashi syndrome. Patients with this syndrome have giant cytoplasmic granules in hematopoietic cells, as easily seen in the neutrophils in this field. Abnormal granules are also present in melanocytes, and many of the patients have partial albinism. The abnormal granules apparently fuse abnormally with phagosomes, with resulting delayed killing of ingested bacteria. Invasive bacterial infection is a frequent cause of morbidity in these patients. If not cured by bone marrow transplantation, patients often terminally develop a lymphoproliferative process (the so-called accelerated phase) that is probably caused by Epstein-Barr viral infection. A morphologically identical disease is seen in mice, mink, cattle, collie dogs, and killer whales. In animals and humans, this is an autosomal recessive disease.

Gene Defects

Molecular Defects in Selected T- and B-Cell Primary Immunodeficiency Diseases

Disease	Mutant Gene Product
B-cell deficiency	
X-linked agammaglobulinemia	Btk
Autosomal recessive agammaglobulinemia	μ heavy chain, λ5/14.1 surrogate light chain, Igα chain, BLNK
Autosomal recessive hyper-IgM syndrome	AID
κ-light chain deficiency	κ-Light chain
T-cell and combined T- and B-cell deficiency	
X-linked SCID	Common cytokine receptor γ chain ($γ_c$)
Autosomal recessive SCID	Janus kinase 3 (Jak3), IL-7 receptor α chain, ζ-associated protein (ZAP-70), CD45 tyrosine phosphatase, Lck tyrosine kinase, RAG1 or RAG2 proteins
Deficiencies of purine metabolism	ADA, PNP
Omenn's syndrome	RAG1 or RAG2
CD3 complex deficiency	CD3γ or CD3ε proteins
MHC class I deficiency	TAP1 or TAP2
MHC class II deficiency	RFXAP, CIITA, RFX5, or RFXANK transcription factors
WAS	WASP
Ataxia telangiectasia	ATM protein
Congenital alopecia and nail dystrophy with SCID	WHN transcription factor
APECED	AIRE protein
X-linked hyper-IgM syndrome	CD40 ligand (CD154)
X-linked lymphoproliferative syndrome	SH2D1A adaptor protein

Figure 26-20.

Genetic basis of selected disorders. This table lists selected gene defects that lead to immunodeficiency from T- or B-cell dysfunction. The classification is based on the cell in which the mutation has its effect and may differ from classifications based on clinical presentation [2–4]. ADA—adenosine deaminase; AID—activation-induced cytidine deaminase; AIRE—autoimmune regulator; APECED—autoimmune polyendocrinopathy-candidiasis-ectodermal dystrophy; ATM—A-T mutated; BLNK—B-cell linker protein; Btk—Bruton tyrosine kinase; PNP—purine nucleoside phosphorylase; RAG—recombinase-activating gene; TAP—transporter protein; WAS—Wiskott-Aldrich syndrome; WASP—Wiskott-Aldrich syndrome protein; WHN—winged-helix-nude.

References

1. Stiehm RE (ed): *Immunologic Disorders of Infants and Children.* Philadelphia: WB Saunders; 1996.
2. Buckley RH: Primary immunodeficiency disease due to defects in lymphocytes. *N Engl J Med* 2000, 343:1313–1324.
3. Frank J, Pignata C, Panteleyev AA, *et al.*: Exposing the human nude phenotype. *Nature* 1999, 398:473–474.
4. The Finnish-German APECED Consortium: An autoimmune disease, APECED, caused by mutations in a novel gene featuring two PHD-type zinc-finger domains. *Nat Genet* 1997, 17:399–403.

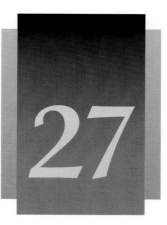

Allergic Drug Reactions

John A. Anderson

Allergic drug reactions are adverse events that occur in an unwanted, often unexpected fashion and differ from the intended therapeutic purpose of the medication. These reactions are caused by either immunologic mechanisms (true allergic reactions) or have clinical features that resemble an allergic reaction (allergic-like reactions) [1]. The manifestations of these reactions include cutaneous reactions, anaphylaxis and anaphylactoid reactions, serum sickness–like reactions, hypersensitivy syndromes, drug-induced autoimmune reactions, and isolated drug fever [2–6]. Allergy consultants devote the majority of their concerns to reactions to β-lactam antibiotics and other antibiotic agents and the prevention of subsequent reactions to radiocontrast media (RCM), local anesthetics, aspirin and other nonsteroidal antiinflammatory drugs (NSAIDs), angiotensin-converting enzyme (ACE) inhibitors, and insulin or other injected proteins.

The history of an unexplained symptom or sign that was related in time to the administration of a medication is the most important issue for the physician when a diagnosis of drug allergy is considered [4]. The likelihood of a drug's causing a specific set of signs or symptoms based on experience published in the medical literature can be helpful to the physician in narrowing the field of possible candidates.

Unfortunately, the list of in vivo and in vitro objective tests to confirm the diagnosis of drug allergy is limited. Use of allergy (IgE-mediated) immediate-reacting skin tests is very helpful in the evaluation of β-lactam antibiotic allergy, but not for most allergic-like reactions to other antibiotics, including sulfonamides [5–8]. Other medications in which skin testing may be helpful are in the case of insulin allergy, allergic reactions to injected enzymes or proteins, and in cases of possible related allergen exposure such as to egg protein in vaccines or to natural rubber latex [4].

Strict avoidance of future contact with a specific drug and use of an alternative therapeutic agent is the usual approach for physicians in most case of suspected drug allergy [6]. Occasionally, however, this course of action can be a problem. This is especially true in the case of a vague history of a mild penicillin rash: an expensive and sometimes toxic alternative antibiotic is often substituted despite experience indicating that penicillin skin test would have had negative results [2,6]. This is also true in patients with unsubstantiated histories of reactions to multiple medications in which alternative drug therapies are limited.

In addition to the possible use of allergy skin testing, the allergy consultant may be able to confirm the safety of the next therapeutic agent by incremental oral drug challenge tests (sometimes termed "test dosing") under controlled conditions [1,4,6,9,10]. Using sequentially subcutaneous administered drugs is the recommended method of determining the safety of a local anesthetic agent [3,4,6].

In the case of a previous allergic-like radiocontrast media (RCM) reaction, the recommendation is to use a low-osmolarity nonionic RCM agent plus a combination of prednisone, diphenhydramine, and perhaps ephedrine before administration of the agent [1,6].

Occasionally, use of alternative medication is not appropriate or possible. In some of these cases, it may be possible to consider drug desensitization [1,6,9,10]. Two typical examples in which the allergist–immunologist might consider desensitization include 1) a patient allergic to β-lactam antibiotics (history and skin test positive) in whom appropriated alternative therapy is not available and readministration of the β-lactam antibiotic may be lifesaving, and 2) an HIV-pos-itive patient infected with _Pneumocystis carinii_ bacteria who also has a history of a rash to trimethroprim-sulfamethoxazole (TMP-SMX), but requires long-term prophylaxis.

Desensitization protocols or references to specific studies using such protocols can be found in the allergy literature [1,6,9,11]. They include well-accepted protocols used in the management of β-lactams, insulin, and heterologous serum allergy plus aspirin, TMP-SMX, and sulfasalazine sensitivity. These references also include desensitization protocols based on very limited experience for drugs such as allopurinol, acyclovir, cytarabine, dapsone, pentamidine, tobramycin, vancomycin, and zidovudine.

Typical Allergic Reactions to Drugs

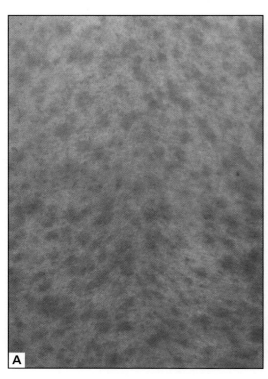 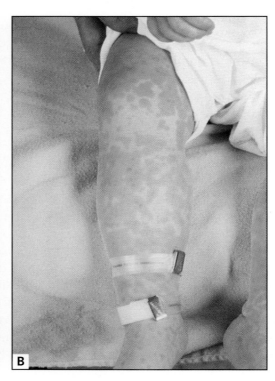

inhibitors are thought to be caused by the release of substance P and bradykinins [3]. Most experts believe that reactions to sulfonamides do not involve IgE [1,2]. Immunologic reactions to local anesthetics are rare [2,6]. The most common manifestation of an adverse reaction to a drug is a rash [3,4,12]. Rashes may occur as frequently as 23% of medical inpatients because of a variety of common drugs. Systemic anaphylaxis and anaphyloid reactions to drugs are estimated to occur at a rate of 0.04% in the same group of patients [4].

A, Maculopapular and morbilliform rash. Most drug-induced skin eruptions can be described as erythemations that are morbilliform or maculopapular in nature [2]. These types of rashes are almost always generalized, are more confluent in the intertriginous areas, and usually spare the face, palms, and soles [12]. Pruritus is a frequent symptom but may be absent. This rash must be differentiated from similar, viral-induced eruptions. It is virtually impossible to identify the causative agent based solely on the morphology of the lesions, and practically any drug can trigger such a reaction [12]. This type of rash is typical of an amoxicillin rash, which occurs in 5% to 13% of patients [6].

B, Amoxicillin rash. A recent Medline search of relevant studies demonstrated that approximately 33% of patients allergic to penicillin (history and skin test positive) presented with such a rash [8]. (**B** _courtesy of_ Paul I. Oh and Neil H. Shear.)

▬ Figure 27-1.

Typical adverse reactions to a drug. In most adverse drug reactions, the exact mechanism is unclear or unknown. Most true drug allergic reactions involve a Gel and Coombs (G-C) type I (IgE-mediated) immune reaction, but the entire spectrum of immunopathologic reactions (G-C types I-IV) may occur. Typical examples are those involving β-lactam antibiotic agents [5]. Other IgE-mediated type I reactions include drug allergy to insulin, enzymes, and heterologous or homologous systemically administered proteins [3,6].

Allergic-like drug reactions are sometimes referred to as "pseudoallergic." Although the exact mechanisms are sometimes unclear, direct mast cell activation and subsequent vasoactive mediator release are often cited for reactions to radiocontrast media, aspirin, and nonsteroidal anti-inflammatory drugs [5]. Allergic-like reactions to angiotensin-converting enzyme

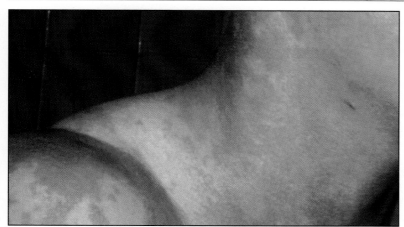

Figure 27-2.

Generalized urticaria (hives). Urticaria is an important manifestation of drug allergy, and pruritus is a frequent symptom. Urticaria with or without angioedema may be associated with systemic anaphylaxis or be part of a serum sickness syndrome. The smooth-surfaced, erythematous papules and plaques are usually palpable, confluent, and generalized. Virtually any drug can induce hives [12]. Acute-onset generalized hives may also be induced by other factors, especially viral infections in children. A history of urticaria with or without angioedema while a patient is taking a β-lactam antibiotic is more likely to be associated with positive IgE immediate reaction skin test result with penicillin than with any other type of rash [6]. Aspirin and nonsteroidal antiinflammatory drugs are frequent drug-induced causes of chronic (and acute) urticaria in adults.

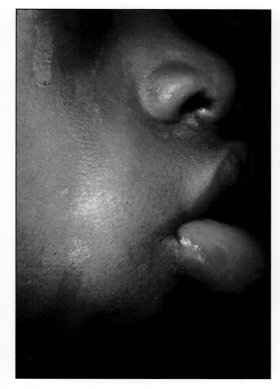

Figure 27-3.

Angioedema of the lips. Swelling of the deeper tissues may accompany drug-induced urticaria about one third of the time. Isolated angioedema occurs in 0.1% to 0.2% of individuals taking angiotensin-converting enzyme (ACE) inhibitors. About one third of individuals who experience these reactions require hospitalization, and 10% of these require intubation because of laryngeal edema [6]. Although symptoms of ACE inhibitor–induced angioedema usually occur early (*ie*, within weeks), late onset episodes (*ie*, occurring within months or years) have been reported and are often repetitive. Hereditary angioedema must be ruled out. This type of angioedema is unaccompanied by either urticaria or pruritus.

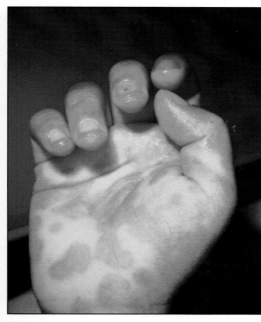

Figure 27-4.

Erythema multiforme, minor. This dermatose consists of multiple, symmetric, persistent macules and papules in which some lesions are "iris" or "targetoid" in appearance. The areas commonly involved are extensor surfaces, palms, soles, and sites of trauma [12]. One mucosal surface may be involved with superficial erosions in approximately 25% of patients.

Most cases are either of infectious (*eg*, herpes simplex) or idiopathic origin [12]. Drugs may be causative in 10% to 20%. The child depicted here had extensive involvement of the trunk and extremities, including the palms (as shown) and soles. In this case, the skin reaction was believed to be associated with phenytoin seizure therapy. (*From* Anderson and Atkinson [13]; with permission.)

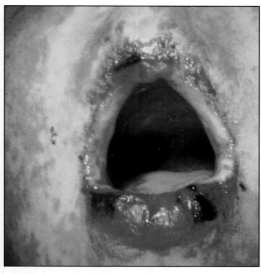

Figure 27-5.

Stevens-Johnson syndrome (SJS), or erythema multiforme, major. In addition to the "target" lesions of erythema multiforme, the skin in patients with SJS is more extensively involved with widespread blistering pruritic macules of the face, trunk, and proximal extremities [6]. At least two mucosal surfaces are involved. The syndrome is usually associated with toxicity, fever, and visceral organ involvement [12,14]. This patient apparently reacted to a β-lactam antibiotic. Note the involvement of the face, mouth, nose, and eyes (not visible).

Drugs are reported to be associated with SJS between 43% to 100% of the time [12,14,15]. The usual drugs identified are antibiotics, including β-lactams, sulfonamides, and now others such as vancomycin and anticonvulsant medications. Mortality has been reported to range from 1% to 5% [14,15].

It has recently been proposed that this syndrome resembles graft-versus-host disease and that it represents an immune reaction directed toward a cell-bound drug metabolite. Although therapeutic use of corticosteroids for patients with this syndrome has been controversial, some experts are strongly committed to their use at the earliest stage of disease as possible [12,14]. (*From* Anderson and Atkinson [13]; with permission.)

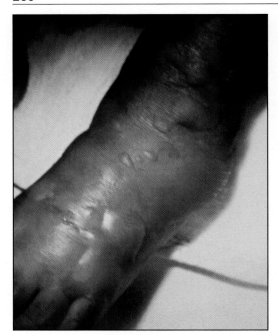

■ Figure 27-6.

Toxic epidermal necrolysis (TEN). Also known as Lyell's disease, TEN generally presents as sudden, widespread erythema and edema that rapidly evolves into bullae formation and subsequent extensive denudation [12]. The involvement is symmetric, total body, but usually spares the scalp. The lesions are very painful. TEN does not have the characteristic target lesions, but it otherwise seems an extension of Stevens-Johnson syndrome (SJS). Mucosal lesions may precede cutaneous involvement. Historically there is a full-thickness separation of the epidermis. The course is fulminate and profound systemic involvement is common, including fever and confusion plus pancytopenia and hepatitis in about 10% of the cases. A mortality rate of 15% to 25% is reported [12].

The same drug spectrum as in SDS is thought to be the predominant cause, if not the only one. This condition must be differentiated from staphylococcal-induced disease. The patient shown here had extensive skin and systemic involvement. Much of the skin of the extremities was denuded. The skin bullae of the syndrome is shown on the patient's foot. The drug that was involved was most likely a β-lactam antibiotic. The recommended management of patients with this condition resembles the management of those with extensive third-degree burns. [12,15]. Experts agree that corticosteroid therapy is not helpful and should be avoided [12,14].

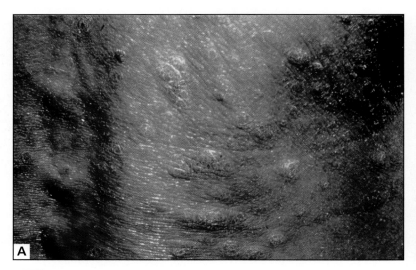

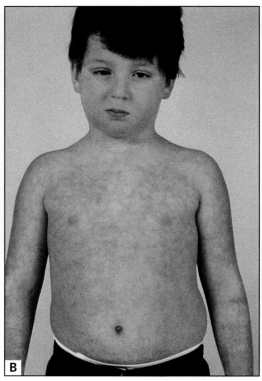

■ Figure 27-7.

Other allergic-like reactions to drugs. The mechanism of other allergic-like reactions to drugs is usually unknown. Type I (Gel and Coombs [G-C]) immune (IgE-mediated) reactions are not involved. These reactions usually are associated with a skin rash, but systemic effects may be present. These reactions include acneiform, eczematous, fixed, lichenoid, photoallergic, phototoxic, or purpuric skin rashes plus systemic vasculitides, drug hypersensitivity syndrome, and isolated drug fever.

A, Lichenoid skin eruption to a drug. This is an example of a drug-induced lichen planus–like skin eruption after intramuscular gold therapy. **B,** Drug hypersensitivity syndrome. This child reacted to phenobarbital. In addition to a generalized erythematous eruption, this hypersensitivity syndrome was associated with fever, lymphadenopathy, and nephritis. (*Courtesy of* Paul I. Oh and Neil H. Shear.)

Antibiotic Allergy

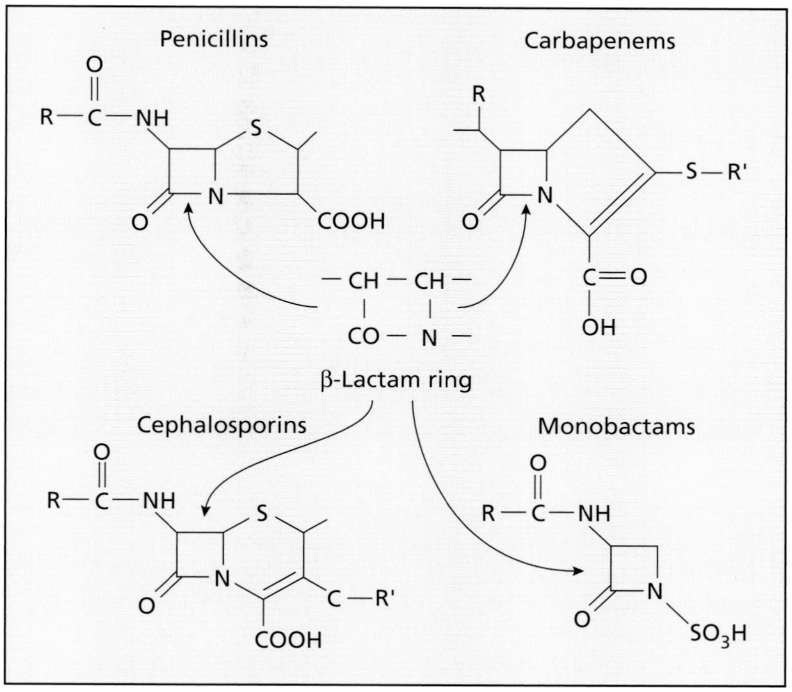

Figure 27-8.

β-Lactam antibiotic allergy. The most important true drug allergy (IgE mediated) and the one in which the mechanism, diagnosis, and optimal management are best understood is that involving β-lactam antibodies, particularly penicillin. All members of this class of antibiotics share a key β-lactam ring, as shown here in the middle and the *dark squares*. Reactions are IgE mediated with antibiotics directed to the β-lactam ring after the parent drug is metabolized and the haptem ring combines with a carrier protein to become a complete antigen [5]. Although reactions caused by IgE antibodies directed to the side chains ("R" in the figure) do occur (especially to ampicillin or amoxicillin as well as some third-generation cephalosporins), they are uncommonly reported in North America [1,6,16].

The chance of developing an allergic reaction differs depending on which β-lactam agent is used. Monobactams carry the lowest risk of reaction, followed by third- and second-generation cephalosporins, carbapenems, first-generation cephalosporins, and penicillin.

The cross-reactivity in a patient allergic to penicillin (history and skin test positive) between penicillin and a second- and third-generation cephalosporin is 2% [6]. However, when a reaction has been reported in such a patient who received cephalosporin, the reaction was usually a case of anaphylaxis. Therefore, the potential risk for a patient allergic to penicillin to take any other β-lactam is 100% [1]. (*Adapted from* Adkinson [5].)

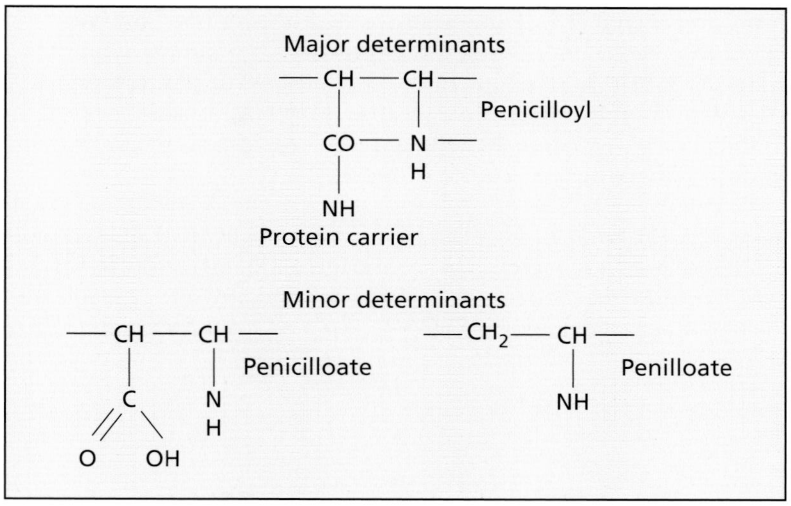

Figure 27-9.

Major and minor penicillin drug determinants. The parent penicillin drug breaks down in humans during metabolism into either a major or minor pathway. In the major pathway, the penicilloyl hapten (*top*) quickly combines with circulating proteins to become a complete antigen, the major determinant.

The haptens penicilloate (*bottom left*) and penilloate (*bottom right*) are examples of products from the minor parent drug metabolism. They may also combine with human proteins to become complete antigens and are called minor determinants [5].

The major determinant is available commercially as PRE-PEN (Kremers-Urban Co., Milwaukee, WI). A minor determinant mixture can be prepared, and some allergy–immunology specialists have done this; however, it is not available commercially [18]. Both of these preparations (PRE-PEN and minor determinant mixture [MDM]) plus the parent drug, penicillin G, are used in IgE skin testing for diagnostic purposes [1,6,17]. (*Adapted from* Anderson [2].)

β-Lactam Antibiotic Allergy Skin Testing

Skin Test Reagent	Dilution	Route of Administration	Test Dose
PRE-PEN* injection, USP	Penicilloyl-polylysine single test dose	Intracutaneous	1 drop
		Intradermal‡	0.02 mL
Potassium/penicillin G	10,000 U/mL	Intracutaneous	1 drop
		Intradermal‡	0.02 mL
Penicillin minor determinant mix†	Individually prepared, containing penicilloate and penilloate, ≤ 0.01 mol/L	Intracutaneous	1 drop
		Intradermal‡	0.02 mL
Other β-lactam antibiotics†	Individually prepared, 0.05, 0.1, 0.5, 1.0 mg/mL	Intracutaneous	1 drop
		Intradermal‡	0.02 mL

*Kremers-Urban Co., Milwaukee, WI.
†Additional skin test if available or necessary.
‡Serial skin testing; lower concentrations may be necessary in very sensitive persons.

Figure 27-10.

β-Lactam antibiotic allergy skin testing. Drug allergy skin testing should be done by allergy-immunology specialists who have a special interest or expertise in this field. Often this is restricted in communities to hospitals, large clinics, and other academic centers that not only have referrals of complicated patients but also have the necessary diagnostic agents [1,3,4,5,6,17].

The risks involved in penicillin skin testing are considered to be low [6]. However, in five trials that involved more than 9000 patients, the collective rate of systemic reactions was 0.11%, a rate higher than that reported with environmental allergen skin testing (0.02% to 0.33%) but lower than that reported with venom skin testing [17].

Faced with a suggestive history of an allergic reaction to β-lactam antibiotics, the key test for the allergy-immunology consultant to verify his or her impression are a battery of IgE immediate-reacting skin tests that use reagents, as shown here. Only skin testing with penicilloyl-polylysine (PRE-PEN USP; Kremers-Urban Co., Milwaukee, WI), penicillin G alone, or in combination with MDM has been validated [1,6,17].

A positive skin test to PRE-PEN correlates best with a history of urticaria or angiodema [2]. A positive skin test result to MDM correlates best with a history of anaphylaxis. Penicillin G contains some—but not all—minor penicillin metabolites [6,17].

If skin test results for a battery of three allergens (PRE-PEN, penicillin G, MDM) or battery of two allergens (PRE-PEN, penicillin G) are negative, (92% to 99%) or (70% to 97%) of the patients, respectively, are expected not to develop an immediate allergic reaction when given the next dose of penicillin [1,2,6,18].

Skin testing with other β-lactam antibiotics (eg, amoxicillin, cephalosporin, carbapenems, monobactams), although it is not validated, may be helpful (if positive) when side chain reactions are being considered [19]. False-negative skin test results, however, may be expected under these circumstances. In a patient who presents with a history of an allergy to cephalosporin, skin testing to penicillin should be done first because most reactions are expected to the penicilloyl major determinant [6]. The results would be helpful in deciding the next course of therapy.

Patient evaluation by *in vitro* assays (eg, enzyme-linked immunosorbent assay [ELISA] or radioallergosorbent technique [RAST]) does not reliably rule out the presence of specific IgE antibiotics to β-lactam agents because they are relatively insensitive and are only available for the major penicilloyl determinant [6]. (*Adapted from* Anderson [1].)

Approach to Patients Suspected of Allergy to β-Lactam Antibiotics (United States)

Clinical Situations	Penicillin Skin Tests	Oral Challenge	Consultants' Report
Rash caused by penicillin	Battery of three:* negative	Not necessary	Not allergic
			Skin test 92% –99% reliable
			Possible minor rash on subsequent administration
Systemic anaphylaxis (asthma, shock, laryngeal edema) caused by penicillin	Battery of three:* negative	Yes	Not allergic if both skin test and challenge test are negative‡
Any reaction to a cephalosporin	Battery of three:* negative	Penicillin: no; Cephalosporin: possibly	Probably not allergic to penicillin; other β-lactam skin tests may be helpful
Any reaction	Battery of two:† negative	Yes or no; yes in all severe cases	Skin test alone only 70%–97% reliable
			Greater risk if challenge test is not done
Any reaction	Positive	No	Avoid all β-lactam antibiotics or desensitize in most situations (see text)

*PRE-PEN (Kremers-Urban Co., Milwaukee, WI), penicillin G, and penicillin minor determinant mix.
†PRE-PEN and penicillin G.
‡Only reliable for next course of β-lactam antibiotic.

Figure 27-11.

Approach to patients suspected of allergy to β-lactam antibiotics in the United States. Most patients suspected of being allergic to β-lactam antibiotics who present to an allergist have a past history of "a rash." The overall likelihood of a patient's having a positive penicillin skin test result is 15% to 20% [6]. The reliability of a battery of three penicillin antigens (ie, PRE-PEN [Kremers-Urban Co., Milwaukee, WI], penicillin G, and the minor determinant mix [MDM]) is up to 99%; therefore, if the test result is negative, the β-lactam agent can usually be safely administered.

Although ideal, the battery of three allergens is frequently not available outside of large medical centers because the MDM is not commercially available [18]. The recently published practice parameters on drug hypersensitivity accept the battery of two skin tests antigens (PRE-PEN and penicillin G) as a suitable substitute and have indicated that 97% of patients with negative skin test results to this battery of two will tolerate penicillin [6]. Other studies would indicate that penicillin skin testing without MDM would only be 70% reliable [1,18]. Most of these patients would benefit from a graded oral challenge under controlled conditions because it would rule out the chance of missing reactions due to antibodies directed to minor determinants [1,18].

If a challenge test is to be done in a patient with these negative skin test results, the new practice parameters recommend a test dose of 1/100 of the desired therapeutic dose followed by a 1-hour wait. If no reaction occurs, the full dose can be safely administered [6]. This initial low dose of 1% is certainly very safe. At the end of the 1-hour wait, however, I would favor a more sequential administration (17%, 33%, 50%) of the total dose over 15- to 30-minute intervals followed by a 2-hour wait in the office [1]. If this test has a negative result, the patient can safely leave the office but should wait 24 hours before continuing the antibiotic therapy.

Patients who present with a history of systemic anaphylaxis to β-lactam agents should be penicillin skin tested. If the results are negative in a battery of two or three antigens, all should be orally challenged to determine the risk of subsequent therapy [1].

Patients with a reaction to cephalosporin and who are penicillin skin test negative should be able to receive penicillin safely, but the cephalosporin should be avoided. Further allergy skin testing with specific cephalosporin antigens (and possible drug challenge) may be helpful in determining the existence of a side chain reaction [19].

In most instances, patients with a history of reaction to β-lactam antibiotics who have positive skin test results to penicillin should be told to avoid all β-lactam agents. If it is necessary to use a β-lactam agent, the patient should be considered for desensitization to the appropriate medication. Although this is the safest approach, some investigators use incremented challenges of third-generation cephalosporins, in select patients with a history of penicillin allergy, who are skin test positive to penicillin [6]. (*Adapted from* Anderson [1].)

Drug Desensitization and Challenge Testing

Drug Desensitization and Challenge Test Principles

The need for drug desensitization or challenge should be clearly established. This includes assuring that the patient is reactive to the drug, needs the drug because there is no suitable alternative therapy, and that drug desensitization or challenge test has been shown to be successful for this medication.

There should be no contraindication for drug desensitization or challenge. This includes (but is not restricted to) history of drug reactions of the following types: Stevens–Johnson syndrome, toxic epidermal necrolysis, exfoliative dermatitis, thrombocytopenia or neutropenia, and drug-induced hepatitis.

The personnel performing these procedures should be skilled in the management of patients with anaphylaxis and other acute allergic-like reactions.

For acute desensitization, the patient should be in the hospital, preferably in an intensive care unit setting. Exceptions include the following:
1. Long-term (over days) oral desensitization or challenge to sulfonamides using protocols that have been successfully done on a outpatient basis.
2. Short-term (over hours) graded oral challenge (test dosing) procedures for other non–β–lactam antibiotics that have been recommended to be done in the clinic or office under controlled conditions (*eg*, appropriate facilities, equipment, personnel, and waiting times).

The patient should be informed. Consent must be obtained before beginning the procedure.

The patient should be as medically stable as possible.

Published protocols for either drug desensitization or challenge should be only used as guidelines and should be adapted to individual clinical circumstances.

Concurrent medications that could exacerbate anaphylaxis (*eg*, β-adrenergic blocking agent) or mask an adverse event during these procedures (*eg*, antihistamines, sympathomimetics, or corticosteroids) should preferably be withheld.

Allergic and other adverse reactions during and after the drug desensitization or challenge procedure should be expected. These reactions should be promptly treated as they occur and necessary adjustments to the protocol should be made.

After successful drug desensitization and subsequent discontinuation of the drug treatment, the patient quickly reverts to his or her previous allergic or reactive state.

Figure 27-12.
Drug desensitization and challenge test principles. Both drug desensitization and incremental drug challenge (test dosing) should only be done under the direct supervision of an experienced allergist-immunologist [6]. Based on limited published data, physicians should expect a reaction to occur during penicillin desensitization about one third of the time [10]. For this reason alone, such procedures are restricted to hospital intensive care settings. Exceptions are long-term oral protocols for trimethoprim-sulfamethoxazole and sulfasalazine, which are usually done on an outpatient basis. Even though incremental drug challenge tests (test dosing) are often done in the clinic or office, proper precautions for a possible adverse reaction should always be in place [1,2,4,6,10].

In patients with certain conditions (*ie*, Stevens-Johnson syndrome, toxic epidermal necrolysis and other blistering eruptions, exfoliative dermatitis, thrombocytopenia or neutropenia, and drug-induced hepatitis), drug allergy skin testing is not expected to be useful, and both desensitization and incremental drug challenge tests are contraindicated because they may exacerbate the condition or be life threatening [6,9,10]. These principles were established by Anderson [10] and generally reflect opinions of experts in current practice guidelines [6] and standard published reviews [2,3,4,5,9]. ICU—intensive care unit.

β-Lactam Oral Desensitization Protocol

Stock Drug Concentration, mg/mL*	Dose Number	Amount, mL	Drug Dose, mg	Cumulative Drug, mg
0.5	1[†]	0.05	0.025	0.025
	2	0.10	0.05	0.075
	3	0.20	0.10	0.175
	4	0.40	0.20	0.375
	5	0.80	0.40	0.775
5.0	6	0.15	0.75	1.525
	7	0.30	1.50	3.025
	8	0.60	3.00	6.025
	9	1.20	6.00	12.025
	10	2.40	12.00	24.025
50	11	0.50	25.00	49.025
	12	1.20	60.00	109.025
	13	2.50	125.00	234.025
	14	5.00	250.00	484.025

*Dilutions using 250 mg/5 mL of pediatric syrup.
†Oral dose approximately doubled every 15 to 30 minutes.

Figure 27-13.

β-Lactam antibiotic oral desensitization protocol. This acute oral desensitization protocol has been successfully used over the past 19 years for patients allergic to penicillin and other β-lactam antibiotic agents but who require these medications, generally to treat life-threatening conditions [2,3,10]. The 10 principles outlined in Figure 27-12 should be considered before attempting desensitization [6,10]. Accumulative reports of adverse reactions during or shortly after the procedure are approximately 36%, but they are usually mild, cutaneous in nature, and manageable [10].

The oral route is preferred over the intravenous (IV) route for this type of β-lactam antibiotic desensitization procedure because experience has shown that most adverse events are mild in nature [6]. However, in some circumstances, the IV route is preferred. An example of a protocol for β-lactam IV desensitization may be found in articles by Anderson [2] and Borish *et al.* [20]. (*Adapted from* Anderson [2].)

Ten-Day Trimethoprim-Sulfamethoxazle Oral Desensitization Protocol

Day	SMX in TMP-SMX Pediatric Suspension or Tablet			SMX Dose, mg/d
	Dose, mL	Stock Concentration	mg/mL	
1	1	1:20	2	2
2	2	1:20	2	4
3	4	1:20	2	8
4	8	1:20	2	16
5	1	FS	40	40
6	2	FS	40	80
7	4	FS	40	160
8	8	FS	40	320
9	10 mL or 1 tablet (80 mg TMP/400 mg SMX)			400
10	1 DS tablet (160 mg TMP/800 mg SMX)			800

Figure 27-14.

Ten-day trimethoprim-sulfamethoxazole (TMP-SMX) oral desensitization protocol. Other than β-lactam antibiotics and sulfonamides, the risk of a serious allergic-like reaction (*eg*, reactions other than skin rashes) to other antibiotics in otherwise healthy individuals is small. Morbilliform or maculopapular rashes are commonly found in patients treated with sulfonamides (*eg*, 3% to TMP-SMX in the general population) [2]. Patients infected with HIV are more likely than the general population to have an adverse allergic reaction to many medications, but particularly to sulfonamides [21].

Commonly, HIV infected patients require treatment or prophylaxis for *Pneumocystis carinii* pneumonia. The agent of choice for this situation is TMP-SMX. However, 18% to 75% of HIV-infected patients treated for pneumonia and 9% to 34% of those placed on prophylaxis with this drug must discontinue it because of an adverse reaction [20].

In these patients, the risk of subsequent exposure to TMP-SMX is unclear [6]. In one well-controlled trial [22], blinded, full-dose readministration of TMP-SMX in this type of patient with a history of a rash with or without a fever, resulted in no reaction to the drug in 50% of the cases. On the other hand, there are case reports [14,23,24] of re-exposure to

TMP-SMX during desensitization procedures that have resulted in life-threatening events.

There are many published protocols [2,6,14,19,26,28–30] for oral TMP-SMX desensitization in the world literature, many of which can be considered for HIV-infected patients who require TMP-SMX. Most of these are long term (*ie*, over days), but they vary in time from 4 hours to 23 days.

Shown is a 10-day protocol that has been proposed by US investigators. Many physicians have had personal experience with the protocol [1,6,15,21]. Only patients with either a simple rash or rash plus fever are candidates for this procedure. It is advisable to wait 1 month or more after the initial adverse reaction has resolved before attempting desensitization [6]. All the principles outlined in Figure 27-12 should be followed. In the initial 1994 report [25] using this protocol, 82% of 28 patients tolerated the procedure. After 20 months, 36% were continuing to tolerate the drug.

Recently, a 5-day protocol was proposed by investigators in Japan [6,9]. This protocol may deserve consideration. The researchers reported on 17 patients in whom a success rate of 88% at 19 months was achieved [23]. These long-term oral TMP-SMX desensitization protocols have been successfully used on an outpatient basis. DS—double strength; FS—full strength. (*Adapted from* Anderson [15].)

Forty-Eight Hour Trimethoprim-Sulfamethoxazole Oral Desensitization Protocol

	SMX in TMP-SMX Pediatric Suspension or Tablet			
Hour	Dose, mL	Stock Concentration	mg/mL	SMX Dose Interval, mg
0	0.5	1:20	2	1
8	1.0	1:20	2	3
16	2.0	1:20	2	4
24	8.0	1:20	2	40
32	1.0	FS	40	160
40	4.0	FS	40	800 to 1600 per day
48	10 mL or one regular or one DS TMP-SMX tablet every day			

Figure 27-15.

Forty-eight hour trimethoprim-sulfamethoxazole (TMP-SMX) oral desensitization protocol. This relatively short-term protocol has been used for 10 years for clinical circumstances when more rapid TMP-SMX desensitization is necessary [24,26]. In the initial study, six of seven patients (86%) were successfully desensitized with an average follow-up period of 6 months. Based on experience, it is best to consider this 48-hour procedure as an acute desensitization on an in-hospital basis after all the principles as outlined in Figure 27-12 because an adverse reaction may occur [14,23,24].

Occasionally, even more rapid TMP-SMX desensitization may be necessary. In 1998, a 6-hour protocol was studied in France that involved 44 consecutive HIV-infected patients with a clear history of a prior reaction to TMP-SMX [24].

The symptoms and signs included a maculopapular rash (88%), fever (30%), and pruritus (25%). All were treated under controlled conditions in a hospital-based outpatient allergy clinic, and 91% were successfully desensitized. However, 25% developed a pruritic rash that the patients were encouraged to "treat through" with cetirizine. In a recent follow-up study [27] of those same patients, all individuals who tolerated the procedure at 1 month were still tolerating TMP-SMX at 1 year. DS—double strength; FS—full strength. (*Adapted from* Anderson [15].)

Local Anesthetic Skin Testing and Graded Subcutaneous Challenge (Test Dosing)

Route	Dilution	Dose
Prick test*	Undiluted	1.0 drop
Intradermal test*	1:100	0.02 mL
SC challenge†	1:100	0.1 mL
SC	1:10	0.1 mL
SC	FS	0.1 mL
SC	FS	0.5 mL
SC	FS	1.0 mL
SC (optional)	FS	2.0 mL

*Skin test with a battery of local anesthetic types (free of epinephrine and parabens).
†Challenge with a single type of local anesthetic (negative result on skin test) sequentially at 15-minute intervals, as recommended by de Shazo and Nelson [29] and Patterson *et al.* [28].

Figure 27-16.

Local anesthetic skin testing and graded subcutaneous challenge (test dosing). Most adverse reactions to local anesthetic agents are caused by nonallergic factors such as vasovagal responses [3,6,27]. These reactions are sometimes complicated by the large amount injected during dental or surgical procedures and side effects of epinephrine, which is usually used with the local anesthetic.

The goal of management for the allergy consultant is to provide information relating to a "safe" local anesthetic for the dentist or surgeon that could be used subsequently in a patient with a history of a prior reaction.

Usually, the patients are skin tested with a small battery of potentially useful local anesthetic agents. Lidocaine is probably the test drug of choice, with nepricaine as a second choice [3]. If paraben preservative sensitivity (rare) is suspected, 1% lidocaine (10 mg/mL) can be obtained in a multiple-dose vial containing 0.1% methylparaben sodium for use as one test agent [2]. This can be compared on testing with lidocaine obtained in single-dose vials containing no preservatives.

The result of skin testing helps in choosing the single appropriate agent for the challenge test. The most important test is the subcutaneous challenge because most reactions do not involve IgE and therefore will not be picked up on skin testing. The top dose injected for the challenge test is usually not more than 1.0 mL [2,3,6]. However, higher doses have been recommended by some investigators [28]. (*Adapted from* Anderson [2].)

Radiocontrast Media Allergy

Reactions to Radiocontrast Media: Premedication Protocol

Time	Medication	Dose, *mg*
13 hours before procedure	Prednisone*	50
7 hours before procedure	Prednisone*	50
1 hour before procedure	Prednisone*	50
	Diphenhydramine hydrochloride	50‡
	Cimetidine†	300‡
	Ephedrine sulfate†	25
Diagnostic procedure	Low-osmolarity nonionic RCM	

*200 mg IV hydrocortisone may be substituted for prednisone.
†Use of either or both cimetidine and ephedrine is optional.
‡May be given intravenously.

Figure 27-17.

Premedication protocol for reactions to radiocontrast media (RCM). Reactions to RCM are allergic-like in nature and do not involve IgE. Some of the symptoms are thought be caused by direct histamine release [1–6]. Patients who have had a prior reaction have a 16% to 44% risk for a repeated reaction if RCM of the high-osmolarity type is used again [6].

Today there are diagnostic alternatives to the repeated use of RCM. However, in patients who require RCM despite the history of a prior reaction, low-osmolarity nonionic RCM can be used. Using this agent reduces the risk of subsequent reaction to 1% [6]. Careful studies over the years have also established a premedication protocol of principally prednisone and diphenhydramine hydrochloride. When these drugs are used (with or without ephedrine or cimetidine) plus low-osmolarity non-ionic RCM, the risk of reaction is reduced to 0.5% or less [2,28]. (*Adapted from* Anderson [1].)

References

1. Anderson JA: Drug allergy. In *Current Review of Allergic Diseases.* Edited by Kaliner MA. Philadelphia: Current Medicine; 1999:193–202.

2. Anderson JA: Allergic reactions to drugs and biological agents. *JAMA* 1992, 268:2845–2857.

3. de Shazo RD, Kemp SF: Allergic reactions to drugs and biologic agents. *JAMA* 1997, 278:1895–1906.

4. De Swarte RD, Patterson R: Drug allergy. In *Allergic Diseases, Diagnosis and Management.* Edited by Patterson R, Grammer LC, Greeberg PA. Philadelphia: Lippincott-Raven; 1997:317–412.

5. Adkinson NF Jr.: Drug allergy. In *Allergy Principles and Practices.* Edited by Middleton E Jr, Reed CE, Ellis EF, *et al.* St. Louis: Mosby-Yearbook; 1998:1212–1224.

6. Bernstein IL, Gruchalla RS, Lee RE, *et al.*: Disease management in drug hypersensitivity: a practice parameter. *Ann Allergy Asthma Immunol* 1999, 83:665–700.

7. Mendelson LM: Adverse reactions to b-lactam antibiotics: *Immunol Allergy Clin North Am* 1998, 18:745–757.

8. Solensky R, Earl HS, Gruchalla RS: Penicillin allergy: prevalence of vague history in skin test-positive patients. *Ann Allergy Asthma Immunol* 2000, 85:195–199.

9. Greenberger P: Desensitization and test dosing for the drug-allergic patient [editorial]. *Ann Allergy Asthma Immunol* 2000, 85:250–251.

10. Anderson JA: *Drug Desensitization in Provocation Testing in Clinical Practice.* Edited by Spector SL. New York: Marcel Dekker; 1995:761–783.

11. Millar M, Grammer LC: Case reports of evaluation and desensitization for Anti-thymocyte globulin hypersensitivity.: *Ann Allergy Asthma Immunol* 2000, 85:311–316.

12. Beltami VS: Cutaneous manifestations of adverse drug reactions. *Immunol Allergy Clin North Am* 1998, 18:867–895.

13. Anderson JA, Atkinson NF Jr: Allergic reactions to drugs and biologic agents. *JAMA* 1987, 258:2891–2899

14. Tripathi A, Ditto AM, Grammer LC, *et al.*: Corticosteroid therapy in an additional 13 cases of Stevens-Johnson Syndrome: a total series of 67 cases. *Allergy Asthma Proc* 2000, 21:101–105.

15. Anderson JA: Antibiotic drug allergy in children. *Curr Opin Pediatr* 1994, 6:656–660.

16. Romano A, Torres MJ, Fernandez J, *et al.*: Allergic reactions to ampicillin: studies on the specificity and selectivity in subjects with immediate reactions. *Clin Exp Allergy* 1997, 27:1425–1431.

17. Macy E: Risks of penicillin skin testing [editorial]. *Ann Allergy Asthma Immunol* 2000, 85:330–331.

18. Macy E, Richter PK, Falkoff R, Zeiger R: Skin testing with penicilloate and penilloate prepared by an improved method, amoxicillin oral challenge in patients with negative skin test responses to penicillin reagents. *J Allergy Clin Immunol* 1997, 100:586–591.

19. Romano A, Mayorga C, Torres MJ, *et al.*: Immediate allergic reactions to cephalosporins: cross-reactivity and selective responses. *J Allergy Clin Immunol* 2000, 106:1177–1183.

20. Borish L, Tamir R, Rosenwasser IJ : Intravenous desensitization to beta-lactam antibiotics. *J Allergy Clin Immunol* 1997, 80:314–319.

21. Beall G, Sanwo M, Hussain H: Drug reactions and desensitization in AIDS. *Immunol Allergy Clin North Am* 1997, 17: 319–338.

22. Hardy WD, Feinberg J, Finkelstein DM, *et al.*: A controlled trial of trimethroprim-sulfamethoxazole or aerosolized pentamadine for secondary prophylaxis of *Pneumocystis carinii* pneumonia in patients with acquired immunodeficiency syndrome: AIDS clinical trials group protocol 021. *N Engl J Med* 1992, 327:1842–1848.

23. Yoshizawa S, Yasuoka A, Kikuchi Y, *et al.*: A 5-day course of oral desensitization to trimethroprim/sulfamethoxazole (T/S) is successful in patients with human immunodeficiency virus type I infection who where previously intolerant to T/S but had no sulfamethoxazole-specific IgE. *Ann Allergy Asthma Immunol* 2000, 85:241–244.

24. Demoly P, Messaad D, Sahla H, *et al.*: Six-hour trimethroprim-sulfamethoxazole gated challenge in HIV-infected patients. *J Allergy Clin Immunol* 1998, 102:1033–1036.

25. Absar N, Daneshvar H, Beall G: Desensitization to trimethroprim/sulfamethoxazole in HIV infected patients. *J Allergy Clin Immunol* 1994, 93:1001–1005.

26. Kletzel M, Beck S, Elsen J, *et al.*: Trimethroprim-sulfamethoxazole oral desensitization in hemophiliacs infected with human immunodeficiency virus with a history of hypersensitivity reaction. *Am J Dis Child* 1991, 145:1428–1429.

27. Demoly P, Messaad D, Reynes J, *et al.*: Trimethroprim-sulfamethoxazole graded challenge in HIV-infected patients: long-term follow-up regarding efficacy and safety. *J Allergy Clin Immunol* 2000, 105:588–589.

28. Patterson R, De Swarte RD, Greenberg PA, *et al.*: Drug allergy and protocols for management of drug allergies. *Allergy Proc* 1994, 15:239–264.

29. de Shazo R, Nelson H: An approach to the patient with a history of a local anesthetic hypersensitivity: experience with 90 patients. *J Allergy Clin Immunol* 1982, 69:275–282.

Index